To Dr. G
May
Live Younger
Longer

Dr. M.

Jan 19, 1987

The Age Reduction System

The Age Reduction System

Dr. Richard Clark Kaufman

RAWSON ASSOCIATES : New York

Library of Congress Cataloging-in-Publication Data

Kaufman, Richard Clark, 1949–
The age reduction system.
Bibliography: p. 285
Includes index.
1. Health. 2. Longevity. 3. Holistic medicine.
I. Title.
RA776.5.K38 1986   613'.0438   84-42933
ISBN 0-89256-285-4

Published simultaneously in Canada by Collier Macmillan Canada, Inc.
Packaged by Rapid Transcript, a division of March Tenth, Inc.
Composition by Folio Graphics Co., Inc.
Printed and bound by Fairfield Graphics, Fairfield, Pennsylvania
Designed by Jacques Chazaud
Second Printing March 1987

To my dad, Jack I. Kaufman

Contents

Acknowledgments

I wish to thank: Elizabeth Backman, my literary agent, for personal guidance and business savvy; Hawkins Cheung, my martial arts instructor, for keeping me in shape; Dan and Enid Faust, for trusting my instincts; Alex Getzy, president of General Research, for information about supplement manufacturing; Theresa Gross at H.I.T. Secretarial, Technical Typing, and Word Processing, for deciphering notes and word processing services; Tom Huber, my computer expert, for helping develop the computer health profile; Harry Langdon, photographer extraordinaire, for a great jacket photograph; Eleanor Rawson, my publisher, for being the best and tough; Toni Sciarra and Grace Shaw, for editorial assistance; Lauren Leigh Taylor, for brilliant ideas; David Wilson at Master File, for helping prepare the manuscript; Dr. David Young, for balancing my energy; Ward Dean, M.D., for his generous advice; finally, my family, colleagues, and friends, for support.

The Age Reduction System

Introduction

May 25, 1975. Brussels, Belgium. It was the kind of sunny afternoon that feels like a holiday, just because you've momentarily abandoned your textbooks. Even running errands is a relief if you're a medical student.

I sat idling on my 750SS Ducati motorcycle at a large intersection. On my left loomed a forty-ton tractor trailer. It cast its shadow, like a net, over me.

I waited for the traffic light to change. When it did, the truck began a right turn, oblivious of my presence. I glanced over my left shoulder just as the steel wall of the rig knocked me off my motorcycle. Time distorted into slow motion as I lay pinned under my motorcycle and watched the rear wheels of the truck roll over my left leg.

I heard a loud crack.

The wheel cleared my leg, and I saw what remained. Shining white bone projected out of my leg. My foot was twisted 180 degrees. Blood was gushing onto the street.

Shock set in immediately, and with it the extreme mental alertness that allows you to take stock of any disaster in a very cold-blooded way.

I realized I was lying in the middle of the road in a foreign country. I was losing a lot of blood. And no one was offering to help me.

Methodically I removed my glasses and zipped them into my jacket, assuming they might get lost in the confusion. Then I started screaming. Frankly, I wasn't in any pain—after a certain point the body administers its own anesthetic. I screamed because I thought I *should* be in pain, and also to try to get some attention.

Fortunately, about twenty-five minutes later a doctor drove by. He gave me an injection for pain and left. Another thirty-five to forty minutes passed. I remained on my back in the middle of the road, vaguely aware that passersby were gawking at me.

Finally an ambulance arrived and scraped me off the road. The public hospital into which I was unceremoniously dumped was one of the filthiest, most unsanitary places—not to mention hospitals—I had ever seen. One couldn't even see out the windows, they were so covered with grime.

I began to worry. I knew just enough about medicine to be scared to death. As I was wheeled into the filthy operating room, I kept having visions of bone infections, foot amputations. I was only twenty-four years old and I couldn't imagine being crippled.

When I awakened from the operation the full implications of my accident began to sink in. I looked down at the long white cast that encased my leg from hip to toe. I felt passive, lethargic, as if my mind and heart had been as effectively immobilized as my body.

I realized that instead of studying to be a doctor, I was going to learn what it was like to be a patient.

Three weeks passed, and I began to worry about the obvious symptoms of infection I was displaying. My parents were able to arrange for my transfer to a Philadelphia hospital near their home. I was relieved to be returning to American medicine.

As I suspected, my leg was infected. The American doctors operated again (the second of many operations over a two-year period) and this time encased my leg in a cast that left the wounded area exposed.

A surgeon appeared periodically over the next six months to scrape away dead and diseased flesh. To prevent infection, my room was specially sterilized and I was kept pumped full of drugs.

At first, I accepted the routine gratefully. I had adopted a "doctor knows best" attitude, so I complied unquestioningly with all the physicians' decisions. I was under the influence of so many drugs at the time—Valium, Librium, Percodan—that it was just too much effort to think for myself.

However, as months wore on with little improvement, my survival instincts began to reassert themselves. I was no longer content to be pacified by drugs and hospital routines. I wanted to take a more active role in improving my health.

I refused to take any more sedatives. As my mind cleared, memory returned, and with it a painful awareness of all I had lost. Skiing, running, martial arts practice—sports that had once been integral to my life now seemed permanently removed from it. Even walking was a challenge I had yet to meet.

Finally, I nerved myself to ask my doctor what I could expect. Would I be able to walk? Run? Resume a normal life? Not entirely, he said. I would probably have to use a cane. It was unlikely I would ever be able to participate in any sports. I would have to adjust to being partially crippled.

Perhaps it was immaturity on my part, but I couldn't accept the idea of being an invalid. I vowed to do everything in my power to become again the person I once had been.

That resolution was my first real step toward health. Choosing life over death, health over sickness, is the first and most important choice you can make.

Does it seem as if the choice should be self-evident? It is not. As any practicing physician will tell you, many patients gratefully surrender to death or sickness, while others cling passionately to life.

The will to live, which doctors feel is so critical to recovery, is comprised of the two most powerful forces in the human mind: willpower and imagination.

It is not enough to passionately want to live; you must also *believe* that you will.

Although these ideas weren't completely clear to me in my hospital bed, I intuitively realized that I must pursue health with every aspect of my being: physical, mental, emotional, and spiritual. I also realized that my doctors, while competent to heal my leg, were ill-equipped to help me regain optimal health—the health of my whole mind and body.

I began to remove the obstacles to my health. The hospital food, for example. By the time it reached my bed, what had once been food had been so manipulated that it had long since lost its ability to nourish me. I asked my parents to bring me fresh fruits, vegetables, nuts, and seeds instead.

I took stock of my physical condition—my muscles were now flaccid. I did sit-ups, push-ups, and every other exercise I could manage in my bed.

I also realized that the greatest atrophy had taken place in my mind, which had lain fallow for almost two years. I began to study health and nutrition and spent countless hours imagining myself whole again, capable of functioning without the use of crutches of any kind.

This vision was a long time arriving.

For two years after my initial release from the hospital, I staggered slowly toward health. I'd like to say I never wavered in my commitment, but that would be a lie. Sometimes I was so frustrated with my slow progress that I wanted to give up and lower my expectations. But after the anger passed, I would pick myself back up again and continue my efforts.

My life was divided among health research, self-prescribed physical therapy, and surgeries. I underwent two additional operations.

I was my first patient. In the name of health, I studied everything from abstract theories of quantum physics to ancient herbal remedies. I learned as much as I could and applied much of what I learned.

By the time I was twenty-nine, four years after the accident, I could walk without the use of cane or crutches. Today I not only walk, I dance. I swim. I bike. I roller skate. And I continue to practice my strenuous and beloved martial arts.

For this I am grateful to Dr. James E. Nixon in Philadelphia, who ultimately and correctly reconstructed my ankle, and to the health program that provided the basis for the Age Reduction System contained in this book.

If the Age Reduction System could restore a half-cripple to vibrant health, just imagine what it can do for you!

The initial choice is yours alone. You must choose to live long and prosper. Commit yourself to that goal. *Believe in it*. My own belief is that you have the power to live *in complete possession of your faculties and physical abilities* for 110 to 120 years.

Together we can slow the aging process so that each year passes gracefully into the next, with minimal concessions to advancing years. We can help you stay mentally alert and physically agile far longer than the average American. And we can create a philosophy that will allow you to extract joy from every day of your life.

Your life is in your hands. If you'll join them with mine, perhaps we can make a better life for both of us.

1

The Emergence of the Age Reduction System

The Age Reduction System is based on the following premises:
- That the whole human organism is greater than the sum of its physical components
- That each part of a human being influences all the other parts
- That health and longevity are the natural result of homeostasis, that is, physical, mental, and emotional balance

To understand how these concepts differ from those of the past, compare them to the tenets of conventional medicine:
- The body and mind are separate entities that do not influence each other.
- The body is comprised of atoms, molecules, and cells, while the mind is comprised of thoughts and emotions, which are considered to be merely electrical transmissions and protein molecule combinations. Modern medicine regards the spirit or soul as a religious artifact.
- It is the doctor's province to treat the body as one would a machine, mechanically repairing any malfunctioning parts.

The primary difference between the Age Reduction System's viewpoint and the historical concept is that the former can best be described as inclusive and the latter as exclusive.

I am willing to explore any theory or therapy that may contribute to health and longevity. I approach new ideas, old ideas, and even so-called proven ideas with the same combination of skepticism and curiosity.

Traditional scientists have tended to try to isolate phenomena from their environment. The validity of this approach has recently been challenged by others who claim it is impossible to be truly "objective" about experiments that rely on the interpretation of an observer. As a result of these challenges, it seems likely that science itself will eventually become more inclusive.

THE SYSTEM'S SOURCES

While obtaining my doctorate in nutrition, I continued to be fascinated by a variety of eclectic studies, theories, and observations. My motorcycle accident had occurred while I was a third-year medical student at the University of Brussels, in Belgium. I had previously received my bachelor's degree in psychology at St. Lawrence University in the United States. Now I wanted to spend time on research and act as a health consultant to business and industry, which would allow me to treat and counsel people with freedom from financial and time constraints.

While pursuing my doctorate, I examined studies about cultures in which it is common for people to be long-lived. I studied ancient methodologies—such as acupuncture and herbal remedies—for examples of noninvasive (i.e., not drug- or surgery-related) therapies that might counteract the damage inflicted by Western society on itself. Clinical studies of humans and animals under controlled conditions offered another abundant source of information. The final source of information was the clinical results that I and other gerontologists have achieved by actually applying anti-aging methodologies.

In my private practice I have used Age Reduction System techniques and information to benefit more than 400 clients. Some of their case histories will be cited throughout the book. In addition, as a health consultant I have been able to influence the treatment of several thousand clients of nutritionists, gerontologists, chiropractors, doctors, psychologists, and other health professionals. The computer profiles that I designed as individual health analysis tools and other age reduction devices have been used by more than 5000 people. All told, about 7000 people have used the Age Reduction System's concepts and techniques to slow and reverse aging.

Since every resource has inherent strengths and weaknesses, I used the technique of cross-field verification—comparing studies conducted by scientists in different health disciplines that nevertheless achieved comparable results—to further ensure the soundness of my Age Reduction System.

How You Can Benefit
FROM THE AGE REDUCTION SYSTEM

What follows are just a few case histories that illustrate some of the benefits you can receive from incorporating the Age Reduction System into your life.

Stress and Success

Steve Nichols was the incarnation of the Great American Nightmare. At forty-five, he had earned all the accoutrements of success: wealth, social position, material possessions. He was also chronically anxious, driven, twice divorced, slightly overweight, uninterested in exercise (except for the occasional tennis match), and ruled by the clock—in essence, a short-lived personality.

By the time Steve came to see me, he had reached the biological age of fifty-five—his body systems operated like those of someone a decade older.

He complained of stomach pains and mentioned that he had already consulted a cardiologist, who told him he had higher-than-normal blood pressure and triglyceride and cholesterol levels. He also diagnosed Steve's stomach pains as resulting from gastritis, a pre-ulcer state caused by inflammation of the stomach lining. The cardiologist recommended a series of drugs to control these problems.

Steve was very reluctant to take drugs. He came to me to see if there were any non-drug therapies that could cure him. He made it clear that he wasn't interested in becoming a health nut; he just wanted to prevent actual illness.

I could see right away that my real work with Steve was going to be reeducation, but I decided to begin from his point of view—by discovering what was physically wrong with him.

Metabolic blood testing confirmed the cardiologist's diagnosis and provided additional information. I discovered that Steve's ratio of HDL (high-density lipoprotein) cholesterol to LDL (low-density lipoprotein) cholesterol was low. These ratios are frequently indicative of risk for heart attack, cardiovascular disease, or stroke.

Once I explained the gravity of his condition, Steve was more willing to cooperate.

We began with the most tangible problem first: the gastritis. Steve was convinced it was caused by spicy foods, but we discovered that he actually ate very few of them. However, several factors in his diet did contribute to gastritis. First, he drank coffee and hard liquor—both irritants to the stomach lining—every day. His diet consisted primarily of refined, low-fiber foods. He ate quickly, sandwiching his meals between all-important business appointments.

I suggested he substitute decaffeinated coffee (from a water-extraction process) for coffee, and wine for hard liquor. I developed a diet that was high in fiber, which seems to protect the body from ulcer conditions. I also recommended a daily dose of pure aloe vera gel, which is protective of the stomach lining.

I asked him to avoid taking aspirin and to use a mild antacid instead if necessary to control pain in the interim. Since his diet was low in magnesium, I suggested he use an antacid with a magnesium base.

I thought his tendency to eat too quickly was symptomatic of stress rather than related to diet. In fact, I believed stress to be the primary cause of his gastritis, as well as of his high blood pressure and cholesterol abnormalities.

This was not welcome news. Although Steve was willing to make minor alterations in diet, he wasn't prepared to consider altering his life-style.

Steve saw stress as a simple fact of life. And he was right. However, there are two kinds of stress: positive and negative. I wanted to teach Steve to seek out positive stress and avoid or reduce negative stress.

The primary difference between positive and negative stress is your internal response to it. Positive stress makes you feel rejuvenated, keenly alert and alive, interested. Negative stress makes you feel anxious, depressed, tense, confused, or paralyzed.

Negative stress triggers the brain to release cortisol, an adrenal gland hormone. Recent research has indicated links between cortisol, degenerative diseases, and death. For example, there is frequently an increase of cortisol in the body one week prior to death. In addition, cortisol is suspected of suppressing the immune system and causing infections and depression. It has been linked to some forty diseases, including Alzheimer's disease, heart attack, arthritis, multiple sclerosis, Parkinson's disease, diabetes, obesity, aging psychosis, cancers, and ulcers.

Since Steve seemed to be more interested in maintaining his life-style than his health, I reminded him that he wouldn't be around long to enjoy one without the other. At the very least, he was on the verge of developing an ulcer. Illness would certainly curtail his work activities.

Finally, once he had allowed himself to overcome his resistance to change, Steve indicated his willingness to work on life-style alterations.

Since changing jobs was out of the question, I devised some stress-reduction techniques that he could use during his workday. These involved meditation and visualizations he could do at his desk.

I encouraged him to delegate as much responsibility as possible. Steve's stress was not just from overwork but also from his almost obsessive need to control other people and events. This gave rise to tremendous resistance from others, resulting in negative stress.

His need to control made him a slave to the second. I recommended that he remove his watch when he was not working. I wanted him to begin to experience time more naturally, rhythmically, as he had been designed to.

Finally, I urged him to exercise regularly. Exercise uses up excess blood fat, cortisol, and adrenaline before any damage is done. I recommended that he play mixed doubles tennis to encourage more social contact and to take long walks so he would have some form of exercise that was *noncompetitive*.

Steve didn't incorporate all these changes at once. The human mind typically resists any change of habit until the new habit has been repeated every day for approximately twenty-one days. We introduced the changes gradually, and gradually Steve began to experience results.

Within only three months, Steve's stomach pains had disappeared. His cholesterol abnormalities, high triglycerides, and high blood pressure all returned to normal ranges. He continues to reduce his biological age.

Achieving Permanent Weight Loss

Susan Peterson came to see me shortly after separating from her husband. Upon recovering from the shock of finding herself suddenly single, she decided to take inventory. She wasn't at all pleased with the results.

Susan was thirty-four years old, but excess fat and lack of exercise had aged her biologically to about forty. She wanted desperately to return to the slim figure she had in her modeling days and before having her two children. She had tried every kind of diet, but to no avail. She simply could not lose weight.

As Susan and I discussed her dieting history, she began to shed light on the source of her problem.

While modeling, Susan had maintained her 115-pound, five-foot seven-inch figure by starving, vomiting, and then binge eating after photo sessions. Although traumatic, the procedure kept her in business for years. In fact, she tried the same approach before coming to see me but found that it no longer worked. Not even starvation could help her shed pounds.

The first step of my analysis was to send her to a lab to have her thyroid gland tested, since thyroid malfunctions can cause weight problems. Had the test revealed any abnormalities, I would have sent her to an endocrinologist. However, the tests showed her thyroid functions to be in the low but normal range.

My next step was a minute analysis of her normal diet, including number of calories, range of nutrients, percentage of protein, carbohydrates, and fats. We created a chart of her activities so we could accurately estimate the number of calories Susan burned each day, compared to the number she consumed.

I then performed a series of anthropometric measurements. These measurements reveal not only the dimensions of one's body but also its deviations from the ideal. By using skin-fold calipers and a computer program I had developed, I was able to compare Susan's present physical condition with a graphic somatagram of her ideal condition. I discovered that of her 140 pounds, 28 to 30 percent was body fat, distributed primarily on her hips, thighs, buttocks, abdomen, and underarm muscles. Her overall muscle tone, with the exception of her arms, was good. We attributed this to recent workouts on Nautilus equipment. However, her muscle definition was blurred by fat padding.

I recommended a goal weight loss of 25 pounds, with a simultaneous body fat reduction to 15 to 16 percent.

I also explained why she had been unable to lose weight.

As Susan had grown older and more sedentary, her metabolism had become less efficient. Since she required less energy, her body had learned to convert food to fat instead of fuel. In addition, her diet was very high in refined sugars, which triggered an excessive release of insulin, a fat-producing hormone. Brown fat, a special kind of fat that turns excess calories into heat when stimulated by the sympathetic nervous system, had also become less efficient.

The overall result was that she was gaining more weight from eating less food.

The first step was not to decrease the number of calories she was consuming but to change their content. Since Susan's personality led her to be more comfortable with a loosely structured program instead of a strict one, I gave her a list of acceptable foods from my "natural foods for longevity." She was allowed to eat 1000 calories a day of any food on that list but had to be sure that specific proportions of those calories were composed of proteins, carbohydrates, and fats.

Susan also had to swear off refined sugars and flours, fruit juices, and dried fruits. These foods are converted into blood glucose so quickly that it causes the pancreas to release excess insulin in response. The insulin mops up the excess glucose by stimulating the cells to absorb it as fat.

Since diet can be controlled more readily through small meals, I recommended that Susan eat three to four small meals each day.

Although Susan's insulin problems were aggravated by diet, I believed that they also were caused by the natural aging process. As you grow older your body becomes less tolerant of glucose and more likely to overreact by producing too much insulin. Consuming natural fibers such as guar gum or psyllium seed husks improves glucose tolerance by slowing the conversion of foods into glucose. Glucose enters the bloodstream more slowly and is less likely to trigger an excessive insulin response.

I also recommended that Susan eat a tablespoon of guar gum and bran fiber in a glass of water about one-half hour before meals for two other reasons. First, guar gum fibers swell when immersed in water or digestive juices, so by the time you sit down to eat you will already feel full. Second, bran increases the speed with which food passes through the intestines, so there is less time to absorb calories from the food you have eaten.

The next step was to alter Susan's metabolism. We stepped up her energy requirements. Aerobic exercises such as walking and bicycling were appropriate because they demand energy without unduly increasing appetite. Exercise began to force Susan's metabolism to become more efficient at producing fuel than fat.

Although she experienced the temporary setbacks so familiar to us all, Susan lost an average of 2½ pounds per week. She achieved her goal weight within three months and has maintained it. In addition, she claims she has more energy and better muscle tone than at any other time in her life.

From her previous biological age of approximately forty, Susan has reduced her age to about twenty-seven.

The Man Who "Grew Younger"

Milton Lawrence should have been dead. His chronological age was 66. His biological age was 75. The average life-span of a white male in this country is 68.7 years.

Milton believed he was living on borrowed time—and he was right.

According to his doctors, Milton had high blood fat, a high resting heart rate, low endurance, a weak circulatory system, and preliminary signs of developmental arteriosclerotic heart condition. In addition, his mental processes, memory, and sexual capacity were impaired, and he suffered from chronic constipation.

To control the symptoms of what his doctors considered the normal aging process, Milton was placed on Inderal, a drug that dilates blood vessels and enhances circulation. Milton said his doctors encouraged him to come to terms with his degenerating condition and to accept the fact that he was aging.

In the midst of this crisis of confidence, Milton began to notice a neighbor—me—who seemed to live on his bicycle. Since it was obvious that my ankle was deformed and equally obvious that that didn't prevent me from staying in shape, he eventually became curious enough to ask me how I did it.

I told him about my accident in Belgium, my research into aging, and my successful efforts to rehabilitate myself. He asked me if I would be willing to work with him.

Although I was extremely busy at the time, I liked him so much I decided to work with him anyway.

We began with a thorough self-inventory. At sixty-six, Milton carried 185 pounds on his five-foot seven-inch frame. He consumed a typical American diet: white flour, high fat, high calories. He slept a great deal, exercised very little, and worked himself to the point of nervous exhaustion. His work as an attorney provided tremendous stimulation, which often translated into negative stress.

By comparison, Milton had been quite fit in his college years. Weighing in at 130 pounds, he was active in track and field, as well as other college sports.

At first, Milton believed those days were gone forever; I was convinced otherwise.

Since I believed his symptoms resulted from years of neglect on a variety of levels, I also believed it was necessary to reverse these processes through a variety of alterations.

First, I developed a diet to lower his blood fat, eliminate constipation, and improve circulation. I limited his fat intake to 10 to 15 percent of his total caloric intake. I reduced his protein consumption and eliminated all sweets. He was permitted 1500 calories per day, which he chose to consume in a series of small meals. I also recommended supplementary dietary fiber and other digestive aids to relieve constipation.

To counter his mental fogginess, loss of memory and sexual abilities, and negative stress, I devised a supplemental program. I recommended B vitamins and amino acid neurotransmitter precursors to enhance neurotransmitter brain function, which controls memory. I devised a biofeedback meditation to increase his sexual capacity and reduce stress. (Zinc, by the way, helps normalize testosterone levels.)

The next level from which we attacked Milton's problems was physical exercise. I knew that consuming the most efficient fuel would do Milton no good if he didn't revitalize his means of converting fuel into energy.

Since Milton was in no condition to undertake a strenuous exercise program, I asked him to walk, walk, walk. We live right next to the beach (probably the only clean air in Los Angeles is within 20 feet of the ocean), so I told him to walk on the sand as much as possible. Beach walking produces a more significant aerobic effect than walking on paved surfaces.

Four years have passed since Milton first embarked on the life-style, diet, and exercise alterations I suggested.

Chronologically, Milton is now seventy years old. Biologically, he's in better shape than most forty-year-olds. He weighs 140 pounds, or 45 pounds less than when he began. His doctors confirm that there has been a marked decrease in arteriosclerotic plaques, total blood fats, blood pressure, and cholesterol. His bowel movement transit time has decreased from an average of one movement every three to five days, to one movement daily.

Although he is now semiretired (Milton says he wanted to devote more time to living), he is both mentally and physically active. He can walk for hours on the beach without tiring, and even includes some jogging in his program.

According to Milton, the two most tangible benefits he earned by following the Age Reduction System are the improvement in his sexual performance and his ability to run the 100-yard dash almost as fast as he did in college.

Other Benefits of the Age Reduction System

While the case histories just presented are representative, they touch on just a few of the benefits that can take place as a result of the Age Reduction System. Others include:
- Transforming the way you experience stress
- Altering your attitudes toward time, money, achievement, and countless other life-style choices

- Reducing or eliminating age-related depression, mental fogginess, loss of physical coordination
- Compensating for the damage imposed by environmental and dietary toxins, or stress factors, among which are air, water, and noise pollution
- Increasing energy, endurance, and strength
- Improving digestion and elimination abilities
- Losing excess fat
- Improving the integrity of immune, nervous, and endocrine systems
- Dramatically slowing skin aging
- Improving appearance
- Enhancing sexual capabilities
- Preventing degenerative disease
- Achieving and maintaining homeostasis (physical, mental, and emotional balance)
- Extending life and reducing biological age

MAKING THE BEST CHOICES
FOR IMPROVING YOUR LIFE

Most of us do not fully realize the tremendous power we exercise over our own well-being. If you chose to die, I believe you could do so in less than a quarter of a second. Your brain would simply release a chemical that would stop your heart from pumping.

On the other hand, your ability to wrench yourself from death's door has been equally well documented.

Your expectations and secret desires or beliefs exercise an important influence on how and when you will age or die. One example of mass consciousness in action can be seen among the American generation now reaching its forties and fifties. In contrast to the previous generation—when most people were expected to develop stiff joints, potbellies, and lined faces shortly after marriage and childbirth—today's maturing generation treats us to a different spectacle. Many prominent men and women in their forties and fifties are more fit and active now than they were in their twenties. Jane Fonda is an outstanding example. Cary Grant, Kareem Abdul Jabbar, Linda Evans, Dick Clark, Jackie Onassis, and Kirk Douglas are others.

You have the ability to slow, halt, and in some cases even reverse aging. This book contains what you need to know to begin such a program today. Not all the information will be appropriate for your individual needs. However, as you gradually become more intimate with the way you function, you'll also become more proficient at analyzing your responses. You'll begin to adapt the Age Reduction System to your needs. NOTE: Do consult your doctor before embarking on the Age Reduction System. This book is not intended to treat illness. It's also possible that your doctor may detect abnormalities that could prevent you from fully benefitting from the Age Reduction System. And always remember that the amounts of nutrients and supplements discussed represent only my personal recommendations: You must check with your personal physician before embarking on any nutritional program.

I am not interested in converting you to blind faith about this system. I want this book to lead you to ask more questions, not fewer. Challenge everything you read in this book—once you have completed it. Pay attention to all your responses as you begin to incorporate its suggestions. Become an active participant in your quest for longevity.

I also urge you to approach these life and death subjects with a little levity. My clinical experience has convinced me that nothing extends life more than laughter. The most obvious example of this is Norman Cousins, who literally laughed himself back to life after a bout with what was supposed to be a fatal illness. Even in everyday life, humor, combined with a perspective of self-acceptance and nonresistance to the ebb and flow of life, is the simplest recipe I know for extending it.

2

Why You Grow Old

Leonard Hayflick, a researcher at the Wistar Institute, Philadelphia, was the first to quantify what many cellular biologists and gerontologists believe to be the maximum human life-span: 110 to 120 years. He based this number—called Hayflick's limit—on his theory, developed in the 1960s, that each of our cells is capable of dividing a prescribed number of times. When the cells can no longer reproduce, death occurs.

In sad contrast to these figures, the average American woman currently has a life expectancy of 77 years; the average American man can expect to live 68.7 years. The oldest American whose age could be authenticated was a former slave by the name of Charlie Smith. He died in a Veterans Administration hospital in 1979, at the age of 138.

Why is there such a wide gap between possible and probable life-spans? The answers are almost as individual as fingerprints. Heredity, environment, attitude, nutrition, exercise, stress, drugs—virtually every aspect of your everyday life influences how and when you will age.

The importance of life-style is indicated by the fact that women in Western societies tend to outlive men by approximately eight years. While there are some physiological reasons for this—women secrete estrogen (a female sex hormone), which appears to protect against certain degenerative diseases, and men are genetically more susceptible to some diseases—the overpowering difference seems to be life-style.

Until very recently, many more men worked outside the home than did women. Work-related stress is considered a factor in the increased incidence of suicide and fatal automobile accidents among men. Stress is also considered a primary factor in the development of degenerative diseases, such as arteriosclerosis and cancer, to which men succumb more often than women.

Other killers primarily of males are cirrhosis of the liver, a common side effect of drinking too much, and respiratory diseases such as emphysema, resulting from smoking or exposure to environmental toxins at work.

However, as women increasingly flow into the workplace, I suspect that their life expectancy will begin to be more closely aligned with men's, unless modifications are made to minimize the damage inflicted by Western work patterns.

Aging is a process that determines not only when you will die but how you will live. The quality of your five senses, the clarity of your mind, the mobility of your body—all will be influenced either subtly or blatantly by aging.

In its most literal sense, aging is the physical deterioration of body functions over time. It is important to realize that your body ages *biologically,* not *chronologically.* The number of years you've been alive—your chronological age—may not correspond with the degree of damage your body has sustained—your biological age.

This is good news because, while chronological age isn't open to negotiation, biological age is. It's just as possible to be a sixty-year-old with a forty-year-old's body as it is to be a forty-year-old with a sixty-year-old's body. *The choice is yours.*

The first step toward reducing your biological age is understanding the process by which the body ages. What follows is a brief description of several theories about aging. Widely accepted though Hayflick's theory is, it is only one among many.

Since scientific research tends to be of a highly specific (and therefore intricately detailed) nature, many of the theories overlap. In addition, it's likely that several theories combined will offer a more accurate assessment of aging than any single theory.

For simplicity's sake, I have described similar theories under a single heading. I also include my own integrated theory of the different reasons why you grow old.

GENETIC CELLULAR AGING THEORIES

Several aging models relate to genetics. The primary one, already discussed, is Hayflick's limit. This theory was developed by testing embryonic human cells in test tubes. It is based on the premise that genes are the primary determinant of longevity.

Each of your genes contains DNA (deoxyribonucleic acid), which in turn contains your metabolic blueprint. A single gene is all that is required to exactly duplicate you. Imagine. A state-of-the-art computer microchip with the greatest possible memory storage doesn't even come close to the capacity of a single moecule of DNA.

According to Hayflick's theory, your genes are preprogrammed to reproduce a specific number of times. When the limit has been reached (between 110 and 120 years), the gene dies—you die.

There is some debate about the validity of Hayflick's limit for every kind of cell. Skin and gut cells, for example, undergo hundreds of thousands of divisions during a lifetime, compared to Hayflick's stated limit of fifty divisions. Cancer cells, too, seem impervious to arbitrary limits.

Hayflick's determination of the maximum division of cells in each species, which he asserts as the basis of genetically determined life-spans, is based in each case on *in vitro* (out of the body) experiments. Who is to say that the time periods between each of these predetermined divisions never vary from individual to individual or according to life-style variables? With the technology available to us today, why can't we make these divisions occur over a longer period of time, thus extending the potential maximum life-span? I believe that the calorie-restricted diet that I talk about in Chapter 10 works by extending the overall time it takes to obtain the maximum number of cell divisions discussed by Hayflick.

Other genetic aging theories focus on damage to the gene itself, or to the transmitter of genetic information, RNA (ribonucleic acid). For example, the "error catastrophe theory," developed in 1973 by Leslie Orgel at the Salk Institute, suggests that when DNA is damaged by changes in enzymes or the external environment, it produces bad information. This bad information is then transmitted by RNA to other cells, which then reproduce incorrectly, creating abnormal cells. As computer programmers say, it becomes a case of garbage in, garbage out.

Other genetic problems that accelerate aging are damage directly to RNA, resulting in inaccurate transmission of information and consequent cell mutation and dysfunction, and the inability of cells to decode transmitted information, also resulting in cell mutation and dysfunction.

The last genetic aging theory we will refer to postulates that since DNA contains a master plan for your construction and operation, it may also contain a preprogrammed master plan for your death.

Non-Genetic Cellular Aging Theories

The primary difference between genetic and non-genetic aging theories is that genetic theories focus on the cell's synthesis, or formation, while non-genetic theories focus on what happens to the cell after it is formed.

The primary non-genetic agents that damage cells and accelerate aging are: free radicals, cross-linkage, and accumulated toxic wastes. Each of the corresponding aging theories is summarized below.

The Free Radical Aging Theory

The free radical aging theory was first introduced in the 1970s by two key researchers, Dr. Denham Harman of the University of Nebraska College of Medicine and Lester Packer of the University of California at Berkeley. A free radical is an immensely reactive (and often deadly) chemical that differs from conventional molecules by possessing an unbalanced electrical charge, a free electron. Free radical reactions are essential to all life processes—energy production, immunity, nerve impulse transmission, hormone synthesis, and muscular contractions. However, excessive free radical levels are deadly. By attaching itself to an otherwise healthy molecule, a free radical creates a cumbersome, nonfunctional molecule.

The short-lived but voracious free radical agents attack the structure of cell membranes, creating waste products called lipofuscins. Lipofuscins bring the cell's normal repair and reproduction processes to a virtual standstill. They disturb DNA and RNA synthesis, destroy cellular enzymes (critical catalysts for chemical processes), and decrease protein synthesis. (More about lipofuscins in the discussion of the accumulated toxic wastes theory later in this chapter.)

Over time, harmful free radical disruption of cell metabolism leads to cellular aging and the production of mutant cells that may cause cancer.

Free radicals also damage collagen and elastin, the tissues that give your skin its structure and elasticity. Free radicals cause collagen and elastin to fray and break so that your skin, instead of clinging to your structure, begins to hang from it. This deterioration is especially noticeable in the face. Wrinkles and folds are largely the work of free radicals.

When combined with protein molecules, free radicals induce aging by causing cross-linkage, an aging phenomenon described immediately below.

Finally, free radicals have been associated with increased risk of cancer, senility, arteriosclerosis, and hypertension.

Sources of free radicals include: by-products from stress, illness, and fatigue; harmful environmental factors such as air pollution, cigarette smoke, ozone, nitrous oxide, and radiation (including sunlight, nuclear wastes, and microwave leaks); oxidized fats (see the discussion of lipofuscins later in this chapter for information on oxidation); chlorinated drinking water; and food additives such as sodium nitrite, sulfur dioxide, and synthetic colors.

The Cross-Linkage Aging Theory

The foremost proponent of the cross-linkage aging theory describes a cross-linking agent as a chemical that seizes hold of two otherwise separate molecules or parts of the same molecule and binds them firmly together.

Molecules thus bound are no longer able to absorb water, oxygen, or nutrients from the blood vessels. Soft contact lenses offer a visual demonstration of what happens to molecules attacked by cross-linkage. When kept in their appropriate saline solution environment, soft contact lenses are about as large as the iris, malleable to the touch, and quickly spring back to their natural conformation no matter how you bend them. Deprived of their natural liquid environment, soft contact lenses quickly become hard and shrink in size, being made utterly nonfunctional. That is pretty much what happens with cross-linked molecules.

Cross-linkage is even more dramatically demonstrated by overly suntanned faces. Sunlight accelerates the cross-linkage process by simultaneously evaporating your skin's natural moisture and cross-linking your skin cells so they can't absorb moisture from the blood vessels. The result is skin that looks tough, weather-beaten, leatherlike. (In fact, the cross-linking process is artificially induced to tan leather hides.)

Cross-linkage of DNA prevents protein synthesis and creates mutated cells that accumulate with age.

In addition to causing cellular and skin aging, cross-linkage has been indicted in the development of atherosclerosis, senile cataracts, osteoporosis, diabetes, and cancer.

While overexposure to sunlight is a primary cause of cross-linkage, other causes include free radicals; pollutants such as ozone and nitrous oxide; heavy metals such as aluminum, lead, and mercury; and antibodies left over from fighting illness or negative stress.

How Accumulated Toxic Wastes
Damage Your Cells

Throughout life, your cells absorb materials from your bloodstream and your skin's surface. Just as a sponge soaks up lighter fluid or grape juice with equal abandon, so your cells soak up toxic substances along with life-giving oxygen, water, and nutrients.

When you are young, your cells' repair and reproduction rates are so fast that poisoned cells are repaired or destroyed before they have a chance to do much damage. As you grow older, however, repair and reproduction rates slow down. Poisoned cells accumulate more poison and reproduce damaged cells that accelerate cellular aging processes.

Your cells collect wastes from two primary sources: environmental pollutants and oxidized fats.

The worst toxic-waste offenders are tobacco smoke, pesticides, mercury, cadmium, nuclear fallout, urban air, and lead (leaded gasoline keeps us well supplied with this poison).

The most common sources of oxidized fats are unrefrigerated margarine, shortening, bottles of liquid oils left open for more than a week, and foods cooked in oils at temperatures higher than 200 degrees Fahrenheit.

When fats are exposed to oxygen or heated to high temperatures, a chemical interaction takes place that combines fat molecules and oxygen molecules. The result is the deadly free radical discussed earlier. Free radicals attack cell membranes, creating waste products called lipofuscins (also mentioned earlier). Colored brown by the pigment melanin, lipofuscins appear on the skin's surface as large brown freckles commonly called age spots. Far from being a harmless phenomenon of old age, lipofucins tell you your cells are stuffed with accumulated waste.

Lipofuscins and other toxic wastes compete within the cell's structure for space and may come to occupy as much as 30 percent of a cell's total volume. Just as you couldn't get enough air if a third of your lungs were filled with a foreign substance, so your cells cannot properly reproduce, repair themselves, or produce energy when they are being smothered by accumulated wastes.

Whether the cause is genetic or non-genetic, cellular aging occurs when the rate of cellular damage exceeds the rate of cellular repair. The causes of cellular damage—bad genetic programming, spontaneous mutation, environmental toxins, viruses, free radicals, cross-linkage, accumulated toxic wastes, etc.—can be attacked and repelled by your body's natural defense and repair mechanisms. For example, your immune system destroys mutant or damaged cells. The naturally occurring antioxidants vitamin C, vitamin E, selenium, and cysteine prevent the formation of free radicals and cross-linkage. DNA repair programs undo cellular damage. However, when your defense and repair mechanisms are insufficient to cope with cellular damage, cellular aging begins.

SYSTEMS-FOCUSED AGING THEORIES

Up to this point, the aging theories discussed could be described as "reductionist." They deal on a molecular level with the activities of a cell or group of cells.

However, many researchers (myself included) believe that cellular aging theories address only a limited spectrum of the phenomena associated with aging. Perhaps at the dawn of evolution one-cell animals did live and die by cellular aging alone. Today, however, evolution has given rise to much more complicated interactions between life and death.

These interactions take place on a *systems* rather than *cellular* level of biological organization. Instead of discussing the role of specific antibodies, for example, we'll be discussing the role of the immune system that produces those antibodies.

Evolution has designed complex control systems to help you maintain a stable internal environment—adequate cell repair and reproduction rates, even body temperature and blood pressure, consistent heart rate, rhythmic flow of chemicals and hormones, strong defense against foreign bodies—

regardless of external conditions. While each of your biological systems contributes to maintaining this internal harmony, four systems are most closely associated with accelerating or delaying the aging process: the reticular activating system (RAS), the immune system, the autonomic nervous system, and the endocrine system. (The nervous and endocrine systems are frequently lumped together as the neuroendocrine system.)

Each of these systems plays a role in one or more of the complex control system's aging theories described below.

Reciprocal Interaction—The Key to Integrated Body Functions

Complex control systems monitor and regulate your internal environment through a communication network called reciprocal interaction or feedback control.

The process begins with the reticular activating system (RAS), your private window to both inner and outer worlds. The RAS operates in much the same way as peripheral vision, in that it is constantly observing and accumulating information without the need for conscious awareness. (Recent hypnosis studies indicate that objects and events seen *only* with peripheral vision actually are recorded more accurately in the subconscious mind than are directly perceived events and objects.)

Your RAS monitors even minute changes in your inner and outer environments. It detects changes in temperature; poisons in the air, food, or water; subtle imbalances in blood chemistry; sudden danger; sexual signals from others; the presence of germs or viruses; and countless other changes.

The RAS then relays this information to the hypothalamus, a pea-sized gland located in the back of your head at the base of your brain. The hypothalamus is the control center of the neuroendocrine system. It acts like a sophisticated switchboard, receiving information from your RAS and triggering the appropriate responses from your pituitary, thyroid, and adrenal glands, as well as other parts of the autonomic nervous and immune systems.

Some potential responses include the release of chemicals and hormones, muscular contractions, nerve stimulation, body temperature and blood pressure elevation, the production of immune system antibodies, and activation of sexual organs and glands.

Here's one example of reciprocal interaction in action. You are outside on a cool, sunny afternoon, wearing a cotton sweater and shirt. The sun sets sooner than you expected, and you find yourself without shelter or additional clothing. Your RAS, having noted the falling temperature, delivers this information to your hypothalamus. The hypothalamus then triggers these responses:

- The release of adrenaline into the bloodstream to increase heart rate and heat production
- Shivering to increase heart rate and heat production
- Thyroid activity to increase the metabolic rate at which food is converted into heat
- Activate brown fat metabolism (brown fat is a special kind of fat that surrounds vital organs, and when stimulated by the sympathetic nervous system, its calories are converted into heat to protect vital organs)
- Contraction of skin pores to minimize heat loss
- Reduce blood flow to hands and feet to conserve heat for essential life processes

When all systems are properly functioning, the interaction is quite elegant. When one or more systems are not working, the outcome is potentially fatal.

Dr. Roy Walford, a research gerontologist at UCLA, was one of the first scientists to discuss the relationship between immunity and aging. His immunologic theory of aging, presented in 1969, postulates that no evolutionary purpose is served in extending life beyond the child-bearing age. He speculates that we sort of "jiggle" apart, with first one system, then another, losing its ability to perform its role.

When Your Immune System Fails

Of all the complex control systems, the immune system offers our primary defense against aging. The immune system eliminates dysfunctional cells, destroys mutant cells, annihilates foreign bacteria and viruses, and generally rescues us from destruction.

However, even the immune system is vulnerable to attack. Too much stress, too much blood sugar, too much blood fat, too many free radicals, and many other factors can depress your immune system and keep it from functioning. Three potential dangers loom:

- The immune system may get lazy and fail to recognize damaged or mutant cells or foreign invaders.
- It may be unable to destroy all deviant cells, harmful bacteria, or other germs.
- It may mistake healthy cells for unhealthy ones, attack them, and thereby ultimately cause a disease.

In the first two instances of immune system failures, it's likely that the deviant cells or foreign bacteria, germs, or viruses will continue to multiply until they create enough symptoms to be called a disease. By then a great deal of cellular damage, leading to premature cellular aging, has been done.

When the immune system attacks healthy cells it creates diseases such as rheumatoid arthritis, multiple sclerosis, AIDS, rheumatic heart disease, SLE (systemic lupus erythematosis) that clearly accelerate the aging process.

Is There a Biological Clock?

Another neuroendocrinological theory, put forth in 1970, relates to the thymus, an important part of the immune system located near the thyroid gland.

According to Sir F. MacFarlane Burnet, of the University of Melbourne in Australia, the thymus may function as a biological clock or pacemaker that determines both the rate and critical stages of aging.

The thymus gland contains t-cells (thymus-derived cells) that circulate through the bloodstream devouring foreign invaders, including cancer cells. Shortly after puberty your thymus gland begins to shrink in size and produce fewer t-cells, increasing your vulnerability to infections and disease.

Negative stress also has a damaging effect on the thymus gland, contributing further to immune system decline, disease, and aging.

A Death Hormone?

Then there is the idea of a "death hormone" that preprograms us to age and die at a certain stage of our development. The best example of such apparent programming is the life and death pattern of the Pacific salmon.

Hatched in streams from the Columbia River and up the west coast of Canada and Alaska, these salmon spend their first six months in gravel river bottoms, the next year or so in lakes, and then drift out to sea. Two to four years later they return, swimming upstream and making heroic leaps up rapids and waterfalls, to the precise place of their birth. Soon thereafter, they spawn. With the birth of the next generation thus assured, the salmon's adrenal glands release a massive amount of corticoid hormones into their bloodstreams, and the fish grow old and die practically overnight.

While only several gerontologists suggest that man releases a similar "death hormone," many neuroendocrinological theories propose that a gradual imbalance of hormones released by the brain induces aging. Others describe an avalanchelike effect. In the example of reciprocal interaction to temperature change, mentioned earlier, the failure of any of the complex control systems would increase your risk of freezing to death.

It's also important to realize that complex control systems are interdependent. Therefore, damage to one may result in damage to all.

For example, age-related chemical and hormone changes have been shown to disrupt the arousal of the RAS. If your RAS is *no longer alert to changes* or *unable accurately to transmit those changes* to the hypothalamus, your hypothalamus will trigger inappropriate and potentially harmful responses. If the RAS, for instance, mistakenly identifies normal cells found in joints as foreign invaders, it will cause your hypothalamus to signal your immune system to attack. The outcome of this misadventure? Arthritis, a degenerative disease of aging.

Nor is the hypothalamus immune to error. Aging may decrease hypothalamic sensitivity to information. And, as you have already seen, misinterpreted information can create premature aging patterns.

Menopause is one (albeit preprogrammed) outcome of hypothalamic decline. In her late thirties or early forties a woman's hypothalamus produces less and less estrogen. As estrogen levels decline, ovulation ceases. Once ovulation stops, the woman is vulnerable to a variety of aging effects. Her calcium metabolism may be disturbed, preventing the formation of healthy bones, leaching calcium from bones and causing osteoporosis. In addition, the calcium may be deposited in soft tissues, causing arteriosclerosis and other sclerotic diseases. The onset of menopause is a key metabolic shift of aging that should be delayed as long as possible. (I'll discuss metabolic shifts in aging in the next chapter.)

3

An Integrated Aging Theory

As you can see from our discussion to this point, no single aging theory adequately explains the aging process, but taken as a whole they begin to reveal certain consistencies and theories that crop up too often to be ignored.

What follows is my integrated aging theory, which I believe addresses the primary aging factors.

I begin with the premise that when one is in a state of homeostasis—perfect physical, mental, and emotional balance—biological aging is slowed or stopped. Anything that disrupts homeostasis induces aging.

Aging is *the gradual disorganization of the orderly processes that create life*. The two key catalysts for creating disorder, disease, and death are:

- Preprogrammed genetic aging patterns
- Self-created premature aging patterns

Each of these aging programs is squared off against anti-aging forces in a war that lasts a lifetime. That aging eventually wins is beyond question; what *is* open to question is when and how you will age.

PREPROGRAMMED
GENETIC AGING PATTERNS

Your progress from birth to death is guided by one fundamental law of nature: *survival of the species*. Nature is not interested in life extension; it's obsessed with reproduction. Consequently, evolution takes a tender interest in your health through the childbearing years, but once that phase is over, that tender interest is over, too. Of course, the magic carpet of anti-aging forces isn't pulled out from under your feet all at once. Even evolution acknowledges the necessity of nurturing the next generation to adulthood. Instead, evolution gradually gives in to the aging forces, weakening the anti-aging response—a little cellular damage here, a little immune system depression there.

From the moment of conception, your genetic aging patterns pre-program your inevitable transition through each of the eight primary stages of life:

- Conception
- Embryonal fetal development
- Birth
- Growth
- Puberty
- Maturity
- Physiological decline
- Death

Most people reach biological maturity by the mid-twenties and remain in this stage until they are about thirty to forty years old. The maturity phase brings into fruition all the fertilization of youth. Rapid cell repair and reproduction rates have allowed you to achieve your full height and weight. Efficient calcium metabolism has helped you build strong bones. Massive growth hormone production and release has helped you build healthy muscles. Carbohydrates supply you with endless amounts of easily manufactured energy. Women produce plenty of the sex hormones estrogen and progesterone to oil their reproductive systems. Most men are easily able to manufacture sperm, produce erections, and experience orgasm. In short, you are exceedingly well prepared to perform the task evolution has set for you: to propagate the species.

However, even as you are experiencing the full bloom of your physical, mental, and emotional flowering, the preprogrammed seeds of self-destruction are slowly germinating within.

Already as you move beyond the age of twenty-five, your biological peak year, subtle changes begin to take place. Your neuroendocrine system produces fewer of the protein enzymes and hormones needed for cell repair and reproduction. The cells themselves lose some of the receptor sites that allow them to use enzymes and hormones. (Self-created aging patterns also influence cell metabolism, but I will discuss these separately.) Consequently, the rate of cellular damage begins to exceed the rate of cellular repair and reproduction. More damage and toxins accumulate and increase the risk of reproducing mutant cells.

Your RAS, hypothalamus, and entire neuroendocrine system are composed of cells, and they suffer from the same cellular aging processes that afflict your organs, muscles, and other tissues. The two-way communication known as reciprocal interaction gradually breaks down. *This breakdown is a major metabolic shift that accelerates aging.* The damaged DNA and RNA of organ (and other) cells are no longer able to *provide* accurate information to create new cells, and the damaged cells of the RAS, hypothalamus, and neuroendocrine system are no longer able to *perceive* information accurately. As a result, the hypothalamus begins to trigger inappropriate responses that create a cascade of aging effects.

The question of which comes first—damaged cells providing bad information or damaged cells misinterpreting information—is a bit like the chicken-and-egg riddle. The truth is as individual as your genetic pattern. However, for simplicity's sake I'll sketch out one scenario in which muscle cell damage creates a cascade of aging effects. Regardless of the catalyst, the aging consequences remain the same.

- Aging muscle cells gradually lose their receptor sites for enzymes and hormones. They also lose their receptor sites for glucose. (Carbohydrate-produced glucose is the primary energy source during the early stages of life.)
- Since your cells no longer absorb as much glucose as before, more glucose remains floating in your bloodstream.
- Your RAS notes the high blood sugar level and informs your hypothalamus.
- Your hypothalamus triggers the release of insulin (a glucose antagonist) to mop up the excess glucose.
- At the same time, these higher levels of insulin create other, less desirable, results. For example, insulin:

   Alters your metabolism so that free fatty acids replace glucose as the primary fuel source. (Excess free fatty acids have been linked to depressed immunity and increased risk of atherosclerosis, blood clots, and cancer. The shift from glucose to free fatty acids as a primary fuel source signals your metabolic shift from maturity to physiological decline.)

   Inhibits the release of growth hormone. (The depression of growth hormone leads to the loss of lean muscle mass.)

   Encourages your metabolism to convert food into fat instead of fuel. (Obesity has lately been categorized as a disease that increases blood pressure and risk of heart attack, accelerates premature aging, and leads to degenerative diseases such as cancer, hypertension, and atherosclerosis.

- Since it is the *balance* of glucose and insulin with free fatty acids and growth hormone that's necessary for blood sugar stability, the excess or insufficiency of either depresses your immune system and leads to the development of adult-onset diabetes, hypoglycemia, and premature aging.

There are many overlapping causes and effects in the aging process. Considered individually, they are not terribly significant. Considered as part of a complex process that ultimately triggers your shift from the stage of maturity to physiological decline, they are incredibly important.

Your brain is the final and most significant control system affected by preprogrammed genetic aging patterns.

The brain is also subject to the cellular aging patterns described earlier. Accumulated toxic wastes (especially aluminum), decrease in energy metabolism, genetically damaged nerve cells, lipofuscin accumulation, loss of nerve cell reactions and chemical signals, and the introduction of a slow-acting virus cumulatively create Alzheimer's disease.

Damaged brain cells contribute to the gradual failure of your RAS and hypothalamus.

The brain also suffers from specific genetic aging patterns that determine whether you will be in any condition to enjoy the later years of your life.

Your mental and physical functions are partly governed by a group of brain chemicals called neurotransmitters. These chemicals are the message carriers of reciprocal interaction. Although there are many different types of neurotransmitters performing a variety of functions, three neurotransmitters are particularly important to aging: acetylcholine, dopamine, and serotonin.

Acetylcholine governs memory, learning, physical movement, and autonomic nervous system balance. The age-related decrease of acetylcholine production creates forgetfulness, difficulty in learning, inability to perform simple motor tasks (such as tying shoelaces), and imbalances in the chemicals and hormones produced by the autonomic nervous system.

Dopamine and serotonin enjoy a yang/yin relationship. Dopamine stimulates your sympathetic nervous system to wake you up in the morning and initiate daytime metabolic processes. Serotonin stimulates your nervous system to induce sleep and initiate cell repair and reproduction activities.

Aging disrupts the correct ratio of dopamine to serotonin. Although production of both neurotransmitters is depressed over time, even less dopamine is produced than serotonin. (Abnormally low dopamine production causes Parkinson's disease.) The imbalance between dopamine and serotonin and cellular damage accelerate aging by altering the sensitivity of your hypothalamus to your body's fine-tuning needs. The influence of the pituitary and other endocrine glands' hormonal secretions is intensified, with damaging effect on target tissues. Diseases of aging develop.

The preprogrammed genetic aging patterns just discussed are ultimately unavoidable. However, *when* these aging patterns take effect and *how severely* you experience their symptoms is mainly up to you.

The self-created premature aging patterns described below reveal just how much control you have over when and how you will age.

YOU CAN CONTROL YOUR OWN
PREMATURE AGING PATTERNS

Each of the premature aging patterns that you create and control is discussed exhaustively in succeeding chapters. We will therefore content ourselves here with a brief overview of the primary self-created premature aging patterns and their effects.

Negative stress is the most significant aging factor within your control. Chronic negative stress triggers the release of cortisol, a hormone associated with the development of more than forty diseases, including cancer, diabetes, hypertension, congestive heart failure, and osteoporosis. Negative stress also weakens the immune system, leaving you vulnerable to degenerative disease.

Mental and emotional states influence the aging process. Studies show that people who are isolated from others, depressed, nonproductive, or lonely are significantly more susceptible to the diseases of aging than are their more involved counterparts.

Body rhythms govern your sleep/wake cycles, hormone/chemical secretions, reproductive cycles, and many other physiological functions. When you are overexposed to negative stress—east/west travel; uneven work, eating, or exercising schedules; social isolation; drugs; or other factors—resultant unbalanced body rhythms accelerate your transition from the maturity stage of life to that of physiological decline.

The environment in which you choose to live can accelerate aging by its proximity to toxic wastes and poisoned air, water, or food; exposure to certain weather conditions such as hot, dry winds or excessive cloudiness; sources and amount of light; and other factors. Poisons that you eat, breathe, or drink cause cellular damage. Hot, dry winds deluge you with positive ions (ions are atoms with an unbalanced electrical charge), which in turn trigger the release of excess cortisol, whose relationship to disease has already been noted. Excessive cloudiness increases the incidence of bone demineralization, leading to fragile, brittle bones. Artificial light deprives you of the full-spectrum light needed to catalyze metabolic processes, while overexposure to sunlight accelerates cellular aging.

A deficient or improper diet causes premature aging because it fails to provide necessary nutrients; burdens your metabolism with too many calories; fails to provide sufficient fiber; and saturates your system with salt, sugar, fat, and protein. Nutritional imbalances (rampant in the United States) disrupt cell repair and reproduction processes and cause vitamin-deficiency diseases such as anemia and pellagra. Deficiencies contribute to degenerative conditions—infertility, congenital defects, psychoses, diabetes, atherosclerosis, hypertension, cancer, heart disease, and osteoporosis. Excess calories cause obesity, a disease whose effects we have already discussed. Insufficient fiber makes the digestive process sluggish, so harmful bacteria have plenty of time to multiply in the beneficial environment of the intestines and colon. Diverticulosis, cancer of the colon, appendicitis, hemorrhoids, hernia, varicose veins, gall stones, colitis, and arteriosclerosis are just a few of the diseases associated with insufficient fiber. Excess salt raises blood pressure and water retention and thereby increases risk of heart attack and stroke. Excess sugar consumption has been reported to contribute to dental cavities, fat gain, muscular degeneration, immune system depression, arteriosclerosis, cardiovascular problems, diabetes, and hypoglycemia. Excess fat leads to cardiovascular disease, heart attack, stroke, arteriosclerosis, and cancer. In addition, oxidized fats damage cells through free radicals and cross-linkage. Excess protein leaches calcium from your bones and strains your kidneys.

Lack of proper exercise accelerates premature aging by reducing lean muscle mass, encouraging your metabolism to convert food into fat instead of fuel, and causing coordination and reaction speed to deteriorate. The loss of lean muscle mass and the accumulation of excess fat is a key metabolic shift that tips you from the edge of maturity to the plateau of physiological decline. Also, when your mind no longer has to fire neurotransmitters (especially acetylcholine) across pathways to initiate physical activity, that contributes to the decline of those neurotransmitters in both number and activity.

By now you must be feeling overwhelmed by all the hows and whys of aging. Don't lose heart. For every theory of aging, there is also a theory of living.

The Age Reduction System is designed to address every aging factor, both preprogrammed and self-created. You'll be amazed to discover just how much you can do to turn back the biological clock, prevent or dismantle the aging processes already occurring, and achieve optimal health and well-being.

We have not yet begun to fight.

Before we do begin, though, I strongly urge you to consult with your doctor. And follow the Age Reduction System only under his or her supervision. The Age Reduction System is designed for use by adults only. It should not be used by children, pregnant women, or individuals with liver or kidney ailments.

I also recommend that you undergo clinical laboratory testing.

- Testing can detect an early warning sign of impending disease that, if left untreated, may shorten life.
- Testing determines nutritional imbalances, exposure to toxins, allergic reactions, and side effects from drugs and supplements.
- Testing reveals success in following the Age Reduction System.
- Testing when you are young develops a reference norm that detects age-related pathology by measuring the deviation in your control systems. This appraises your body's condition and reveals aging disorders that you should correct with the Age Reduction System.

Test yourself when you begin the Age Reduction System, and repeat these tests on a regular basis—perhaps once every two years—throughout your life. Some of the tests that I recommend are:

Reason for Test

Prediagnostic Testing	Predicts future problems and current degree of pathology (See Chapter 12 for details)
Electroacupuncture (see Chapter 12)	Pinpoints nutrient requirements, allergic and side reactions to drugs and supplements
Bioilluminence photography (see Chapter 12)	Measures stress, autonomic nerve system reactivity, and organ function
Urine Testing	Determines problems in your kidney, prostate, and blood. Monitors vitamin and mineral status, hormone activity, liver and gall bladder function, hormonal balance, and nutrient metabolism
Multistix—urine dipstick available for home use (about $35.00 for 100) (pH, protein, glucose, ketone, bilirubin, occult blood, nitrates, urobilingen, ascorbic acid)	Measures nine functions
Microscopic examination	Measures/checks for substances indicating body and metabolic functions noted above
Hematology	Routine blood testing often performed on automatic counter produces information about blood and other systems
Complete blood count	
Red blood count and Hematocrit, Hemoglobin	Tests oxygen transport system, determines anemia, drug toxicity, kidney and organ problems
White blood count and differential	Tests immune system function, infections, stress, cancer, allergic reactions, and hormonal imbalances
Iron and total iron-binding capacity	Measures iron toxicity and requirements for supplemental iron
Energy Balance	
Growth hormone	Determines hyper- or hyposecretion of growth hormone from the pituitary gland
Fasting blood sugar	Detect abnormal sugar regulation and insulin secretion; confirm hypoglycemia or diabetes
Glucose tolerance test	
Diastix (self-testing glucose kits available for home use)	
Total blood cholesterol	Determine heart and blood vessel disease, bowel nutrition, liver problems, and kidney damage; measure central control problems in energy metabolism
HDL/LDL cholesterol	
Triglycerides	
Lipoprotein electrophoresis	

| Body fat percent | Determines metabolic efficiency, caloric imbalance, necessity for dieting, and risk of aging disorders |

Adaptive Systems

Dexamethasone suppression test	Measure hypothalamic–pituitary gland–adrenal cortex system balance, indicate stress reactivity
Plasma cortisol	
17 hydroxycorticosteroids	
17 corticosteroids	

Thyroid Balance

T3	Indicate hyper- or hypothyroid activity and central control problems of thyroid balance
T4	
Blood TSH	

Reproductive System

FSH	Detect infertility, climacteric, sexual system hormonal imbalance; pinpoint need for hormone replacement therapy in women
LH	
Testosterone	
Progesterone	
Estrogen	

Kidney Function Tests

Blood urea nitrogen (BUN)	Evaluate kidney function and dysfunction
Serum creatine and creatinine	
Uric acid	
Creatinine clearance	

Liver Function Tests

| Bilirubin tests (total, direct, indirect) | Evaluate liver function and dysfunction |

Enzyme Tests

LDH	Reflect tissue damage and organ malfunction
SGOT	
SGPT	

Electrolytic Balance

CO_2 (carbon dioxide)	Assess fluid balance, acid-base balance, organ function, and control mechanisms; evaluate bone, adrenal, kidney, bladder, and bowel functions
Chloride	
Sodium	
Potassium	
Inorganic phosphorus	

Miscellaneous Tests

Breast self-examination	Detects development of breast cancer. (Women should examine breasts once a month for lumps, wrinkles, dimples and discharges.)
Oral vitamin C test	Determines need for vitamin C
Exercise stress test Blood pressure and pulse rate	Evaluates heart and circulatory system, autonomic nervous system function, exercise's stress reactivity. (Learn to measure your pulse rate at home with a stopwatch. Monitor your own blood pressure with a sphygmomanometer.)

NOTE: Some of the test names used here may not be fully understandable to you, but your doctor will know them well. Feel entitled to request a full explanation of the tests from your physician.

Longevity: Attitude, Life-style, and Environment— They All Make a Difference

4

The Basic Steps Toward a Longer, Healthier Life

Much has been written about the importance of diet and exercise in encouraging long life. Obviously, this is not much ado about nothing. I cover this connection myself in later chapters.

However, recent research has revealed some inconsistencies in the relationship between living right and living long.

For example, a study commissioned by the Committee for an Extended Lifespan (and reported by UPI in 1979) examined common characteristics among people who lived to be more than 100 years old. A. Stuart Otto, the San Marcos, California, minister who founded and ran the committee, said: "At the beginning of this study we thought they would have long-lived parents, that they would not smoke or drink; they would be vegetarians, and so on. We were wrong on all counts."

Of more than 1000 centenarians investigated, many were poor, smoked, drank, ate meat freely, and were descended from ancestors who did not live very long lives.

However, Otto said that many of them had these factors in common:

- They did all things in moderation. They might drink, but were never drunks. Smokers tended to smoke cigars or pipes; if they smoked cigarettes, they did not inhale.
- They tended to get up early in the morning, which usually meant they went to bed early at night.
- They were devoutly religious and accepted the trials of life as "God's will."
- They were busy people, hard workers with a penchant for action instead of contemplation.
- They were "self-protective," refusing to allow the problems of life to distress them.

• They were frequently self-employed and therefore free of the stress of working for a boss.

My own research corresponds with these findings. It is interesting to note that each of these six common factors relate to *attitude and life-style,* rather than to diet and exercise. Particularly interesting are the third and fifth factors: accepting the trials of life as God's will and being self-protective. Either indicates a willingness to accept rather than resist, to bend rather than break. This is an all-important attitude, which we will discuss thoroughly in another part of this chapter.

In a separate study, *Prevention* magazine sponsored a Louis Harris survey of 103 leading health experts. The experts were asked to vote on what they thought were the twenty most important things people could do to live longer. The results, reported in the 1985 *Prevention Index,* were surprising.

Here are the experts' recommendations, listed in order of importance:*

1. Not smoking
2. Avoiding smoking in bed
3. Wearing seat belts
4. Not driving under the influence of alcohol
5. Living in a home or apartment with a smoke detector
6. Socializing regularly
7. Exercising strenuously
8. Keeping alcohol consumption moderate
9. Avoiding home accidents
10. Restricting dietary fat
11. Maintaining a normal weight
12. Obeying speed limits
13. Having blood pressure checked at least yearly
14. Controlling stress
15. Consuming adequate fiber
16. Restricting dietary cholesterol
17. Getting adequate vitamins and minerals
18. Having periodic dental exams
19. Restricting sodium
20. Restricting sugar
21. Sleep seven to eight hours

Of these twenty-one items, *fully 60 percent are life-style* choices that have nothing to do with diet or exercise. Fifty percent involve safety measures. The moral of the survey is that both good sense and good health are prerequisites for long life.

That's why the first section of the Age Reduction System is devoted to attitude, life-style, and environment. In the larger sense, of course, diet

* From *The Prevention Index, 1985.* Emmaus, Pennsylvania: Rodale Press, 1985.

and exercise also are life-style choices. However, your attitudes, values, and beliefs exert a tremendous influence over your body's aging mechanisms.

Before we begin, I'd like to share with you a Zen koan (*koan* means story or riddle).

An English professor of Oriental philosophy invites a Zen master to his home for tea and discussion of mutual interests. When the Zen master arrives, the professor greets him warmly, sits down in front of a tea service, and begins waxing eloquent about his extensive interest in and knowledge of Zen philosophy. The Zen master asks if he may pour the tea; the professor readily acquiesces. As the professor continues to expound, the master quietly fills the professor's cup. He keeps pouring the tea, even though the cup is overflowing. The professor, eventually distracted by the sight of tea spilling over his Oriental carpet, remarks in consternation, "Sir, excuse me, but you are spilling the tea. The cup is overfull." The Zen master replies, "So it is with your mind. It is already so full of opinions that it has no room for anything I might offer you. You must empty the cup first."

Will you empty the cup of your preconceptions now?

And now let's begin our work together with a self-evaluation. Before you can determine where you want to go, you must know where you are.

In the next section of this chapter, you'll read a comparison of typical long- and short-lived personalities. As you read this, consider which category you fall into for each of the characteristics. This profile will reveal the primary factors that you should alter to reduce your biological age.

A LONG LIFE OR A SHORT ONE?
PERSONALITY PROFILES

In the United States only four or five people out of every 100,000 will live more than 100 years.

In isolated portions of the Russian republics of Azerbaijan, Georgia, and Armenia, as well as Vilacamba in the Ecuadorian Andes, more than ten times as many people will live to be more than 100 years.

Consistent overestimation of ages in centenarian communities has cast doubt on the authenticity of their actually being so long lived. Accurate birth records are kept in these primitive cultures, but past the age of seventy it is common to add extra years with each subsequent birthday since in these societies appearing older increases status and respect.

While these centenarians don't live beyond Hayflick's limit of 110 to 120 years, overall they significantly outlive us. These elderly men and women are much more physically and sexually active than we are in the later years. They suffer far less heart disease, atherosclerosis, cancer, arthritis, hypertension, and osteoporosis than do our elderly.

What causes this statistically significant difference?

By examining the various cultures and comparing them to our own, we can arrive at reasons relevant to age reduction.

Six primary factors—present in every society—influence longevity. They are:

- Attitude, personality, and philosophy
- Social and cultural life
- Geography, climate, and environment
- Diet and nutrition
- Physical and sexual activity
- Heredity

As you read these profiles, circle the traits in each column with which you identify. In some cases you will probably see yourself in both lists at once. That's fine. Human beings are complicated. Then take note of the short-lived personality traits that you circled. These are the areas in which the Age Reduction System will prove most relevant to extending your life.

A long-lived personality	A short-lived personality
Sees life as a series of endless, rhythmic cycles	Sees life as a linear path filled with obstacles that must be overcome
Happily anticipates a long life marked by the changes of the seasons and the birth of younger generations	Expects to grow old and die shortly after retirement
Does not understand the concept of retirement but rather adjusts his/her work load to slowly declining abilities	Looks forward to retirement as a relief from an unhappy occupation
Is noncompetitive	Is highly competitive
Is equally interested in the process and the goal	Is only interested in achieving results; views process as only a means to an end
Is flexible about altering decisions or goals that are no longer appropriate	Is inflexible about changing his/her mind, which he/she views as a sign of weakness
Lives and works in the same geographical area throughout life	Frequently changes jobs or moves to new locations
Prefers quality to quantity	Prefers quantity to quality
Measures time by sunsets and seasons	Measures time by a stopwatch
Has a strong will to live	Has a strong fear of death
Loves to play	Doesn't have time to play
Is emotionally stable, with few prolonged highs or lows	Is emotionally unstable, wavering between euphoria and depression

A long-lived personality	A short-lived personality
Views work as natural and necessary, but no more so than marriage and family and play time	Views work as both monster and mistress, at once too demanding and also perhaps the only rewarding aspect of life
Is active within the community throughout life	Is isolated from the community, participating less and less with advancing years
Lives in a culture that reveres and respects the aged, frequently seeking them out for counsel	Lives in a culture that despises old age and treats the elderly as if they were childish or useless
Has children who remain close throughout life	Has not had children, or is estranged from them
Is quite social, frequently walking in the community to visit neighbors	Is introverted and tends to hide from the world behind closed curtains
Lives in a rural environment	Lives in an urban environment
Breathes pure air, drinks pure water, eats organic foods	Breathes polluted air; drinks polluted water; eats processed, refined, degraded foods
Lives at fairly high altitudes, where the air is cool and temperate	Lives at low altitudes, subject to extreme changes of weather, high pressure, dry winds, and temperature inversions
Lives in fairly simple conditions, relying on natural resources such as sunlight, wood, and water, for light, fuel, and liquid needs	Lives in a high-technology environment, surrounded by power lines, electrical appliances, artificial light, and computer monitors
Consumes between 1200 and 2000 calories per day	Consumes between 2000 and 4000 calories per day
Eats a diet high in complex carbohydrates, low in animal protein and fat	Eats a diet high in refined carbohydrates, fat, and animal protein
Eats foods primarily in their natural state, fresh and uncooked	Eats foods that are refined, processed, canned, frozen, and otherwise manipulated
Consumes very little refined sugar or salt	Consumes an average of 125 pounds of sugar and about 8 pounds of salt per year
Drinks a moderate amount of alcohol distilled from grains, fresh vegetables, fruits, or dairy products	Drinks an excessive amount of hard liquor
Has no concept of exercise as a separate activity, since it is of necessity a major part of life	Conceives of exercise as an unwelcome fad; dreads the idea that it might be necessary
Is involved in agricultural work and physical labor throughout life	Has a desk job
Walks and rides bicycles or animals as primary means of transportation	Drives a car to the corner store
Uses his/her body rhythmically and economically for long hours, never reaching the point of exhaustion	Uses his/her body as little as possible. Any exercise is sporadic and frantic, producing exhaustion and sore muscles

A long-lived personality	A short-lived personality
Dances regularly as a member of community gatherings	Socializes in sedentary ways
Experiences few sexual inhibitions or obsessions	Is inhibited, compulsive, anxious, or obsessive about sex
Perceives sex as a simple, natural extension of life, interconnected with social and familial values	Perceives sex as a physical activity separate from the rest of life, including relationships and children
Enjoys sex throughout life, sometimes siring children when as old as eighty or bearing them when as old as fifty	Experiences a declining sexual appetite and ability with advancing years
May have inherited a predisposition for long life from mother's side	Was conceived by parents with a consistent history of degenerative diseases, such as cancer, heart disease, or stroke

You probably found yourself identifying more closely with short-lived than long-lived personality traits. That isn't surprising in a culture as mobile, competitive, and "civilized" as ours.

When I first began to introduce the Age Reduction System concepts into my life, I was shocked to discover how many unhealthy habits I had acquired over the years. Some were unconscious childhood habits, such as adding salt and fat to foods. Others were the inevitable result of conscious choices, such as breathing polluted Los Angeles air. Still others were deeply ingrained behavior patterns created in childhood and compounded over the years that did not support health and longevity. For example, I used to cope with negative stress by internalizing my feelings until they erupted in a cold, flu, or other illness. Now I've learned to minimize my exposure to negative stress, express my feelings more easily, and, when all else fails, take out my frustrations by kicking a punching bag in my martial arts class.

I adopted the Age Reduction System as I discovered it—over a period of years. Although you are receiving this information all at once, I suggest that you, too, allow yourself at least a year to incorporate its recommendations gradually. The mind rebels at too many changes all at one time.

The first step is to identify your primary short-lived personality traits. Having completed this, you may want to make a short list, in order of priority, of those traits you are most willing or able to change. I recommend that you review the entire Age Reduction System before adopting any of its suggestions. (Your priorities or approach to age reduction may change.) Then incorporate one set of suggestions at a time. For example, if your list of short-lived personality traits includes being ruled by the clock, being isolated from others, and eating too much fat, take steps to deal first with your compulsion about time before attempting to create new bonds with other people. Excessive change creates negative stress. Too desperate an effort at cure can kill the patient.

Before you embark on the Age Reduction System, let me offer an important piece of advice: Be kind to yourself. Humor, patience, and self-acceptance are qualities that add years to your life *and* life to your years.

5

The Awesome Power of Your Mind

Perhaps the most important unexplored frontier of our time is the human mind. Brain/mind researchers may argue over whether we use 10 or 20 percent of it on a conscious basis, but they all agree that the functions of the remaining 80 to 90 percent are largely mysterious. Research into brain function is continually leading to new discoveries, many of which explode previously accepted theories.

For example, brain/mind researchers once believed that memory was located in a particular part of the brain. By selectively inducing brain damage in monkeys, they believed they could eliminate memory. What they discovered instead was that the brain has an awesome ability to relearn and restructure memory in other parts of the brain.

Contrary to expectations, the human brain/mind cannot be neatly and automatically divided into different parts with specific functions. The human brain is a gestalt. The thoughts, emotions, chemicals, hormones, cells, tissues, and other factors that influence brain/mind function are constantly changing and interacting with each other. If one portion of the brain is damaged, the rest responds by nurturing the damaged area and simultaneously attempting to reapportion the functions of the damaged area to other parts of the brain. Brain-damaged monkeys suffering from memory loss relearn those memories even if the damaged brain tissue dies.

One thing seems certain: The capacity of our minds to influence our physical, mental, and spiritual well-being is staggering.

What follows is one example of the human mind in action.

A MIND-INDUCED WORK ALLERGY

Rita Stravos was a reader at a prominent Hollywood movie studio. Her work consisted of reading and analyzing screenplays submitted to the studio for development.

When Rita came to see me, she complained of terrible headaches, nausea, and itchy, puffy eyes. I asked her whether she had made any major changes in her life recently. She said no, she had held the same job for five years, lived in the same apartment in North Hollywood, remained single. When I asked if she was happy, she shrugged her shoulders and said, "I'm surviving."

"Tell me what doesn't work about your life," I asked.

After some coaxing, she began to describe her work. "When I first started my job I was very starry-eyed about Hollywood. I hoped to work my way up to being a studio executive in charge of developing projects.

"After the first year or so, though, the fun started wearing thin. All I did all day was sit in my office, read scripts, and write analyses. When I was allowed to attend story meetings, I began to understand why great movies rarely get made. The politics! Everyone sitting around holding their breath, waiting to see who's going to venture an opinion. It made me sick."

I glanced up from taking my notes at this point. Our eyes met for a silent few seconds. I continued taking her history, then recommended a series of laboratory tests.

The results were ironic, to say the least. Rita had acquired a violent allergy to ink—printer's ink, typewriter ink, any kind of ink at all.

It was no wonder she experienced most of her attacks at work, where she spent her day inhaling the fumes of typewritten scripts and printed books.

Even Rita had to laugh at the thoroughness with which she had boxed herself in. She said, "You know, if you had suggested that my problems were stress-related and that I look for another kind of work, I would have said, 'No way. I can't afford it. I won't even consider it.' But now I really don't have a choice about it. I can't very well continue to work in an environment that makes me violently ill."

Once Rita accepted the fact that change was required, she had to consider what she might like to do instead.

First, Rita decided that she no longer wanted to live in Los Angeles. She hated the smog and the crowds and the crime. She decided to move to the country. Having made that decision, she also realized that she disliked the loneliness of just reading and writing. She wanted to work with people. So, she decided to renew her teaching certificate and see if she could find work in a country school.

Perhaps you are wondering how Rita could teach if she couldn't read school books. An interesting dilemma. At first, Rita proposed to resolve it by laminating the pages of her school books so the fumes couldn't escape. This solution proved unnecessary, however. Within two months of Rita's resignation as a reader, her allergy to ink had disappeared.

How Does the Mind Do It?

Nobody really knows how the human mind translates such intangibles as disliking one's work into physical symptoms such as allergies. We've only begun to learn how the mind influences the brain and the brain influences the body.

What follows is a summary of what we do know about the relationships among brain/mind function, health, and longevity.

For the purposes of this explanation, we'll define the mind as that part of each of us that feels, perceives, thinks, wills, and reasons. The brain, on the other hand, is the organ of thought and neural coordination. The reticular activating system (RAS), which includes the hypothalamus and pituitary glands, mediates between the mind, the brain, and the body.

In the past, researchers tended to view the nervous system and the higher centers of the brain as a series of separate circuits, each performing a particular task. However, more recent evidence seems to indicate that the mind and body function as a unified, holistic system.

The RAS is one of the best pieces of neurophysiological evidence for a profound interconnection between mind and body.

The RAS functions as a kind of two-way street, carrying messages from the mind (or higher awareness centers) to the organs and muscles, and also relaying muscular and organic messages to the cerebral cortex. Whether the messages are intangible, such as thoughts, or tangible, such as the communication of cell or muscle damage, the result is the same: Neurophysiological responses are triggered. These responses include the release of chemicals and hormones by the hypothalamus or pituitary gland, the depression or activation of the immune system, the manipulation of electrical currents within the body.

Neurophysiological responses in turn trigger physical changes. They may alter your mood, whet or depress your appetite, increase or decrease your energy level, create ulcers or headaches or allergies, or set the stage for degenerative disease.

Perhaps the most drastic neurophysiological response has to do with disruption of the body's electrical currents. At its most extreme, this disruption can cause sudden death syndrome. Sudden death syndrome is defined as an unexpected natural death occurring within about six hours after the onset of acute symptoms or signs. (Often death is instantaneous.) For example, Lyndon Johnson suffered a fatal and entirely unexpected heart attack the day after President Nixon announced his intention of dismantling Johnson's Great Society program.

There is considerable evidence indicating that sudden death syndrome is caused by cardiac arrhythmia, which means that the electrical currents in the heart have gone haywire.

What causes the currents to go haywire? According to recent evidence: stress. Chronic, prolonged stress (which will be more precisely defined later in this chapter) causes the sympathetic nervous system to overload the heart with an increased pulse rate and blood pressure, causing the electrically regulated contractions to become irregular.

Each year in the United States, about 450,000 people succumb to SDS, accounting for 25 percent of all deaths. It is the leading cause of mortality in the twenty-to-sixty-four age group and approximates the annual toll exacted by all malignancies.

The following case history (reported in the April 1979 issue of *Psychosomatics* magazine by Dr. Patrick T. Donlon, Dr. Arnold Meadow, and Dr. Ezra Amsterdam, all associated with the University of California School of Medicine at Davis) illustrates the differences between physical and emotional stress as they relate to cardiac arrhythmia and sudden death syndrome. This account is condensed and paraphrased.

GUILT: A SELF-DESTRUCTIVE FORCE

Walter Parkinson was a thirty-eight-year-old, tall, slender, twice married engineer. When he entered treatment with doctors Donlon, Meadow, and Amsterdam, he had recently experienced a "mild heart attack."

Prior to this attack, Walter had displayed no cardiac symptoms. His general health, as well as that of his parents, was excellent. He didn't smoke, rarely drank alcohol. However, he had experienced a great deal of emotional stress the week prior to the attack. He spoke of problems with his supervisor over a contract deadline, of rejection by a friend and marital friction.

Upon recovering from acute symptoms, Walter resumed his normal activities. Physical exercise had been one of his sole forms of relaxation before the cardiac episode, and he found he could return to it without experiencing any cardiovascular symptoms. In the succeeding year he learned to ski, frequently backpacked into the high mountains, and helped farm friends do heavy labor, such as throwing bales and cutting wood.

In contrast, Walter reported that emotional distress frequently triggered irregular heartbeat and angina. Six weeks after his attack, he sought psychiatric help. He was afraid that emotional factors might provoke another "heart attack."

In interviews, Walter described himself as "hard-working, overly honest but full of guilt and unable to express feelings." He had married his wife—who was pregnant at the time—out of a sense of guilt and obligation, only to lose the child to congenital heart disease at the age of two. He said the marriage had quickly soured, and he now found himself disgusted at his wife's developing alcoholism.

Work relationships proved equally stressful. Walter described his supervisor as "critical, guilt-provoking, and frustrating" with respect to his own career aspirations. Although Walter frequently worked sixty hours a week, he claimed his supervisor was unhappy with his overall performance, and that any attempts to increase productivity went unrewarded.

The interviewers characterized Walter as having a "high level of anxiety and tension, isolation of affect, and moderately depressed mood."

During therapy, Walter described a confrontation with his supervisor the previous day. The supervisor had found fault with a major proposal Walter was finishing. Walter said he reacted at the time by withdrawing into politeness, but when he recalled the incident in therapy his reaction was markedly different. Tension, an unsteady yet controlled angry voice, sweating, a strained facial expression, pallor, and rapid respiration were obvious. It was then Walter experienced chest pains, which were relieved by nitroglycerin. He said he experienced similar chest pains when confronted with friction at home.

According to doctors Donlon, Meadow, and Amsterdam, "Continuous cardiac monitoring of hospitalized patients who experience sudden death demonstrates that death is most commonly preceded by arrhythmias, especially ventricular fibrillation" (irregular heartbeat).

In Walter's case, stress was the primary cause of the irregular heartbeat that made him vulnerable to sudden death syndrome. The fact that the source of stress was emotional rather than physical may give you some idea of the power of the human mind. Clearly, what Walter needed was a way either to reduce emotional stress or to cope with it more effectively.

Herbert Benson, researcher at the Harvard School of Medicine and author of *The Relaxation Response,* writing in the 1975 issue of *Lancet,* states: "Passive relaxation, meditation, and sleep decreases neural sympathetic stimulation of the heart, and reduces ventricular premature beat frequency [irregular heartbeat]." We'll discuss these methodologies in greater detail later in this chapter.

STRESS: THE INVISIBLE INFLUENCE

Based on the case history you've just read, you may have concluded that stress, any kind of stress, is an enemy agent.

Remember, however, that Walter Parkinson, in the example cited above, was actually rejuvenated and relaxed by physical stress such as skiing and hiking.

So what do we learn from this?

Perhaps the first thing we learn is that *stress is an active force*. It is a catalyst. It motivates you to get up in the morning, to take risks, to learn new things. It also can make you want to avoid getting up in the morning, make you fearful about taking risks, and prevent you from learning new things.

Positive and negative stress are two sides of the same coin. To a large degree, *you* determine the flip of the coin. Your attitude, your viewpoint determines whether you will respond to stress with fear or excitement, uncertainty or equanimity.

Before we discuss some of the solutions to negative stress, let's understand how your body experiences it.

Stress Types and Their Consequences

Negative stress can be divided into two categories: acute and chronic.

Acute stress occurs when you are facing an immediate threat, such as an impending automobile accident. Messages are sent to the brain within milliseconds of perceiving the threat; the brain responds by releasing massive doses of adrenaline or noradrenaline activating fight or flight responses. The phenomenal burst of energy and mental clarity provided by these hormones is responsible for "miracles" of survival, such as the feat of strength in which a woman lifted a car off her husband, who was trapped underneath. These hormones are also responsible for the shakes you may experience when an impending accident or disaster is narrowly averted. Acute stress responses are survival-oriented and necessary.

On the other hand, chronic stress, such as you might experience when working in a noisy, smelly factory or a high-pressure stock exchange, is prolonged and unabated. In fact, according to stress researchers, subliminally perceived stimuli, such as white noise (e.g., a refrigerator hum), noxious odors, or gory photographs can produce anxiety in a person without that person's knowing why he or she is anxious. Chronic stress activates a different hormone, called cortisol. The raw material for cortisol is cholesterol.

In an article titled, "Stress, Cortisol, Interferon and Stress Diseases," published in the 1984 issue of the journal *Medical Hypotheses,* Dr. Alfred Sapsie enumerates some interesting characteristics of cortisol. He cites studies indicating that death is often preceded for two to seven days by increased cortisol levels. Sapsie hypothesizes that increased cortisol levels may *predict* death rather than *result* from it.

In addition, Sapsie associates elevated cortisol levels with a number of degenerative diseases, including:
- Hypertension
- Ulcers
- Myocardial infarction (a precursor of sudden death syndrome)
- Diabetes
- Infections
- Alcoholism

- Obesity
- Chronic painful organic diseases such as arthritis
- Cerebral vascular accidents
- Psychosis of the aging
- Skin diseases such as psoriasis
- Acne
- Eczema
- Parkinson's disease
- Multiple sclerosis
- Alzheimer's disease

Sapsie suggests that stress reactions, in the form of excess cortisol, promote the development of degenerative diseases by:

- Interfering with the immune system
- Actively encouraging the development of disease

Cortisol is considered a potentially powerful immune system suppressor. When produced in excessive amounts, it not only inhibits the production of antibodies, it may kill antibodies already in existence.

Sapsie also suggests two ways in which elevated cortisol levels promote the development of disease.

His first premise is that elevated levels of cortisol *precede* certain diseases, rather than follow them. To support this premise, he cites studies of cancer, recurring herpes genitalis, and diabetes, in which cortisol was found to influence the onset of disease. For example, a study by Dr. Stanley Bierman of 375 herpes patients reported that "emotional stress induced a reactivation of genital herpes recurrences in 86 percent of the cases." (Bierman has a private practice in Los Angeles; his survey results were reported in Sapsie's article.)

Recent research seems to support Dr. Sapsie's claim. Apparently, a loss of cortisol receptors in your brain from aging causes excess cortisol and degenerative disease.

Sapsie's second premise is based on the side effects of corticosteroid therapy. Used to treat inflammatory diseases such as arthritis, kidney disease, and bronchial asthma, corticosteroid therapy has been found to produce symptoms of "chronic diseases" in patients. When corticosteroid therapy was discontinued, the "chronic disease" symptoms would disappear.

Obviously, excessive cortisol levels aren't desirable. But how can you prevent them?

I have found two methods that are useful:

- Ingesting nutrients and drugs that are antagonistic to cortisol
- Altering neurophysiological responses so your body doesn't overproduce cortisol.

These are the anti-cortisol nutrients and drugs I recommend:

- Vitamin C—1 to 2 grams per day

• Aspirin—Two tablets in the morning and two tablets at night. In place of regular aspirin use Encaprin, encapsulized aspirin that is released in your intestines and doesn't produce gastric distress.

• Procaine (the active ingredient in GH-3, an anti-aging drug discussed in Chapter 13)

• Ginseng, which may be your best way to control stress and cortisol. Ginseng contains steroid chemicals such as panaxatriol, similar in their structure to adrenocortical hormones. These substances prevent overstimulation of the adrenal gland, stimulate other organs, and balance your neuroendocrine system. Siberian ginseng, available from supplement suppliers in Chapter 9, is a very potent stress control supplement. (See Chapter 9 for warnings on who *should not* take ginseng and on avoiding the Ginseng Abuse Syndrome.)

Another important method of reducing cortisol is to eat less cholesterol-rich foods such as egg yolks, high-fat dairy products, organ meats, shell fish, shrimp, and fatty meats. In retrospect, the success of the Pritikin program may result from its reduction of cortisol.

Birth control pills are hazardous. They contain high amounts of estrogen and progesterone that increase cortisol and disease. The lifelong process of replacing estrogen and progesterone that I describe in Chapter 13 lowers cortisol.

For complete instructions on proper use of supplements see Chapter 9.

Stress and Your Personality Type

Almost everyone has heard about the Type A personality—the individual who is aggressive, ambitious, impatient, obsessive. Type A's try to control things—their schedules, environments, diets, friends. They usually have a compulsion to dominate life, to try to bend it to their will. They tend to explode easily, confronting conflicts with their fists up. Not surprisingly, Type A's are more likely to experience hypertension, ulcers, heart attack, stroke, and depression than other people.

But what about Type B or Type C? Seen many headlines about these types lately? When I describe them you will understand why they don't receive more special attention.

Type C is the flip side of Type A. Where Type A is extroverted, Type C is introverted. Where Type A tries to control life, Type C feels controlled by it. Type C's probably experience the same degree of frustration as Type A's, but they turn this destructive force inward, rarely revealing the storm that lies beneath the surface. In their mild-mannered way, Type C's are just as self-destructive as Type A's. However, they typically display diseases other than heart attacks to express this destruction, among which are cancer, viral infections, and colds. Interestingly, Type C's don't produce quite as much cortisol as Type A's, but they often have an impaired interferon (immune) response, resulting in increased risk of degenerative disease, especially cancer.

Type A's take it out on the world.

Type C's take it out on themselves.

Type B personalities, as you may have guessed by now, tend to strike a harmonious balance between Type A and Type C characteristics. The long-lived personality factors described previously offer an excellent profile of a Type B personality. The primary characteristic of this personality is the ability to control stress and benefit from it. Because of this, the Type B personality is not associated with any particular degenerative disease.

Transforming Personality Types

The key question is: How do you transform a Type A or C personality into a Type B, thereby reducing the aging factors of stress?

Work with my own clients has revealed that the answer is simple but not necessarily easy: Analyze your own stress reactions and alter those that don't work.

There are several methodologies for achieving this goal, which we will discuss fully in the next sections of this chapter:

1. Discover precisely how you respond to stress.
2. Determine which of your reactions are useful *and which are not.*
3. Learn how your stress reactions travel through the body and what havoc they wreak.
4. Understand how the autonomic nervous system works and why its balance is important.
5. Determine whether your sympathetic or parasympathetic nervous system dominates and what you can do to equalize their activity.
6. Learn how to achieve altered states to improve your stress reactions and reduce your biological age.
7. Consider altering the attitudes that increase aging and adopting those that reduce it.

Now it's time to implement Step 1 of this list by taking the assessment that follows. From there we will discuss techniques you can use to alter your less healthy responses to stress.

A Stress-Response Questionnaire

I designed the following questionnaire to help you discover how you typically cope with stress. Respond to the following hypothetical situations by circling the answer (A, B, or C) that most closely corresponds to what you would do. For the questionnaire to be useful, you *must* be relentlessly honest in your answers. We're trying to discover how you *do* respond, not how you *should* respond.

When you have completed the questionnaire, read the analysis of your responses.

1. You are ready to leave for the airport to catch a flight to Minneapolis, but your taxi is twenty-five minutes late. You would:
   A. Call the cab company in a rage, scream at them to have a cab there on the double, then wait impatiently outside.
   B. Avoid calling the cab company for as long as possible while being extremely anxious about missing your plane.
   C. Call the cab company as soon as you realize it's late, and inquire whether it's on its way. If you don't feel confident it will get there on time, you quickly make other arrangements.
2. You've been feeling fragmented as a result of overbooking your social calendar and are looking forward to spending an evening at home alone. However, just as you're settling into a good book, the phone rings. An out-of-town business acquaintance is in town overnight and would like to have dinner. You would:
   A. Reply that you would very much like to get together; however, you've already made plans for the evening. If he/she isn't available for lunch tomorrow, the visit will have to wait for another trip.
   B. Decide an evening alone isn't so important. Who knows? This business acquaintance could turn out to be an important contact.
   C. Change your plans to see your acquaintance while secretly resenting the imposition.
3. Your spouse claims that he/she doesn't feel loved enough by you. You would:
   A. Withdraw into feelings of helplessness and inadequacy. After all, if he/she doesn't already feel loved, what can you do about it?
   B. Realize that, regardless of what you consider the truth of the matter, your spouse's feelings are real and should be taken seriously. So, you would probe a little deeper, hoping to discover why he/she doesn't feel loved, what would make him/her feel loved, and whether you are willing to do that.
   C. Counterattack by claiming that your spouse expects too much from you. Why should he/she need constant protestations of love? You married him/her, didn't you?
4. Your work supervisor chooses in an office meeting to criticize your work or behavior unfairly. You would:
   A. Listen without comment, swallowing your anger and humiliation until such time, if ever, you think it's appropriate to express it.
   B. Quickly replace shock with anger and defend yourself, giving at least as good as you got.
   C. As soon as you recognized the supervisor's intentions, interrupt in a firm but polite manner: "I don't think it's very useful to discuss my work here. However, I'd be glad to meet with you privately whenever it's convenient." If the supervisor continues to be abusive, you would excuse yourself and leave the room.

5. You're on an ocean cruise to Hawaii. The travel brochures have filled you with fantasies of exquisite weather, exotic foods, beautiful shipmates. The reality, however, is that it's been raining since you left port; the over-rich food is making you fat; your shipmates are too old, young, fat, thin, or the wrong sex. You would:
   A. See the ship's captain and demand a refund, while lamenting the waste of your time and money.
   B. Retreat to your cabin, where you can commiserate with yourself over the fact that you've been taken again. '
   C. Abandon any expectations you had for the trip, then look for ways you can amuse or enlighten yourself.

6. You are scheduled to begin an important business trip tomorrow. Your plan calls for you to make five air trips to as many cities in as many days. The day before your departure, you come down with a terrible head cold. You would:
   A. Revise or cancel the trip until you had recovered.
   B. Vow that you couldn't allow a cold to interfere with your plans, and leave as scheduled.
   C. Resent the fact that you had to take the trip, load yourself up with medications, and drag yourself to the airport.

7. You have just discovered that your spouse has lied to you about a matter of some importance. You would:
   A. Be hurt and distressed and angry. You would confront your spouse and express your feelings. However, that done, you would be willing to consider your part in the lie—how you might have made it necessary by being unwilling to hear the truth.
   B. Never mention it to your spouse. Instead, you would inwardly nurse your grievance and take it out on your spouse in a variety of indirect ways.
   C. Fly into a rage that would expend itself on whatever was available: the furniture, the dog, your spouse.

8. You started a mail-order business ten years ago, based on a concept and series of products that really appealed to you. However, as times has passed your interest has diminished. Lately you've noticed that your profit margin is slipping, and the most recent set of books shows you're bordering on bankruptcy. You would:
   A. Be deeply shocked and frightened. After a cursory glance at the figures, you would lock the books away, telling no one what they contained. Then you would retreat into your private world to worry and wonder what to do.
   B. Explode in anger at the figures, then move heaven and earth to find a way to save your business.
   C. After allowing the initial knot in the stomach to loosen a bit, ask yourself the following questions: *Why did I set my business up to*

fail? What do I learn from this? Do I still truly want the business to succeed? Is financial failure my only permissible escape from this business? Is there some other way to set up the business so I could both enjoy it and profit from it? Based on your answers to these questions, you would devise a plan for resolving the situation.

Stress-Response Analysis

Your answers to these hypothetical situations indicate whether you are primarily a Type A, B, or C personality in terms of stress response. You may have circled responses that fall into more than one category. In this case, simply identify the category that predominates.

Type A	*Type B*	*Type C*
1. A	1. C	1. B
2. B	2. A	2. C
3. C	3. B	3. A
4. B	4. C	4. A
5. A	5. C	5. B
6. B	6. A	6. C
7. C	7. A	7. B
8. B	8. C	8. A

Remember that Type A is aggressive, ambitious, impatient—he or she prefers the fight of a fight-or-flight response. Type C is the opposite: introverted, easily intimidated, unable to express anger. Type C's opt for flight instead of fight. Type B is the type who (magically?) manages to maintain that all-important position we keep talking about: balance. Type B's are capable both of experiencing emotion and expressing it and simultaneously able to observe the experience and learn from it.

Type B's differ from A's and C's primarily in their willingness and ability to accept life on its own terms. In a later section of this chapter, we will discuss resistance versus acceptance and what you can do to embrace a more life-enhancing attitude.

However, since most of us are either Type A or Type C (or some combination thereof), it might be useful first to understand how our stress reactions travel through the body, what havoc they wreak, and how you can minimize the damage through neurophysiological intervention.

The Biology of Stress Responses

Stress reactions are provoked primarily by the hypothalamus through its control over the autonomic nervous system and endocrine system. The autonomic nervous system is comprised of the sympathetic and parasympathetic nervous systems. In simple language, the sympathetic system stimulates aggressive responses; the parasympathetic system stimulates relaxation responses. As I will show, balancing these two nervous systems can help you inhibit the release of damaging hormones and protect yourself from the aging influence of stress.

Stress, whether internal or external, physical or conceptual, is first perceived by the reticular activating system. The RAS transmits stress messages through neurotransmitters to the hypothalamus, a small volatile structure located at the top of your brain stem. The hypothalamus is the critical link in understanding stress reactions because it controls the two primary physiological systems activated by stress: the autonomic nervous system and the endocrine system.

The sympathetic and parasympathetic nervous systems ideally coexist in a kind of yin/yang balance.

As you will see from the table that follows, the sympathetic nervous system fires as a unit, quickly stimulating many organs at once. It tenses and constricts muscles and blood vessels, increases heart rate, produces instant energy, triggers the endocrine system to release hormones such as adrenaline and cortisol, and produces fear reactions such as clammy hands and a pounding heart.

The parasympathetic nervous system is organized for local discharges. It generally relaxes the muscles and blood vessels, slows the heartbeat and respiration, lowers blood pressure, stimulates digestive processes, and produces more pleasurable reactions, such as warm, dry hands and a heart that is full of pride and joy.

Although it is convenient to imagine the two nervous systems as mutually exclusive, it is not entirely accurate. Some functions do overlap and intertwine. The systems are interdependent, very complex, and equally important.

Sympathetic dominance sometimes results from a weakened parasympathetic system rather than its more common cause—overactivity of the sympathetic system.

Parasympathetic dominance is usually due to sympathetic system exhaustion as a result of chronic, long-term stress rather than overstimulation of the parasympathetic system. Since the parasympathetic nerves work independently, you rarely see all the signs of parasympathetic dominance occurring together.

Perhaps the simplest way to describe the duality of the sympathetic and parasympathetic nervous systems is through the concept of stress and rest. The sympathetic system fires you up to cope with any and every form of stress; the parasympathetic system provides you with the nutrition of relaxation. Both are equally necessary.

Most Americans, however, are conditioned to live in a chronic state of siege. Both Type A and Type C (and that's most of us most of the time) are

TABLE 1

Nervous System Dominance Characteristics

Sympathetic Dominance	(Characteristic)	Parasympathetic Dominance
"Trembling with fear" "Cold feet" "Chills up and down my spine" "Racing heart" "Knot in my stomach"	(Verbal descriptions)	"Warm-hearted" "Flushed with excitement" "My heart goes out to you" "Filled with pride"
Tall and slender	(Body build)	Short and stocky
Tense neck and upper back Shoulders hunched	(Muscles)	Relaxed and loose
Forms goose bumps easily "Cold sweats" Cold and clammy extremities Pale skin	(Skin)	Doesn't form goose bumps easily Perspires easily Warm and dry extremities General flushing
Large pupils Little winking Dry eyes	(Eyes)	Small pupils Frequent winking Plentiful tears and secretion
Pale color	(Ears)	Normal or flushed
Dry mouth Little saliva Gagging tendency Tight throat	(Mouth and throat)	Watery mouth Excess saliva Little gagging
Dry mucous membranes of mouth, nose, and throat	(Mucous membranes)	Moist membranes of mouth, nose, and throat
Rapid heartbeat Pounding sensation High blood pressure**	(Heart and blood)	Slow heartbeat Irregular heartbeat Low blood pressure**
Rapid	(Respiration)	Irregular
Sluggish Poor appetite Little stomach acid	(Digestion)	Rapid Healthy appetite Excess stomach acid
Easily startled Irritated by bright lights and loud noises Anxiety prone** Mentally alert	(Nerves)	Sluggish responses Insensitive to surroundings Serene Thoughtful
Slow to heal Acid pH Low blood calcium Responds to cold weather, high pressure	(Metabolism)	Quick to heal Alkaline pH Normal or high blood calcium Responds to warm weather, low pressure
Heart attack Ulcer Hypertension Stroke	(Disease vulnerabilities)	Cancer Colds Viral infections Arthritis**

**Especially strong indicator

constantly buffeted by time pressures, conflicting emotions, and other debilitating situations that trigger the overstimulation of sympathetic or parasympathetic response. Rarely do we allow ourselves to surrender to relaxation, which we consider more optional than necessary.

The results of this kind of imbalance are devastating. Here are just a few I've observed:

- The immune system breaks down.
- The body retains sodium (and thus water) and chloride and loses potassium.
- Blood pressure increases.
- The potential for kidney damage is increased. (Kidneys play a crucial role in maintaining health by regulating chemical composition and water content of the blood.)
- Increased levels of adrenaline and cortisol may make the heart more vulnerable to cardiac arrhythmias, perhaps increasing risk of sudden death syndrome.
- The complex control systems malfunction and trigger a metabolic shift from glucose to free fatty acids as primary fuel source. (The aging effects of this metabolic shift were noted in Chapter 2.)

Fortunately, several methodologies are available for balancing the autonomic nervous system. Before we discuss these alternatives, please take a few moments to reexamine Table 1, "Nervous System Dominance Characteristics." You will probably identify with traits on both sides of the table. If you identify equally with both sides, then you are probably Type B, extraordinarily well balanced, and can skip to the next section. If, however, you notice that you identify predominantly with one system or the other, you should turn to the recommendations that follow for balancing the autonomic nervous system.

Recommendations for Balancing Sympathetic Dominance

Life-style

- Slow down, pursue more relaxing activities—long walks, deep breathing exercises.
- Practice meditation or hypnosis.
- Consider living in a warm, low-pressure climate.
- Consult an acupuncturist (see Chapter 12).

Visualization

- See exercise titled "To Balance a Sympathetic Dominance" later in this chapter.

Diet

- Eat at least two servings of fruit each day.

- Eat at least two servings daily of foods rich in potassium—leafy dark green vegetables, seeds and nuts, beans.

Supplements*
- Basic nutrient supplements. (See tables 26, 27, and 28 with accompanying text in Chapter 9.)
- Bupleurum and Dragon Bone Combination (traditional Chinese herbal formula)—Bupleurum (5 gm), rhubarb (.5 gm), jujube (2.5 gm), oyster shell (2.5 gm), hoelen (3.0 gm), cinnamon (3.0 gm), ginseng (2.5 gm), Dragon Bone (2.5 gm), Pinellia (4.0 gm), scute (2.5 gm).

Recommendations for Balancing Parasympathetic Dominance

Life-style
- Become more physically active in strenuous, stimulating activities.
- Express yourself outwardly.
- Consider living in a cold, high-pressure climate.
- Consult an acupuncturist (see Chapter 12).

Visualization
- See exercise titled "To Balance a Parasympathetic Dominance" later in this chapter.

Diet
- Make sure that grains and cereals account for at least 70 percent of total daily calories.
- Increase protein consumption up to 20 percent of total daily calories.

Supplements*
- Basic nutrient supplements. (See tables 26, 27, and 28 with accompanying text in Chapter 9.)
- Chinese herbal formulas prescribed for your symptoms by a qualified herbal doctor. (See Chapter 9.)

ALTERED STATES CAN ALTER
YOUR STRESS REACTIONS AND AGING

You may not be familiar with the recommended technique of mental visualization. This potentially powerful process travels under many names: altered state of consciousness, hypnosis, meditation, mental movies, creative visualization, and mental visualization. Each of these

* See the Age Reduction Supplement Guide in Chapter 9 for a list of supplement suppliers and complete instructions on the correct and safe use of supplements.

names describes what is essentially the same process: inducing an altered state of consciousness and then using this trancelike condition to achieve deep relaxation and program the mind to alter behaviors or involuntary responses.

Regular use of altered states of consciousness has been found to exert a powerful and positive influence on stress reactions, aging, and longevity. What follows is a brief summary of a few of these studies.

In the journal *Psychosomatic Medicine* (volume 35, 1973) researcher Orme Johnson reported his finding that people who use altered states restored internal balance more quickly after exposure to a stress such as a loud noise than did a control group.

Another 1973 study, by Johann M. Stoyva and Thomas H. Budzinski, of the University of Colorado Medical Center, showed that people trained in the use of altered states can decrease the amount of sympathetic arousal caused by stress. This involves higher-brain–initiated cortical interventions that alter (and balance) the autonomic nervous system.

In addition to improving stress responses, altered states can also be used to reduce your biological age. In a recent British study by Michael Toomey and colleagues, subjects who regularly used altered states were examined for measures of biological age, including systolic blood pressure and vision and hearing acuity. The subjects' average chronological age was about thirty-one years. Average biological age was about seven years younger than average chronological age.

In a later study of the same group, average biological age decreased from seven years younger than chronological age to about ten years younger. The length of time subjects practiced altered states appeared to be correlate with the result.

A United States study of Transcendental Meditation and aging, reported in the *International Journal of Neurosciences,* 1982, supports this finding. The average biological age of short-term (less than five years) meditators was five years below chronological age. The average biological age of long-term (more than five years) meditators was twelve years younger.

The Kung Fu masters with whom I train every day are a living example of the benefits of altered states. Since Kung Fu requires the mastery of both physical and mental disciplines, both of my instructors have spent years performing deep breathing exercises, employing meditation and visualization techniques, refining control over both voluntary and involuntary muscles, and developing an awareness of the internal flow of energy through techniques such as Tai Chi. As a result, they look younger, react more quickly, and have more energy than most people ten to fifteen years younger.

Whether you know it or not, you alter the state of your consciousness at least twice a day—when you fall asleep at night and when you awaken in the morning. At these times your brain activity either slows down or speeds up, passing through these levels of brain-wave activity:

Beta: Full consciousness
Alpha: Crossing over into sleep at night
        Awakening in the morning
        Hypnosis
        Meditation
Theta: Early stages of sleep
        Deep hypnosis
        Deep meditation
Delta: Deepest sleep or unconsciousness

I would define an altered state as the relaxed concentration of attention on just one idea, image, or emotion.

Think about how you feel just as you are slipping into sleep at night. Your body is relaxed; your mind relaxes. At the same time, you are still aware of sounds in the room around you. If the telephone rang, you would hear it. You might not feel motivated to answer it, however.

Different people perceive information differently while in an altered state. You may *see* pictures—either moving, as in a film, or still, as in a slide show. Or you may be one of those people who *hear* information through voices that seem to be talking inside your head. (I tell you this so you won't panic at the thought of "hearing voices.") Some people won't see or hear anything but will simply become *aware* of information. And still others will not see or hear or be aware but will *feel* a variety of emotions relating to the subject on which their attention is focused.

Regardless of the manner in which you perceive information, visualization can help you gain insights into and actually alter your internal world.

Meditation or Hypnosis: Which Should You Use?

Much has been made of the differences between meditation and every other form of altered state. The implication is that meditation takes you to some higher place, resulting in a superior experience. Not true. As I've already explained, the only levels through which your brain travels are Alpha, Beta, Theta, and Delta.

However, there is one distinctive characteristic of meditation it may be useful to understand.

Once you have achieved an altered state, you may take a passive or an active approach to its use. Traditionally, meditation is more passive, focusing more on emptying the mind of tail-chasing thoughts and creating a state of deep relaxation. Hypnosis or mental visualization is more active, suggesting specific ideas on which to concentrate or goals to be achieved.

If, in the previous section, you discovered that you are strongly sympathetic dominant, meditation probably would be a better choice. To balance your autonomic nervous system you need to learn to surrender, to relax. Meditation is ideal for this.

If, on the other hand, you discovered you are parasympathetic dominant, hypnosis or other mental visualization techniques might prove more useful. You need to activate and stimulate yourself into responding more effectively to your environment.

No matter which avenue you choose, regular use of altered states will improve your ability to cope with stress.

Here are just a few of the techniques I've used with my clients to induce an altered state of consciousness and recreate stress reactions.

To Induce an Altered State of Consciousness

1. Lie down in a comfortable position in a quiet room. (Some people also prefer darkness.)
2. Begin to hush the constant babble of your conscious mind by focusing on your breathing. If distracting thoughts intrude, don't resist. Simply acknowledge the thought, promise yourself you will deal with it after completing this altered-state exercise, then deliberately refocus your attention on your breathing. Take several slow, deep breaths, inhaling through the nose, exhaling through the mouth.
3. Once you feel your mind beginning to lose its grip on daily trivia, use your imagination to relax your body deeply, one part at a time. Start with your toes and gradually work up to your head, focusing your relaxed attention on each part. It might be helpful to imagine a warm fluid or light slowly filling your body.
4. When your body feels loose and relaxed, begin to focus your attention on a single idea, sound, or emotion. You may want to chant a simple phrase over and over (some meditators use their own mantra, a word chosen to "vibrate" harmoniously with their own energy). You may choose to concentrate on counting slowly forward or backward while imagining yourself in a physical situation relating to the count. (For example, you may see yourself floating or flying up or down, walking up or down steps.) The point of this imagery is to engage your imagination and help you focus your attention.
5. Since it's possible to be in Alpha or even Theta while still maintaining conscious awareness, you can gauge the depth of your "trance" by looking for the following signs of an altered state of consciousness:
   Your breathing is shallow and slow.
   You can feel your pupils moving quickly beneath closed eyelids in response to your mental imagery.
   You feel completely relaxed, both mentally and physically.
   Your body feels slightly heavy and somehow disconnected from your mind.
   It is easier to concentrate on one idea at a time instead of chasing endless, overlapping ideas.
   You experience a deep feeling of peace and serenity.

Once you're in an altered state, you're free to create almost any experience you choose. What follows is a brief summary of some of the meditations or visualizations you may want to use.

To Create Rejuvenation

This exercise is useful both on its own and as a prelude to other exercises. For the greatest benefit, you should precede it with a thorough body relaxation such as has been already described. However, you can also use it to instantly restore peace of mind during highly stressful situations. Simply remove yourself to some quiet place (a bathroom, for example) where you won't be disturbed for a few minutes. Close your eyes, take several deep breaths, and imagine the following situation.

You are in an environment that is utterly peaceful to you. Create every detail in your mind:

- Whether you are indoors or outdoors, in the city or the country
- What you are wearing
- What you are doing
- Who, if anyone, is there with you
- What it smells like and sounds like
- Most important, how you feel. (You should feel completely relaxed, at peace with yourself, filled with quiet joy.)

To Balance a Sympathetic Dominance

Before beginning this exercise, isolate three different circumstances in your life with which you associate negative stress. Some examples are: work or social pressure; activities you feel obligated to do but don't enjoy; unhappy relationships with your spouse, boss, child, or relative.

Once you are feeling completely relaxed, bring these stressful circumstances to mind, one at a time. Notice your internal responses to these ideas. Do your muscles tense? Does your heart beat faster? Do you feel yourself mobilizing for self-defense?

When you have become acutely aware of your neurophysiological responses, take a deep breath. Tell yourself to relax. Send your mind into each of the affected areas and consciously direct your heart to slow down, your muscles to relax. While continuing to imagine these stressful situations vividly, create an equally vivid image of yourself responding assertively to the situation but without the corresponding negative emotions you usually feel. Continue working with this exercise until you can face any of these situations in your mind with calm detachment. Repeated use of this exercise will improve your ability to face these situations in real life.

To Balance a Parasympathetic Dominance

Since you are more likely to deal with stressful situations by ignoring them, falling asleep, or refusing to recognize your feelings consciously, this exercise is designed to activate awareness and responsiveness. Before beginning this exercise, isolate three sets of circumstances that trigger the responses already described.

After following the directions for inducing an altered state, bring to mind one of the stressful situations you've chosen. Notice your internal responses. Does your mind recoil from thinking about it, try to distract you with other subjects, or make you desperately sleepy? Do you notice a familiar sense of numbness, helplessness, or impotence? Allow this to continue until you feel sure you understand exactly how your responses feel.

Now let go of these ideas, and conjure up instead a completely dissimilar experience, one in which you feel safe and powerful and free to express yourself. Do this with every ounce of imagination and emotion at your disposal. Really get your juices flowing.

When you are completely filled with these positive feelings, reach back for the stressful situation you were considering earlier. But this time imagine responding to the situation with all the power and positivity you're now experiencing. Recreate the stressful situation so that you're aware of its implications and are able to respond appropriately.

The more you work with this exercise, the greater the results you will experience in real life.

Returning to Full Consciousness

When you have completed any of the exercises already described, you can awaken yourself to full Beta consciousness by telling yourself, "On the count of five, I will be wide awake, remembering all that has transpired." Then count slowly from one to five while consciously arousing your heartbeat, blood circulation, and body awareness.

You should awaken feeling totally relaxed and refreshed.

ATTITUDE: AN ANTIDOTE FOR AGING

Warning: A negative attitude may be hazardous to your health.

I realize that you've already waded through an enormous amount of evidence proving the mind's power over your physical well-being. However, the public has also been presented with abundant evidence that smoking causes lung cancer, yet despite that information, many smokers continue to ignore the Surgeon General's warning. It takes more than awareness of evidence; it takes a receptive attitude toward implementing change in the direction indicated by the evidence. That attitude in connection with longevity is best summarized in the words *love of life.* Bear with me while I present just a few of the studies linking longevity with a love of life.

- The importance of social ties and "life satisfaction" to longevity was highlighted in a study of nearly 5000 men and women conducted by

Dr. Lester Breslow and colleagues at the University of California in Los Angeles. It found that the death rate was more than double among the men and nearly triple among the women with the fewest social connections, as compared to those who had the most. A similar increase in mortality was noted among those who expressed the least satisfaction with life.

- A Duke University study suggests that men who are cynical and hostile are more prone to heart disease and die earlier. The 255 men who participated in the study had all been graduated from medical school between 1954 and 1959, at which time they were classified as either "cynical, high hostile" or "non-cynical, low hostile," based on their responses to a series of questions. By 1980, 16 of the cynics had died, compared to only 3 of the "non-cynics."

- An earlier study, also conducted by Duke University, showed that hostility can harm the heart as much as smoking, cholesterol, or high blood pressure.

Clearly, attitude is important. But what kind? Some important clues can be discovered by rereading the longevity personality profiles included at the beginning of this section.

Perhaps the most important difference between the two personality types can be summed up as *acceptance versus resistance*.

Long-lived personalities tend to accept life on its own terms. They live in the present rather than *for* the future or *because* of the past. They laugh when they're happy, cry when they're sad, and accept, even cherish, the unexpected.

Long-lived people intuitively understand that everything in life is essentially transient, impermanent. They embrace change, recognizing that life's happiest miracles are often unexpected, its worst tragedies largely unavoidable.

Above all, long-lived people love life. They are intrinsically connected to it by their community, family and love relationships, by their work, by the harmonious progression of internal and external cycles. Who has time to die when there's the birth of a grandchild to witness, a community dance to attend?

Short-lived personalities, in contrast, are willing to accept life only on *their* terms. They live and work as a means to an end, rather than as an end in itself. They have goals and plans and schedules for achieving them. They hate surprises, even pleasant ones, because these interfere with the illusion that they are in complete control.

Short-lived people tend to be ruled by fear: fear of death, fear of life, fear of success or failure, fear of not being enough. They react to this fear by compulsively seeking the symbols of security: money, status, recognition. They seek security in the possession of objects rather than in the possession of self.

Short-lived people perceive life as a linear path strewn with obstacles. Once they set their sights on a particular goal, they grit their teeth and plow over, under, or through any obstacle. Never mind what they might have learned by examining the obstacle. Short-lived people do not want to be confused by new facts. They're extremely reluctant to change their minds or adopt another approach.

Thinking about these two personality types reminds me of the parable of the reed and the oak tree. The reed is a slender, flexible plant that grows in the water. The oak is among the staunchest of trees. According to the parable, the two struck up a conversation. The oak tree admonished the reed, "Why do you sway with the slightest breeze? You should be strong like me. I stand firm against even the heartiest wind." The reed replied, "But I do not have your strong roots or your mighty limbs. If I didn't bend, I'd break." The oak tree smiled to itself and allowed as how that was probably true.

One day, a mightier wind blew than had ever blown before. The delicate reed was all but flattened against the surface of the water. It watched as the mighty oak tree groaned and creaked, trying to hold its own against the wind. In silent horror, the reed watched as the oak's ancient roots were slowly pulled out of the ground. "Bend, bend!" he cried to the oak tree. The oak tree groaned in reply, "It's too late," and with a final wrench fell to the ground.

Similarly, short-lived people tend to resist the winds of change until one day they are felled by them.

Prescription for Achieving a Long-Life Attitude

Wouldn't it be wonderful if you could just pop a vitamin pill or ingest an herb to alter a lifelong attitude?

Unfortunately, since it was you who adopted the attitude in the first place, you will also have to be the one who changes it.

You might find the following techniques useful. I do caution you, however, to be patient with yourself. You didn't accumulate your attitudes overnight, and you're not likely to change them overnight either. Try out your new attitude in small ways first. Over time you'll find you are able to sustain your positive outlook for longer and longer periods until finally that positive attitude becomes an integral part of your emotional makeup.

1. Begin by taking a self-inventory. Sit down and make a list of different subjects that affect your everyday life, such as time, work, play, relationships. You may not want to tackle all these subjects at once. For each you do tackle, simply concentrate on it in a relaxed way, then write down all the beliefs that pop into your head.

2. If you find that negative thoughts occur much more often than positive ones, you may want to practice a simple thought-substitu-

tion technique. Every time you catch yourself thinking a negative thought, quickly replace it with a positive one that you *truly believe* on the same subject. Eventually this procedure becomes a reflex action that tips the balance in favor of a positive attitude.

3. If you don't feel capable of altering all your negative attitudes on your own (few of us truly are capable of this), consider seeking professional counseling.

4. Use the hypnosis or meditation exercises already described to recreate your attitudes.

5. Deliberately create circumstances in your life that make you laugh. Read humorous books. See funny movies. Watch the antics of children or animals.

6. Increase your connectedness to other people. Let your friends and relatives know you love and need them. Allow yourself to develop more intimate, nurturing friendships.

7. Remember that few things are ever as important as they seem.

6

How Your Life-style Affects Your Longevity

Life-style choices reflect attitudes.

If you believe that getting ahead is the most important thing in life, then you devote your time and attention to this goal to the exclusion of anything else. If, on the contrary, you believe that the process of life itself is more meaningful than building up a list of accomplishments, you divide your life more harmoniously between work and play, exertion and relaxation.

If you believe that time is an enemy to be outwitted, you are reluctant to sacrifice much of it to sleep or relaxation. Instead, you rise by the alarm clock, work by stopwatch, socialize until you drop from exhaustion. If, however, you believe that life creates and requires its own rhythms of stress and rest, you surrender to it more gracefully and benefit more fully. You rise by the sun, work steadily without exhausting yourself, and go to bed relatively early.

If you believe that life is stressful, difficult, or overwhelming, you may compensate by drinking too much coffee or alcohol, taking drugs, or smoking cigarettes. If, instead, you find life fulfilling, manageable, and enjoyable, you may still indulge in moderate drinking or smoking, but you will be motivated by the desire for pleasure rather than by the need for a crutch.

The key to life in life-style choices is rhythm and balance—not too little, not too much. That may sound simple, but it's not necessarily easy—not in a society that was brought up to believe that anything worth doing is worth doing to excess.

According to research conducted by Lester Breslow and M. B. Belloc, at the University of California, Los Angeles, School of Medicine, the key to longevity is moderation. In a five-year study of 7000 adults, published in 1972–73, Breslow and Belloc identified seven key factors favoring longevity. They are:

- Eating three meals a day, with no snacking
- Eating breakfast
- Exercising moderately two to three times per week
- Getting adequate sleep
- Not smoking
- Maintaining a moderate weight
- Consuming little or no alcohol

Breslow and Belloc concluded that someone who practices six of these suggestions will live, on average, eleven years longer than a person who only practices two or three.

Rhythm, moderation, balance. These are the most important keys to reducing your age.

YOUR INTERNAL BODY RHYTHMS

The idea that we are rhythmic, cyclical creatures was first formally advanced in 1959 by a researcher named Franz Halberg of the Chronobiology Laboratory at the University of Minnesota. He introduced the term *circadian* (from *circa,* a Latin word meaning about, and *dies,* another Latin word, meaning day) to describe internal body rhythms that are based on an approximate twenty-four–hour schedule. These rhythms include blood pressure, body temperature, sleeping/waking, digestion, energy, and mental alertness.

Circadian rhythms are only one of many clocks governing our internal progression from birth to death, from well-being to illness. *Ultraradian rhythms* describe shorter-than-twenty-four-hour cycles. *Infraradian rhythms* are based on weekly or monthly cycles. And *circannual rhythms,* as you may imagine, govern annual alterations. Table 2 (next page) lists each of these rhythms and the body functions they control.

Your internal body rhythms directly affect the rate at which you will age. When they are synchronized with each other and your environment, aging is slowed. When they are desynchronized, premature aging is induced. All cycles interact. Disturbances in the daily cycles may ultimately shorten your life cycle. For example, continually prolonged daily lighting can disturb the female monthly menstrual cycle. Menstrual difficulties are the first sign of female sexual aging.

Body rhythms influence aging primarily by upsetting internal clocks that govern metabolic shifts and the timely release of chemicals and hormones. (Metabolic shifts are thoroughly explored in Chapter 12.)

Body rhythms are inborn. Researcher Christian Poirel of the Laboratory of Neurophysiology and Experimental Psychopathology at the University of Quebec, Canada, postulates that circadian rhythms are created by DNA/RNA protein programs. However, the rhythmic flow of energy through acupuncture channels discovered thousands of years ago by the

TABLE 2

Body Rhythms

Ultraradian (less than 24 hours)	Circadian (24 hours)	Infraradian (weekly/monthly)	Circannual (yearly)
Heart rate	Blood pressure	Monthly ovulation and menstruation in women	Life-span: birth, growth, puberty, maturity, decline, death
Respiration	Body temperature		
Brain waves	Sleep/wakefulness		Female reproductive cycle: beginning menstruation, pregnancy, menopause
Urine output	Digestion		
	Physical energy		Cell division
	Mental capacities and learning		
	Endocrine hormones secretion		

Adapted from C. Ehret. *Overcoming Jet Lag*. New York: Berkley Books, 1983. © 1983, Berkley Publishing Corporation.

Chinese and confirmed by modern instruments may influence the DNA/RNA programs that create your daily rhythms. (See Chapter 12.)

Circadian rhythms are also in part dependent on external cues. It is these cues that you can control and use to prevent the aging effects of irregular rhythms.

Some of the primary external cues or factors that can desynchronize your inner time clocks are:

- Insufficient, excessive, or irregular sleep
- Travel, particularly across time zones
- Stress
- Overexposure to artificial light
- Uneven work or eating schedules
- Inappropriate choice of foods
- Lack of social interactions
- Inconsistent periods of physical exertion
- Overconsumption of alcohol
- Use of other drugs

So what happens when an imbalance occurs?

First, your hypothalamus goes haywire. It destroys autonomic nerve system balance. It sends all the wrong signals to your pituitary, which in turn triggers the release of the wrong kind of chemicals and hormones at the wrong times. Some of the symptoms of unbalanced body clocks include:

- Mental fogginess and confusion
- Memory loss
- Decreased appetite
- Off-schedule bowel movements, diarrhea, or constipation
- Fatigue
- Insomnia
- Slow reflexes
- Loss of endurance, muscle tone, and coordination
- Headaches

The long-term aging effects of disrupted body rhythms are even more serious than the temporary discomforts. Some of the premature aging patterns associated with unbalanced body rhythms include:

- Degeneration of the female sexual organs, leading to menstrual difficulties, premature menopause, and aging
- Disturbed thyroid gland activity, causing abnormal metabolic rate
- Reduced stress-handling capabilities, resulting in the myriad aging effects discussed in Chapter 6
- Decreased production of growth hormone and excess production of insulin and free fatty acids, triggering a premature shift into physiological decline, accumulation of excess fat, and loss of lean muscle mass
- Irregularities in blood pressure and body temperature, forcing adaptive systems to work overtime
- Abnormal eating behaviors that tax the digestive system and supply infrequent and inadequate nutrients to the cells
- Brain dysfunction that leads to neuroendocrinological aging

The sleep/wake cycle offers a dramatic example of how body rhythms rely on both internal cues (such as hormones) and external cues (such as the light/dark cycle) to maintain consistency. Here's how it works.

At sunrise your hypothalamus increases dopamine activity to wake you up and perform daytime metabolic processes. At sunset, your hypothalamus increases serotonin activity to induce sleep and perform nighttime metabolic processes. It is the *balance* of sunrise and sunset, the dopamine and serotonin systems, that is necessary to keep your sleep/wake cycle on schedule.

According to Donald L. Tasto, Michael J. Colligam, and associates (researchers at Stanford Research Institute), people who chronically disrupt normal sleep/wake cycles by working on night or graveyard shifts have more frequent illnesses, accidents, behavioral abnormalities, fatigue, and menstrual problems than workers on normal schedules. I believe this is because these workers' internal clocks, governing (among other things) the cyclical release of dopamine, serotonin, and other hormones, are out of synch with the demands of their external environment.

Dopamine and Serotonin:
A Yin/Yang Balance

Since the dopamine/serotonin cycle is probably the most significant body rhythm in terms of aging, let's pause for a moment and examine exactly how it works. What follows is a simplified linear explanation of the activities, sources, and aging effects of dopamine and serotonin.

Dopamine, noradrenaline, and adrenaline are related signal carriers in the catecholamine system* that I call the dopamine system. Dopamine is a neurotransmitter found in your brain, peripheral nerves, adrenal gland, blood, and other organs. Adrenaline is the principle hormone released from your adrenal gland and a messenger for the sympathetic nervous system. Noradrenaline is the neurotransmitter in sympathetic nerve fibers.

Dopamine is synthesized in a series of steps from the dietary amino acids phenylalanine and tyrosine, then converted into noradrenaline and adrenaline.

The dopamine system stimulates your sympathetic nervous system and maintains the proper function of your hypothalamus, reproductive organs, coordination centers, and energy processes.

Serotonin is a blood vessel constrictor and neurotransmitter. Milk and fruits such as pineapples and bananas contain serotonin as well as dopamine. Serotonin is the major transmitter in the serotonin system.

Serotonin is synthesized from the dietary amino acid tryptophan. Two percent of dietary tryptophan is converted into serotonin. Ninety percent of your body's serotonin is synthesized and found in the intestines. Different regions in your brain also synthesize and contain serotonin, and it is present in other tissues, bound with other substances and located in cells such as blood.

Serotonin pathways in your brain control sleep/wakefulness and act as a time clock for your other body rhythms. Serotonin increases cortisol. Serotonin reactions in other body sites alter your heart rate, respiration, blood coagulation, circulation, and gastrointestinal activity.

Since dopamine/serotonin levels fluctuate drastically depending on the time of day and the function of individual cells, it is impossible to measure an individual's dopamine/serotonin levels precisely or state a "correct" amount or ratio. What is important is the *balanced, rhythmic ebb and flow* of these two cycles. Dopamine dominates during the day; serotonin holds sway at night.

Aging causes your body to produce substantially less dopamine and somewhat less serotonin as you pass from maturity to the physiological decline stage of life.

---

* Catecholamines are a class of neurotransmitters. Some texts use the term *norepinephrine* and *epinephrine* for noradrenaline and adrenaline, respectively.

Declining levels of dopamine and/or serotonin in your hypothalamus decrease the hypothalamus's control over your body. Incorrect signals are transferred through your autonomic nervous system, pituitary and other glands, and other signal pathways to peripheral organs and tissues throughout the body. Rhythmic integrity is lost, neuroendocrinological aging is accelerated, and degenerative diseases develop in compensation for these metabolic shifts, according to Dr. V. M. Dilman, one of the chief researchers at the Petrov Institute of Oncology in the Soviet Union and one of the world's foremost authorities on neuroendocrinological aging.

The relationship between dopamine and serotonin is very complex and mostly antagonistic, like that of feuding lovers. What follows is a list of the most common symptoms and results of dopamine/serotonin imbalance on different bodily functions.

TABLE 3

Roles of Dopamine/Serotonin Imbalance in Aging

Function	Dopamine	Serotonin
Sleep	Inadequate amount decreases energy during the day, contributes to daytime sleepiness.	Inadequate amount produces insomnia and sleeping difficulty. Excess causes grogginess.
Autonomic nervous system	Inadequate amount decreases sympathetic nerve activity, inhibits correct adaption to changes.	Excess amount prevents dopamine from working correctly and depresses autonomic nervous system.
Stress	Stimulates pituitary gland hormone to stimulate adrenal gland and increase cortisol.	Stimulates pituitary gland hormone to stimulate adrenal gland and increase cortisol.
Reproduction	Inadequate amount inhibits sexual functions (especially in women).	Excess amount inhibits reproductive function and lowers testosterone in men.
Growth hormone release	Inadequate amount decreases growth hormone during the day.	Inconclusive. Tends to decrease growth hormone at night.
Movement	Inadequate amount produces a loss of coordination, leads to Parkinson's disease.	Imbalance causes both inhibition and stimulation of movement.
Mental state	Inadequate amount causes depression, contributes to senility.	Inadequate amount causes depression. Severe psychological disturbances are associated with serotonin imbalances.
Appetite and eating	Inadequate amount increases appetite and food consumption.	Inadequate amount increases appetite and cravings for carbohydrates.

Out of Step: A Case History

The patient whose history I'm about to relate epitomizes the disasters that can result from desynchronization.

Barry Roberts not only marched to the beat of a different drummer, he slept, ate, and worked to it.

When I first began working with Barry, he had no such thing as a daily routine. Sometimes he would stay awake for as long as forty-eight hours; then he might sleep for eighteen hours. Next he might remain conscious for twenty hours, then sleep for another fifteen hours. Barry believed that his sleeping habits were dictated by his moods, which were prone to wild swings. When depressed he was capable of sleeping for twenty to thirty hours straight. When excited, elated (even manic at times), he could stay awake for more than forty-eight hours.

Barry's sleep/wake cycle was only one of his many desynchronized rhythms. His eating habits were equally bizarre. Instead of eating approximately every six hours, as most of us do, he might neglect to eat for twenty hours while conscious, fall asleep, then wake up after six or eight hours, eat an enormous meal, and go back to sleep. In addition, Barry usually preferred to binge on one food for a few days at a time until he grew sick of it and then switch to another food for another binge.

Barry described his closest social contact as his television set. He had no girl friend, no close friends, no family ties. He hadn't exercised since college, had no hobbies, no passions. He was virtually disconnected from human life as we know it.

With one exception: his work.

Barry conducted business seminars. He loved his work and was extremely good at it. Consequently, when his schedule was booked full of seminars, he was happy and hyperactive. When no seminars were scheduled, he was depressed and semicatatonic.

The effects of these excesses were not immediately apparent. His overall health was good. He didn't drink, smoke, or use drugs. Yet he looked at least ten years older than his thirty-five years. He was forever at the mercy of his moods. And he was unable to function in normal society.

I began by explaining why body rhythms are necessary and useful. Sleep, I told him, is a neurological, physiological, and psychological restorative. During sleep the body releases growth hormones to build new cells and repair damaged ones. Protein, DNA, and RNA synthesis peak during sleep. Sleep also helps conserve energy, prevent wear and tear, and maintain metabolic balance.

However, more than enough sleep is too much. The primary benefits of sleep are generally bestowed between midnight and 4:00 A.M. A few extra hours on either side is fine—sleep requirements do vary—but thirteen hours is deleterious. It causes your body to overproduce serotonin, resulting in euphoria followed by exhaustion; irritability; sore throat; runny nose; chills; sweats; swelling; oversensitivity to light, sound, and smell; depression. Lactic acid accumulates in your muscles, creating stiffness and soreness. And your metabolism is unbalanced, leaving you low on energy . . . and just about everything else.

Other inner time clocks are equally important. Digestion is based on an approximate twenty-four–hour schedule to maximize the amount of nutrients absorbed. Irregular and incorrect eating habits cause food to be improperly digested, causing allergic reactions, abnormal behavior, depressed immunity, and cellular aging.

I believed that Barry's unbalanced life-style was just as likely a cause of his unbalanced moods as the reverse. In addition, I suspected that disproportionate release of chemicals and hormones was speeding up his neuroendocrinological aging.

It took two full years to make all the necessary adjustments in Barry's life-style. Since I understood that his mind would rebel at too many simultaneous changes, we tackled them one at a time.

Barry's sleep habits were the most wildly variant of his routines, so I suggested that he begin to rise at the same hour every morning, even if he was still sleepy. I recommended that he take a 1500-milligram daily dose of supplemental L-tyrosine to increase the amount of dopamine produced by his brain. As I mentioned earlier, dopamine increases alertness and stimulates daytime metabolic activities. I also suggested high-protein breakfast menus. (See "Barry Roberts' Menu" immediately following for one example.)

Getting Barry to bed at a reasonable hour was more difficult. He simply wasn't sleepy. I suggested that he take a minimal dose (500 milligrams) of supplemental L-tryptophan, an amino acid that is converted into serotonin in the brain, and more when he was suffering from insomnia. As we've noted, serotonin induces sleep for nighttime cell repair and reproduction. I also recommended that he increase his serotonin at night by eating high-carbohydrate dinners. ("Barry Roberts' Menu" offers one example.)

Next I recommended that he adopt a daily exercise program. I wanted to accustom his body to undergoing similar metabolic changes at the same time each day. Barry chose to take up jogging and weight-lifting.

Once Barry began to feel more confident on his ability to cope, I urged him to abandon his television set in favor of friends. I asked him to mke commitments to see people, to socialize, to participate in group activities.

Two years later, Barry is nearly normal. Although he still occasionally strays from a twenty-four–hour to a thirty-hour schedule, he now has the tools to adjust quickly. He has lost more than twenty pounds without dieting and currently runs five to ten miles per day. Perhaps most important, he feels much more emotionally stable and optimistic about the future.

Barry Roberts' Menu

Morning	Midday	Evening
4 oz. of protein (fish, chicken, etc.)	2 servings of milk or dairy product (1 cup milk, 4 oz. yogurt, 1 oz. cheese)	5 to 6 servings of complex carbohydrates
1 slice of bread		2 cups of vegetables or salad
	2 cups of vegetables	
1 teaspoon of butter		1 to 2 cups of sliced fruit or whole fruit
	1 to 2 cups of cooked vegetable or salad	
Carbohydrate-free beverage (herbal tea, decaffeinated coffee)		1 tsp. of butter or 2 Tbsp. salad dressing
	4 portions of complex carbohydrates (1 slice of bread, ½ cup of cooked pasta)	
		Fruit juice or vegetable juice
	1 tsp. of butter or 2 Tbsp. of dressing	
	1 piece of fruit	
	Beverage (herbal tea and fruit or vegetable juice)	

RESETTING YOUR INNER TIME CLOCKS

The Age Reduction System is designed to help you keep your inner clocks in order. By following my recommendations you will restore synchronicity to your inner and outer environments.

In the best of all possible worlds, you would live as centenarians do—rising with the sun, working and playing at the same unhurried pace, retiring soon after sunset. Resetting inner time clocks would be unnecessary, since you'd never get out of synch in the first place.

In the real world of late twentieth-century America, that kind of life just isn't possible for most of us. So the Age Reduction System compensates by providing general guidelines to stay synchronized, describing each of the primary unbalancing factors and how you can compensate for them.

General Strategies for Staying in Synch

- Make sure your evening meal includes no more than one-third of your total daily protein allowance and as much as two-thirds of your daily carbohydrate allowance.
- Minimize east/west air travel. When unavoidable, at least allow yourself time to recuperate. As a rule of thumb, your body requires one day of adjustment for each time zone you've traveled through. For example, a trip from New York to Los Angeles, which crosses three time zones, would require three days to adjust.

- Avoid taking drugs, if possible, or drinking more than two alcoholic drinks each day.
- Mitigate weather sensitivity by using a humidifier in dry areas and maintaining an indoor temperature of between 68 and 72 degrees Fahrenheit.
- Eliminate environmental toxins where possible (more on this in Chapter 7).
- Consult a physician about respiratory or allergy problems. They disturb your precious sleep.
- Increase physical exercise to regulate body rhythms and stimulate daytime metabolic activity such as energy production and digestion.
- Avoid spending your evenings in nightclub-like atmospheres. Bright, artificial lights, overcrowding, and harsh, loud noises stimulate your sympathetic nervous system to release adrenaline, which disrupts normal nighttime body rhythms.
- Maintain a happy balance between time spent alone and with significant others. Try to spend at least ten hours each week completely alone and engaged in some occupation you find absorbing and relaxing. Also try to spend at least ten hours each week with people whose company you find nourishing and invigorating.
- Consult an acupuncture energy doctor. He or she can resynchronize your body by creating a smooth flow of energy through it. (Read Chapter 12 for more details.)
- Increase dopamine during the day and serotonin at night by ingesting dietary amino acids at the time of day suggested below.

Increasing Dopamine and Serotonin Levels

Increasing dopamine and serotonin levels can make a great contribution to keeping your inner time clocks synchronized. Remember that these levels must be in balance. Avoid boosting one or other in such fashion as to create an imbalance. Excess serotonin may prematurely age your body.

Supplement	Amount	Effects
L-tyrosine	500–1500 mg. on an empty stomach early in the day	Increases dopamine and energy during the day
Vitamin B-6 Vitamin C	20–30 mg. 500 mg. with the L-tyrosine	Help convert L-tyrosine to dopamine
L-tryptophan	200–800 mg. in the evening and before bedtime	Increases serotonin; aids sleep
Vitamin B-6 Vitamin C	20–30 mg. 500 mg. with the L-tryptophan	Help convert L-tryptophan to serotonin

See the Age Reduction Supplement Guide in Chapter 9 for a list of supplement suppliers and complete instructions on the correct and safe use of supplements.

The EAV (electroacupuncture according to Voll) machine discussed in Chapter 12 will pinpoint your requirement for these nutrients at the appropriate time of day by measuring changes in bioenergy.

You can, however, approximate your own requirement without instrumentation:

- Begin by taking 200 milligrams of tyrosine each morning.
- Gradually increase the amount by increments of 200 milligrams up to 1500 milligrams per day over the course of several months. (Monitor your blood pressure. Dopamine usually normalizes blood pressure, but not always.)
- Begin taking 200 milligrams of L-tryptophan at night when using more than 600 milligrams a day of L-tyrosine if the L-tyrosine produces insomnia.
- If increasing L-tyrosine produces insomnia, compensate by increasing the amount of L-tryptophan up to 1000 milligrams per day until the insomnia disappears.
- If you crave carbohydrates, increase L-tryptophan.
- If you feel depressed, increase either L-tyrosine or L-tryptophan—or both.
- If L-tryptophan causes morning fogginess, you are taking too much; reduce your intake.
- The idea is to find the right balance for your body by only taking just enough L-tryptophan to prevent insomnia and keep you synchronized. Creating excessive serotonin may accelerate aging, not delay it!

Sleep Disturbances
and How to Deal with Them

Aging fragments sleeping patterns. A majority of the elderly have problems in initiating sleep and remaining asleep. Lack of sleep causes cell wear and tear, lowers cell repair rates, and decreases protein synthesis.

Insomnia is a circadian rhythm disturbance that is typically caused by:

- Physical or psychological illness or pain
- Anxiety or stress
- Depression
- Jet lag
- Drugs
- Alcohol
- Weather sensitivity
- Environmental toxins
- Respiratory problems
- Allergic reactions

Excessive sleep is characterized by undesirable daytime sleepiness, increased sleeping time, difficulty waking up, and an inability to stop napping. Like insomnia, excessive sleep occurs as a result of disturbances in your rhythmic balance. In fact, excessive sleepiness may result from a lack of sound sleep at night and the same factors that typically cause insomnia.

The need for sleep varies among individuals. One person may need six hours, another may need twelve hours. The minimum nightly requirement for most people is about five hours, the maximum about eleven hours. Your need for sleep decreases as your age increases. If you're an average twenty-five-year-old, you'll require seven to eight hours, while if you're an average fifty-year-old, you'll need only six to seven hours of sleep.

If you suffer from insomnia or other sleep disturbances and are not sure of their cause, I strongly urge you to consult your physician and/or psychiatrist. Sleep disturbances frequently mask some more serious ailment, such as cardiovascular disease, chronic obstruction of the pulmonary system, brain or thyroid dysfunction, or psychological disturbances.

If, however, you recognize yourself to be affected by the less drastic factors in the list of causes above, you may overcome insomnia by following these recommendations:

- Follow my general recommendations for synchronizing your body rhythms.
- Use the mental visualization techniques recommended in Chapter 5 to reduce anxiety and stress.
- Refer to Table 4 for natural herbal or nutrient combinations you can take to help you sleep. When taken during the day, these herbs and nutrients also calm a stressed body and overactive sympathetic nervous system.

Caution: Don't use L-tryptophan at night as a sleep aid unless you take L-tyrosine during the day. Excessive serotonin may accelerate aging, not delay it!

TABLE 4

Sleep Aids

	Daily Amount	*Effect*
Herbs		
Passion flower	(at bedtime)	Promote natural sleep
Valerian root	500–1000 mg. each, equal	
Lady slipper	amounts of powdered herbs	
Scullcap		
Nutrients		
GABA (gamma amino butyric acid)	1000–2500 mg.	Stimulate the sleep cycle at bedtime
Inositol	2000 mg.	

See the Age Reduction Supplement Guide (Chapter 9) for a list of supplement suppliers and complete instructions on the correct and safe use of supplements.

East/West Travel

Jet lag results from the desynchronization of circadian rhythms caused by rapid flight across time zones. As a result of more than twenty recent studies, these consequences of jet lag have been identified:

- Memory loss
- Fatigue
- Disorientation
- Reduced mental alertness
- Loss of physical coordination/reflexes
- Upset stomach
- Constipation or diarrhea
- Insomnia
- Loss of appetite
- Headache
- Muscular atrophy
- Shortened attention span

The severity and duration of the symptoms depend on the direction of travel and the number of time zones crossed. Resynchronizing yourself can take as long as twelve days. (See C. Ehret and L. Scanlon, *Overcoming Jet Lag,* New York: Berkley Books, 1983, for programs intended to prevent or overcome jet lag.)

Too Much Caffeine Can Disrupt Your Mind and Body

Before you indulge in your next wake-up cup of coffee, consider this: While you are resorting to caffeine to stimulate alertness, you are preventing your body from releasing natural chemicals that would achieve the same result.

One hundred milligrams of caffeine, the amount contained in less than one cup of coffee, can disrupt body clocks in sensitive individuals by delaying the release of dopamine, the hormone responsible for promoting alertness.

The rush of energy created by caffeine through its overstimulation of the sympathetic nervous system is very short-lived. Within ninety minutes, your metabolism has gone on a roller-coaster ride that ends with a whopping crash. Here's how it works:

- Caffeine stimulates the liver, which is why you usually need to urinate within ten minutes of drinking a cup of coffee.
- The irritated liver releases its supply of stored glucose. That's when you experience the rush of warmth and energy associated with coffee drinking.
- The RAS (remember this "window on the world" from Chapter 2?)

notifies the hypothalamus that there is excessive glucose in the bloodstream.

- The hypothalamus triggers the release of insulin to mop up the glucose.
- The insulin is so efficient at mopping up the glucose that you're actually left with a lower blood sugar (and therefore energy) level than before you drank your coffee. It's at this stage that you may experience fatigue, tremors, irritability, and insecurity.

By now you've begun craving the ten o'clock coffee break, which, unfortunately, only creates yet another rush and crash.

Caffeine has another curious effect on circadian rhythms. When consumed in mid-morning, caffeine overstimulates the sympathetic nervous system and causes its daytime dopamine cycle to peak early, around three o'clock in the afternoon instead of seven at night. This causes the serotonin cycle to kick in early, causing excessive late afternoon drowsiness and the untimely release of nighttime chemicals and hormones. When caffeine is consumed after five o'clock in the afternoon, it artificially prolongs the dopamine cycle and delays the onset of the serotonin cycle, resulting in insomnia, excessive amounts of adrenaline and cortisol in the blood, and depressed cell repair and reproduction rates.

In addition to disrupting circadian rhythms, overconsumption of caffeine (more than one cup a day for sensitive individuals) has been linked in other research studies to these emotional and physical problems:

- Irritability and hostility
- Mood swings
- Anxiety, depression, and jittery nerves
- Insomnia
- Diarrhea
- Increased cholesterol
- Heart disease risk
- High blood pressure
- Peptic ulcers
- Overstimulation of the sympathetic nervous system
- Rapid pulse
- Uneven heartbeat
- Hypoglycemia
- In pregnant women, increased risk of birth defects
- In many women, fibrocystic disease (benign fibrous breast tumors)

Caffeine is by no means the only culprit causing these disorders. It is only one of a group called the xanthine drugs, which stimulate the sympathetic nervous system and create symptoms similar to those described above. Other xanthine drugs are theophylline and theobromine. Tea is a common source of theophylline and caffeine; cocoa contains theobromine and caffeine. Table 5 tells you the typical amount of this drug in common beverages.

Caffeine tolerances vary widely among individuals. Some people experience symptoms after just one cup of coffee; others can drink as much as four cups a day without ill effect. (It's important to realize, however, that circadian rhythms can be disrupted and aging accelerated without the manifestation of symptoms.) As a rule of thumb, you should limit your coffee consumption to one cup of drip coffee, two cups of instant, or one and one-half cups of percolated coffee each day. If you drink teas with caffeine, limit yourself to two cups of brewed (or tea bag) tea each day.

TABLE 5

Caffeine Content of Beverages

Beverage (5-ounce cup)	Caffeine (milligrams)
Prepared coffee	
Instant	60
Percolated	109
Drip	150
Decaffeinated Coffee	1–4
Tea	
1-minute brew	10–30
3-minute brew	20–40
5-minute brew	20–50
Tea bags	10–40
Carbonated cola drinks	15–30
Cocoa/Hot Chocolate	11

Like most drugs, caffeine can be both useful and harmful. Consumed in moderate amounts, caffeine can help you control or lose weight. As I've already mentioned caffeine stimulates the sympathetic nervous system. The sympathetic nervous system in turn stimulates the metabolism of brown fat surrounding your heart, liver, and other organs to burn up calories as heat (more on this in Chapter 8). That's why you feel a rush of warmth soon after drinking coffee. Two cups of coffee consumed before an athletic event increase the serum level of glycerol and the release of free fatty acids, which can be used as an initial energy source. Since carbohydrates provide the main source of energy in the long run and can only be stored in limited quantities, running on fats delays the depletion of carbohydrates and thus extends endurance.

Here are some ways you can benefit from caffeine while curbing its negative impact:

- Gradually reduce your coffee consumption to one cup of coffee or tea per day. If you suffer from headaches during withdrawal, relieve them with pure aspirin or non-aspirin pain relievers. (NOTE: Some pain relievers contain caffeine, so be sure you read the labels.)

- To avoid disrupting circadian rhythms, drink tea or coffee in the middle of the afternoon, which is when the British take their highly caffeinated tea.
- See Table 6 for a list of supplements that will help you painlessly conquer your caffeine addiction.
- Substitute carob for chocolate or cocoa.
- Substitute decaffeinated for caffeinated coffee. However, try to find out if the coffee is decaffeinated by *the water extraction process*. The solvent extraction process leaves residues that are low-grade carcinogens.
- Substitute herbal teas for caffeinated tea or coffee. I make my own tea out of wood betony, rose hips, chamomile, cinnamon bark, lemon grass, peppermint, papaya, Pau D'Arco, anise, orange peel, ginger, cinnamon oil, and orange oil. Voila! Great-tasting, no-caffeine tea.
- Drink sodas that are caffeine-free.

TABLE 6

Caffeine Addiction Aids

Supplement	Amount	Effect
B vitamins (especially B-1 and B-2)	10–60 mg. (B-1) 10–35 mg. (B-2)	Compensate for lost nutrients and ease withdrawal symptoms
Vitamin C	1–2 gm.	
Zinc	30–50 mg.	Compensates for cadmium found in caffeinated beverages

See the Age Reduction Supplement Guide (Chapter 9) for a list of supplement suppliers and complete instructions on the correct and safe use of supplements.

Too Much Alcohol Can Be Lethal

Alcohol holds the dubious distinction of being the world's number one recreational drug.

When consumed in small quantities, alcohol can be beneficial. One to two drinks per day can relieve anxiety; they can also help protect against cardiovascular disease by positively altering blood fat ratios and the ratio of HDL cholesterol, which protects the heart, to LDL cholesterol, which attacks and damages the coronary blood vessels. Almost half the centenarians in primitive cultures drink a little of the local brew on a daily basis.

When consumed in large quantities, alcohol can be lethal. Don W. Walker and fellow researchers in the Neuroscience Department of the University of Florida College of Medicine have recently reported conclusive evidence that *alcohol is directly responsible for brain damage*. It reduces the amount of the neurotransmitter acetylcholine, thus causing impaired mental function and poor memory. The Florida study, done with rats and translated into human terms, suggests that consuming one-third of one's daily calories as alcohol is sufficient to cause defects in residual learning and memory. Acetaldehyde, alcohol's first by-product, causes free radical and cross-linkage damage, which in turn promotes cellular aging. Alcohol's sedating nature disrupts circadian rhythms. Liver damage, malnutrition, anemia, sexual impotence and sterility, degeneration of the nervous system, muscle wasting, senile dementia, hepatitis, liver fat deposits that can cause brain and blood clots, cardiac failure . . . the list of potentially fatal consequences goes on and on.

If you consume more than two alcoholic drinks per day, you risk increasing your biological age. If you consume more than sixty drinks per month, feel compelled to drink, or are encouraged by others to cut down on drinking, it's possible you are an alcoholic.

Please remember that alcohol is a drug, and alcoholism is a disease. If you think you might be an alcoholic, I strongly urge you to seek professional help. Overcoming an alcoholic addiction is no easy matter. Withdrawal symptoms include delirium tremens, psychosis, and other serious difficulties.

If you drink any alcohol at all, you should protect your body with the cell aids and brain and nerve enhancers discussed in Chapter 13.

Abuse of Other Drugs

Drugs, whether prescription, nonprescription, or illegal, interact in complicated ways with your body. Many factors influence the outcome of this interaction, including your age, the state of your health, the time of day the drug was taken, the kind of food (or other drugs) consumed simultaneously.

While current research is insufficient to spell out exactly how your body reacts to every drug, one fact is clear: *Each drug you take affects more than just the problem for which it is targeted.* And many drugs have an adverse effect on aging.

Physicians prescribe drugs because they believe that, in specific circumstances, the benefits outweigh the risks. In many cases that is undoubtedly true. The right drug can mean the difference between life and death today; in the future, it may also prevent or control aging.

Taking drugs can cause you to age prematurely by:
- Disrupting the sensitive and sophisticated systems your body normally uses to keep itself in perfect physical balance
- Triggering one or more aging mechanisms
- Creating toxic side effects that can actually cause disease and death. (Remember Thalidomide babies?)

• Decreasing bioenergy

• Altering the metabolism of nutrients and supplements.

It's been estimated that 10 percent to 35 percent of drugs produce side reactions. In an evaluation of 1000 patients, the anti-diabetic drug tolbutamide was shown to produce a significant increase in deaths and cardiovascular disease.

Stimulants—amphetamines, cocaine, and appetite suppressants, for example—interfere with circadian rhythms by delaying fatigue and interfering with sleep.

Corticosteroids such as prednisone, cortisone, hydrocortisone, and betamethasone, when taken in doses of 40 milligrams or more for a period of more than four weeks, can cause neuroendocrinological aging by altering the action of the hypothalamus and the pituitary gland, stressing your body and depressing your immune system. In addition, corticosteroids can create toxic side effects such as diabetes, hypoglycemia, insomnia, hypertension, osteoporosis, cataracts, and cancer.

Drugs such as Desyrel and fenfluramine stimulate excess serotonin production, destroying the important serotonin-dopamine balance discussed earlier. Serotonin drugs also create side effects such as cardiovascular stress, anxiety, hot flashes, head pains, depression, and breathing problems.

Some drugs induce aging by interfering with DNA or RNA synthesis or by damaging chromosomes. Cancer chemotherapy agents such as actinomycin and mytomycin fall into this category.

Drugs also affect your nutritional balance. Table 7 lists some common drugs and their potential side effects on nutritional balance.

TABLE 7

Common Drugs That Affect Nutrition

Drug(s)	Major Side Effects	Nutrient Effects
General		
Antacids	Constipation, diarrhea, nausea, vomiting	Altered calcium/magnesium/phosphorus ratio, increased phosphates, depleted thiamine, reduced vitamin C absorption
Antibiotics	Severe allergic reactions, intestinal tract irritation, muscle and nerve problems	Decreased vitamin K
Anticonvulsants	Nerve disturbance, intestinal disorders, skin rashes	Decreased folic acid, vitamin B-12, vitamin B-6
Corticosteroids	Abnormal weight gain; insomnia; increased risk of diabetes, hypoglycemia, cataracts, cancer, osteoporosis	Decreased calcium, phosphorus, zinc, biotin; increased excretion of vitamins, calcium, potassium, zinc, amino acids

Drug(s)	Major Side Effects	Nutrient Effects
Diuretics	Allergic reaction, excessive fluid loss	Increased excretion of calcium, magnesium, potassium
Diuretics (mercurial)	Allergic reactions, mercury poisoning, intestinal irritation, alkalosis	Nutrient effects are the same as those for nonmercurial diuretics, above
Mineral oil	Pneumonia, abnormal defecation and rectal itching	Reduced absorption of vitamins A, D, E, K and phosphorus and calcium
Oral contraceptives	Weight gain, headaches, nausea, breast discomfort, irregular menstrual bleeding, moodiness, increased risk of cancer, diabetes, hypertension	Vitamin C and vitamin B-6 decrease
Steroids	Adverse hormonal effects dependent on steroid type	Reduced absorption of calcium and potassium; increase protein metabolism
Specific		
Achromycin	Gastrointestinal systemic irritation, skin rash, rise in blood urea nitrogen (BUN), stained teeth	Reduced absorption of calcium, magnesium, and iron
Aldactazide	Drowsiness, lethargy, mental confusion, gastrointestinal irritation, menstrual irregularity, headache	Reduced potassium excretion
Aldactone	Drowsiness, lethargy, mental confusion, gastrointestinal irritation, menstrual irregularity, headache	Reduced potassium excretion
Apresoline	Headache, palpitations	Vitamin B-6 depletion
Atromid-S	Nausea, vomiting, loose stools, abdominal stress	Reduction in circulating vitamin K levels
Azo Gantanol	Headache, nausea, vomiting, skin rash	Folic acid deficiency
Azulfidine	Allergic reaction, hemolytic anemia, urinary tract disturbances, blood disorders, and many other untoward effects	Reduced folic acid absorption
Bentyl with Phenobarbital	Dry mouth, fatigue	Accelerated vitamin K metabolism
Betapar	Fluid retention, muscle weakness, gastrointestinal hemorrhage, convulsions	Zinc and potassium deficiency, accelerated B-6 metabolism

Drug(s)	Major Side Effects	Nutrient Effects
Brevicon	Thrombophlebitis, pulmonary embolism, cerebral thrombosis, nausea, vomiting, rash, mental depression	Vitamin B-6 and vitamin C depletion
Bronkotabs and Bronkolixir	Nervousness, restlessness, sleeplessness	Accelerated vitamin K metabolism
Butazolidin	Edema, gastrointestinal distress, rash, confusion, vertigo	Folic acid deficiency
Cantil with Phenobarbital	Dry mouth, blurred vision	Accelerated vitamin K deficiency
Chardonna	Dry mouth, blurred vision	Accelerated vitamin K metabolism
Chlorthalidone	Excess blood sugar	Increased zinc excretion
Cholestyramine	Constipation	Reduced absorption of vitamins A, D, K, B-6, folic acid, fat, iron, calcium
Colbenemid	Headache, gastrointestinal distress, urinary frequency, dizziness	Decreased absorption of lactase, fat, sodium, potassium, and vitamin B-12
Colchicine	Headache, gastrointestinal distress, urinary frequency, dizziness	Decreased absorption of lactase, fat, sodium, potassium, and vitamin B-12
Cortisone	Hirsuitism and supraclavicular fat pads, diabetes, cataracts (*See also* Corticosteroids above)	Vitamin B-6 deficiency; accelerated vitamin D metabolism; zinc, potassium, and vitamin C deficiency
Cortisporin	Systemic intolerance	Reduced lactase levels; vitamin K, B-12, and folic acid deficiency
Cycloserine	Insomnia, headaches, tremor, dizziness, confusion, nervousness, psychosis	Reduced protein synthesis, reduced calcium and magnesium absorption, circulation decrease of folic acid and vitamins B-12 and B-6
Diethylstilbestrol	Nausea, vomiting, vertigo, anxiety, thirst, rashes	Vitamin B-6 depletion
Diupres	Nausea, vomiting, diarrhea, dizziness, vertigo	Increased magnesium and potassium excretion
Diuril	Nausea, vomiting, diarrhea, dizziness	Increased magnesium and potassium excretion
Doriden	Skin rash	Folic acid deficiency
Glutethimide	Dependency, gastric irritation, headache, skin rashes	Accelerated vitamin D metabolism and bone resorption

Drug(s)	Major Side Effects	Nutrient Effects
Hydralazine	Headache, diarrhea, nausea, vomiting, urination difficulty	Vitamin B-6 depletion
Hydrotensin Plus	Headache, palpitations	Vitamin B-6 depletion
Indocin	Gastrointestinal bleeding, headache, dizziness, anorexia, edema, skin rash	Accelerated vitamin K metabolism
Lidosporin	Overgrowth of nonsusceptible organisms	Malabsorption of vitamins B-12, K, and folic acid
Mycifradin	Nausea, diarrhea	Reduced lactase levels, vitamin K deficiency, malabsorption of vitamin B-12 and folic acid
Mycolog	Localized atrophy	Reduced lactase levels, vitamin K deficiency, malabsorption of vitamin B-12 and folic acid
Neo-Cortef	Miliaria, folliculitis	Reduced lactase levels, vitamin K deficiency, malabsorption of vitamin B-12 and folic acid
Neomycin	Nausea, vomiting, nephrotoxicity	Reduced lactase levels, vitamin K deficiency, malabsorption of vitamin B-12 and folic acid
Neosporin	Overgrowth of nonsusceptible organisms	Reduced lactase levels, vitamin K deficiency, malabsorption of vitamin B-12 and folic acid
Norinyl	Thrombophlebitis, pulmonary embolism edema, gastrointestinal upset	Vitamin B-6 and vitamin C depletion
Orasone	Exaggerated hormonal effects	Increased vitamin B-6 requirement, increased vitamin C excretion, zinc and potassium deficiency
Os-Cal-Mone	Uterine bleeding, mastodynia (breast pain)	Vitamin B-6 depletion
Para-amino salicyclic acid	Diarrhea, stomach pain, painful urination, low back pain, chills	Reduced vitamin B-12, iron, folic acid absorption
Penicillamine	Rash, itching, joint pain, fever	Vitamin B-6 depletion, increased B-6, zinc, and copper excretion
Phazyme	None	Accelerated vitamin K metabolism
Phenophthalein	Rectal irritation, allergic reactions	Reduced absorption of vitamin D
Polysporin	Overgrowth of nonsusceptible organisms, including fungi	Malabsorption of vitamins B-12, K, and folic acid

Drug(s)	Major Side Effects	Nutrient Effects
Prednisone	Exaggerated hormonal effects (*See* corticosteroids)	Increased vitamin B-6 requirement, increased vitamin C excretion, zinc and potassium deficiency
Premarin	Uterine bleeding, loss of libido	Folic acid deficiency, reduced calcium excretion
Pro-Banthine	Dry mouth, blurry vision, urine retention	Accelerated vitamin K metabolism
Ser-Ap-Es	Increased gastric secretion, angina-like pain, depression, deafness	Vitamin B-6 depletion
Sterazolidin	Edema, gastrointestinal upset	Increased vitamin B-6 requirement; increased vitamin C excretion; folic acid, zinc, and potassium deficiency
Sumycin	Gastrointestinal upset, vomiting, anorexia, nausea, diarrhea, dermatitis	Reduced absorption of calcium, magnesium, and iron
Tetracycline Tetracyn	Gastrointestinal upset, anorexia, nausea, vomiting, diarrhea, dermatitis	Reduced absorption of calcium, magnesium, and iron
Triameterene	Nausea, vomiting, leg cramps, dizziness, excess fluid loss	Decrease in circulating level of folic acid, increased calcium excretion

Adapted from *Index of Nutritional Abnormalities Induced by 50 Commonly Prescribed Drugs.* La Jolla, California: Intermarketing Association, 1978.

7

Your Environment
Is a Factor
in Aging

Four and a half billion of us coexist on an island surrounded by space. We can't get off the island—at least, not many of us and not for long—but that doesn't stop us from spoiling our own and only home.

Just like you, the planet Earth has finite resources for supporting life. Just like you, the planet must have clean air to breathe, pure water to drink, and wholesome food to eat in order to sustain all the creatures who share its life. And just like you, the earth is capable of just so much adjustment. When the demand for adaptation exceeds its ability to adapt, the planet will die. And you'll die, too.

Historically, industrialized nations have contributed the lion's share of pollution and suffered the lion's share of consequences. Not so today. Now, third-world countries are rushing headlong toward industrialization, but are producing more pollution than profit. And even the countries that haven't joined the race are experiencing its consequences. Astronauts circling the earth have sighted pollution in places where no factory has ever existed.

Since I've lived in the United States all my life, I've witnessed firsthand its reluctant attempts to grapple with pollution problems. In developing countries, however, systematic efforts to control pollution simply don't exist.

On a recent trip to Mexico City I learned that it is six times more polluted than any other city in the world. Experts estimate that if no measures are taken by 1995, citizens of Mexico City will suffer a 30 percent mortality rate from air pollution alone.

Even in the United States, pollution controls don't begin to keep pace with the problem. In 1970 more than 90 percent of the water supplied in the United States did not meet federal standards for purity. Pollutants in the environment include industrial wastes such as mercury, cadmium, and flouride; agricultural wastes such as phosphates and nitrates; radioactive waste material; and microorganisms, including bacteria and viruses. Although some of these pollutants are immediately toxic, others accumulate quietly for years with no symptoms but ultimately result in such insults as a congenitally damaged baby or an early death.

Asbestos poisoning has reached near epidemic proportions. According to one study, asbestos-induced growths were found in the lungs of two-thirds of 3000 consecutive autopsies performed in New York City—and the study is nearly fifteen years old! Think of how pollutants have increased since then.

And pollution is only one of many environmental factors in aging. You are also influenced by your geographical and topographical location, the climate, certain weather conditions, your home and work environment, and countless other factors.

Before we discuss each environmental problem and its Age Reduction System solution, I think it would be useful to isolate the primary environmental aging factors currently influencing your life and health. The checklist that follows will help you do just that. The Age Reduction System suggests solutions to each factor in this chapter.

ENVIRONMENTAL AGING FACTORS—A CHECKLIST

This checklist will help you determine which environmental aging factors are currently operating in your life. In many cases, more than one response to each statement will apply to you. Simply check every response that applies. When you have completed the checklist, use the answer key to score yourself.

1. I live:
   A. In the city
   B. In the country
   C. In the suburbs
   D. In a small rural town
2. I work:
   A. In the city
   B. In the country
   C. In the suburbs
   D. In a small rural town
3. The altitude where I live is:
   A. Between sea level and 500 feet
   B. From 500 to 1000 feet
   C. From 1000 to 5000 feet
   D. Greater than 5000 feet
4. The topography of the area in which I live is typically:
   A. Desertlike
   B. Mountainous

    C. Near or on the ocean
    D. A tropical jungle
    E. A valley surrounded by mountains
    F. Open plains
    G. Rolling green hills with forests of deciduous trees

5. The climate where I live is:
    A. Warm-to-hot and dry year-round, with little rainfall
    B. Cool-to-cold and dry year-round, with little rainfall
    C. Moderate in temperature and humidity, with few seasonal changes
    D. Cool-to-cold and moist year-round, with frequent rainfall
    E. Warm-to-hot and wet year-round, with frequent rainfall
    F. Subject to extreme temperature changes, hot in the summer and cold in the winter.

6. The place where I live is subject to:
    A. Hot, dry winds (called Santa Anas or Chinooks)
    B. Extremely hot weather
    C. Extremely cold weather
    D. Excessive sunlight
    E. Excessive cloudiness
    F. None of the above

7. In my home I have:
    A. Floors or walls covered by synthetic fabrics
    B. Floors or walls covered by natural fabrics, wood, or stone
    C. Furniture made of particle board or plastic
    D. Furniture made of natural materials, such as wood, stone, glass, or natural fibers
    E. Furniture covered by synthetic fibers
    F. Painted walls and/or ceilings
    G. Insulation that contains asbestos
    H. Air-conditioning
    I. Electric, forced-air, or gas heating
    J. A fuel-burning fireplace
    K. Solar heating
    L. Poor air circulation
    M. Excellent air circulation
    N. An air ionizer and filter system
    O. Many plants
    P. Predominantly artificial lighting
    Q. Predominantly natural lighting
    R. Many electrical appliances, such as a refrigerator, stove, washer/dryer, microwave oven, television, computer
    S. Frequent loud noises or consistent low noise
    T. Many detergents, cleansers, polishes, waxes, varnishes, air fresheners, disinfectants

U. Aluminum cookware, utensils, or foil for heating or storing food
V. Automobile fumes
W. Tobacco smoke
X. Residues from home pesticides or insecticides

8. I spend most of my working hours:
   A. In a controlled, indoor environment (e.g., an office building, home, car, or airplane)
   B. In a factory
   C. Outdoors, in the city
   D. Outdoors, in the country

9. The air pollution where I live is considered:
   A. Nonexistent
   B. Minimal
   C. Moderate
   D. Severe

10. When I work I am exposed to:
    A. Floors or walls covered by synthetic fabrics
    B. Floors or walls covered by natural fabrics, wood, or stone
    C. Furniture made of particle board or plastic
    D. Furniture made of natural materials, such as wood, stone, glass, or natural fibers
    E. Furniture covered by synthetic fibers
    F. Insulation that contains asbestos
    G. Painted walls and/or ceilings
    H. Air-conditioning
    I. Electric, forced-air, or gas heating
    J. Solar heating
    K. Poor air circulation
    L. Excellent air circulation
    M. An air ionizer
    N. Many plants
    O. Predominantly artificial lighting
    P. Predominantly natural lighting
    Q. Electrical or electronic equipment such as typewriters, photocopiers, adding machines, computers, word processors
    R. Heavy machinery such as printing presses or factory equipment
    S. Frequent loud noises or constant low noises
    T. Automobile fumes
    U. Tobacco smoke
    V. Chemicals from typewriter ribbons, carbon paper, ink, photo development chemicals, dyes
    W. Industrial pollution such as ozone, smog, sulfur oxides, fuel combustion, carbon monoxide, hydrogen sulfide, soot, or quartz
    X. Industrial wastes such as mercury, cadmium, and fluoride

    Y. Agricultural wastes such as phosphates and nitrates

11. My home or workplace is located near:
    A. Power lines or transformers
    B. An airport
    C. A toxic waste dump
    D. An electrical, gas, or nuclear power plant
    E. None of the above

12. My primary means of transportation is:
    A. Car, bus, or subway
    B. Airplane
    C. Bicycle or foot

13. Most of the food I eat:
    A. Contains additives such as chemicals added for color, flavor, preservation, or processing (sprays, waxes, emulsifiers, etc.)
    B. Is free of additives
    C. Contains contaminants such as pesticides, fertilizers, antibiotics, and hormones (used to treat meat, fish, and poultry)
    D. Is free of contaminants
    E. Is cooked at high heat or for long periods
    F. Is fresh, raw, or lightly cooked

14. Most of the water I drink is:
    A. Tap water
    B. Distilled water
    C. Mineral water
    D. Fresh water from a pure source

15. Most of the clothes I wear are:
    A. Made from synthetic fibers
    B. Made from natural fibers
    C. Dry cleaned only
    D. Machine washable

16. I am exposed to sunlight:
    A. Very little
    B. Occasionally
    C. Frequently

17. I use a sunscreen:
    A. Never
    B. Seldom
    C. Usually
    D. Always

ANSWER KEY

1.	A.	10	7.	A.	2	10.	A.	2	13.	A.	6
	B.	−10		B.	−2		B.	−2		B.	−6
	C.	7		C.	2		C.	2		C.	8
	D.	3		D.	−2		D.	−2		D.	−8
				E.	1		E.	1		E.	7
2.	A.	10		F.	1		F.	6		F.	−7
	B.	−10		G.	6		G.	1			
	C.	7		H.	4		H.	4	14.	A.	4
	D.	3		I.	3		I.	3		B.	−2
				J.	2		J.	−6		C.	−4
3.	A.	7		K.	−6		K.	5		D.	−8
	B.	4		L.	5		L.	−5			
	C.	−7		M.	−5		M.	−10	15.	A.	2
	D.	0		N.	−10		N.	−5		B.	−2
				O.	−5		O.	6		C.	2
4.	A.	5		P.	6		P.	−6		D.	−2
	B.	−5		Q.	−6		Q.	3			
	C.	−2		R.	3		R.	7	16.	A.	4
	D.	7		S.	5		S.	5		B.	−4
	E.	7		T.	1		T.	4		C.	6
	F.	−1		U.	1		U.	4			
	G.	−2		V.	1		V.	2	17.	A.	10
				W.	5		W.	8		B.	7
5.	A.	6		X.	1		X.	9		C.	−3
	B.	−6					Y.	9		D.	−10
	C.	−2	8.	A.	8						
	D.	3		B.	8	11.	A.	3			
	E.	6		C.	6		B.	7			
	F.	8		D.	−10		C.	10			
							D.	7			
6.	A.	8	9.	A.	−10		E.	−10			
	B.	6		B.	−5						
	C.	6		C.	5	12.	A.	8			
	D.	8		D.	10		B.	7			
	E.	6					C.	−6			
	F.	−8									

What Your Score Means

After arriving at your composite score, read the categories below to see which applies to you. Then go back to your answer key and circle the responses that were given a score of more than 3. These are the environmental aging factors that are most important for you to address.

−141 to −60: Congratulations! You have achieved a degree of environmental purity common to centenarians. Chances are you will experience little or no aging effects from your environment.

−60 to 0: This is also a very good score. Although you are somewhat affected by the polluted environment in which most of us live, it's clear that you are already following many of the Age Reduction System's recommendations for cleaning up your environment. You will experience minimal aging effects from environmental factors.

0 to 100: You should make substantial changes in your environment to avoid premature aging. If you continue this range of exposure, you can expect to experience prematurely aged skin; respiratory ailments; fatigue; irritability; watery, red eyes; immune system dysfunction; and premature cellular aging.

100 to 265: You are literally poisoning yourself with every day you spend in this environment. Drastic measures are necessary to prevent premature aging, disease, or death. I urge you to study your responses with care to discover the primary offenders and consider ways to remove them. Incorporate into your life as many of the Age Reduction System's environmental recommendations as you possibly can.

TOPOGRAPHY, CLIMATE, AND WEATHER SENSITIVITY

Cultures famous for longevity share several common topographic and climatic traits:
 • Moderately high altitude (1000 to 5000 feet)
 • Mountainous topography that has rocks and soil containing life-sustaining nutrients in forms readily released into the air, water, and food
 • Cool air in constant motion
 • Low humidity with little rainfall
Structurally, the western Rocky Mountains share a common geographic origin with the land of the centenarian communities in the Soviet Union, Pakistan, and Ecuador. This region includes the mountainous areas of Arizona, New Mexico, Nevada, Utah, Colorado, Idaho, Montana, Wyo-

ming, British Columbia, and Alberta. Settling down in a rural farm valley surrounded by these mountains with hard water and low humidity, and at an altitude of 3000 to 5000 feet may increase your life-span. Unfortunately, it is not common to find this optimum combination of factors in the western Rockies.

Statistically speaking, the counties east of the Rocky Mountains in the north central United States running from central Wisconsin to eastern Colorado have the longest-lived people in America. Their enhanced longevity occurs from a rural life-style and environment.

Although trying to choose the perfect Shangri-La is problematic, you should be aware of the region of the United States with the least longevity: the Southeast. Living in the area from Alabama to Kentucky may decrease your life-span.

The ideal environment we have just described promotes longevity because it offers clean air with an appropriate balance of positive and negative ions, pure water with protective minerals and nutrients, and fresh produce that contains all the life-sustaining nutrients. The long-life environment does not require your body to make a lot of adjustments. The climate is temperate and dry year-round. In addition, the long-life environment does not include any of the extremes associated with the development of degenerative disease.

Extremely cold weather, for example, is considered a contributing factor to heart disease, strokes, embolism, respiratory and rheumatic diseases. Cold weather also increases blood pressure, stimulates the sympathetic nervous system, constricts blood capillaries, and increases the survival time of bacteria and viruses, resulting in flus, colds, and pneumonia.

Extremely warm weather is also associated with heart disease. However, it is more likely to wreak havoc with your neuroendocrine system. By altering the secretion of hormones in your pituitary gland, thyroid gland, pancreas, and adrenal gland, warm weather affects your energy, emotions, and fuel consumption.

Excessive cloudiness increases the incidence of bone demineralization; excessive sunshine leads to skin aging and skin cancer.

Even more than climate, specific weather conditions can influence the rate at which you age.

Fully 50 percent of the adult North American population is highly sensitive to weather conditions. The nine most common complaints resulting from weather sensitivity are:

- Fatigue
- Ill-humor
- Headaches
- Dislike of work
- Insomnia
- Difficulty concentrating
- Nervousness
- Bone-fracture pain
- Forgetfulness

One way to determine your degree of weather sensitivity is to examine your reactions to weather changes. Does scorchingly hot weather leave you sapped of energy, while freezing cold makes you hyperkinetic? Do you recall ever feeling peevish and unbalanced just before a thunderstorm? Or exhilarated when the thunderstorm is over? Do hot, dry winds make you feel irritable, tired, or overly sensitive? Does damp, cold weather make old bone fractures ache?

If you answered yes to most of the above questions, chances are you are weather sensitive.

If you are weather sensitive, it's because your autonomic nervous system has difficulty adjusting to weather changes. Your nervous system becomes unbalanced, alternately allowing your sympathetic or parasympathetic system to dominate. And as you already know, an unbalanced autonomic nervous system leads to neuroendocrinological aging.

Maladjustment to weather changes generally shows up in one of three ways:

- The brain and other organs overproduce serotonin, causing insomnia, irritability, tension, vomiting, sore throat, oversensitivity to light, fatigue, apathy, and low blood pressure.
- The sympathetic nervous system overactivates the thyroid gland, which causes hyperactivity, tension, and vomiting.
- The neuroendocrine system generates excessive or insufficient amounts of several hormones. For example, maladjustment to cold weather may stimulate overproduction of adrenaline and cortisol, two stress-related hormones. After a few years the adrenal gland may become exhausted, leading to total exhaustion. Excessive positive ions increase production of sex hormones, which may account for premature puberty in cities with hot, dry climates. Sensitivity to changing weather causes histamine to be released from your tissues

TABLE 8

Factors Influencing Weather Sensitivity

More Sensitive	Less Sensitive
Female	Male
Lean	Muscular
Tall	Short
Slender	Stocky
Introverted	Extroverted
Emotional, nervous, or high-strung	Calm and relaxed
Unstable	Stable
Sensitive	Insensitive
Lower class	Middle class
Upper class	White collar worker
Professional	Middle management
19 to 30 years of age	30 to 49 years of age
50 or more years of age	

and blood cells, which in turn causes irritation and allergic reactions such as hives and rashes. Other hormones influenced by weather sensitivity include growth hormone, which supports the immune system and builds muscles; pancreatic hormones (e.g., insulin and glucagon), which aid digestion and food metabolism; and the hormones of the parathyroid gland, which control calcium metabolism.

To prevent premature aging from topographic, climatic, or weather-related factors, the Age Reduction System recommends that you:

- Choose to live in an environment that simulates the long-life environment already described
- Modify your diet. During cold weather you should eat slightly more proteins and fats in relation to carbohydrates. Protein contains L-tyrosine, which converts in the brain into dopamine. As noted earlier, dopamine stimulates energy and heat production. Recent studies show that fats help you maintain a constant body temperature. During hot weather, increase your intake of carbohydrates, fruit and vegetable juices, and water. Carbohydrates do not stimulate heat production, so it's easier to stay cool. Leafy green vegetables and most fruits contain water-soluble vitamins that are lost through perspiration. Juices and water help keep perspiration—your body's main cooling agent—flowing. Remember to drink water every hour to replace the water lost in perspiration. Cold, nonsweet fluids will rehydrate you most quickly.
- Follow the exercise recommendations in Chapter 11. Exercise improves your ability to adapt to weather changes by improving your heating and cooling systems just as it improves muscle tone, heart and lung capacity, and blood circulation.
- Dress appropriately for the climate. Wear layered cotton or wool garments in the cold and light cotton garments in the heat.
- Avoid the antiperspirant type of deodorant that is advertised as keeping you dry. By blocking normal perspiration, it may interfere with body temperature regulation.
- Try not to rely overmuch on heating or air-conditioning. Both devices decrease the body's ability to adjust when exposure is necessary. (Remember central heating and air-conditioning also increase positive ions.)
- In cold or dry climates, use a humidifier.
- Install an air ionizer in your home and office (to be explained thoroughly in the next section).
- Refer to Chapter 5, "Recommendations for Balancing Sympathetic/ Parasympathetic Dominance" for a list of helpful supplements. Table 9, which follows, also provides helpful recommendations.
- Take the basic nutrient supplements listed in Chapter 9 and the supplemental nutrients for the brain and nervous system listed in Chapter 14.

TABLE 9

Supplementing Weather Adaptation

Supplement	Daily Amount	Effect
Phosphatidyl choline (lecithin)	5–15 gm	Increase the brain chemical transmitter acetylcholine
DMAE (dimethylaminoethanol)	100–300 mg.	to help regulate temperature
Aconite	0.5–1.0 gm	Traditional Chinese "Aconite Combination" formula.
Astractylodes	5.0 gm	Treats sensitivity to cold—cold hands and feet,
Hoelen	4.0 gm	chills, arthritis, numbness
Ginseng	3.0 gm	
Peony root	4.0 gm	

See the Age Reduction Supplement Guide in Chapter 9 for a list of supplement suppliers and complete instructions on the correct and safe use of supplements.

Positive/Negative Ions: The Unseen Influence

Positive ions make you feed bad; negative ions make you feel good. A puzzling fact but true.

Air ions are atoms with an unbalanced electrical charge. Positive ions have an extra electron; negative ions are missing an electron.

Positive ions are created by the friction of hot air passing over surfaces. Hot, dry winds such as the Santa Anas in California or the Chinooks in the Rockies create a massive imbalance of positive to negative ions. Heating and air-conditioning units, especially those with long shafts, are formidable generators of positive ions. Pollution attracts positive ions, as do synthetic fabrics, electrical appliances (e.g., television sets, computers, typewriters), and tobacco smoke. Negative ions are primarily created by natural environmental causes: a thunderstorm, a green forest, ocean spray, a tumbling brook. The primary man-made generator of negative ions is the air ionizer, invented to compensate for the myriad of man-made positive ion generators.

Excessive positive ions trigger your neuroendocrine system to release excessive serotonin, which has been linked to heart disease and premature aging. In addition, positive ions may cause an overproduction of adrenaline, noradrenaline, or cortisol, whose connection to stress reactions and aging has already been noted. The primary symptoms of positive ion sensitivity are exhaustion, depression, irritability, anxiety, and insomnia.

Large doses of negative ions create a feeling of well-being; reduce allergy, sinus, and respiratory problems; and have been shown in experiments to increase tissue repair rates and decrease risk of infection in burn patients.

If you live or work in a controlled indoor environment or in a city (especially a polluted one), are surrounded by synthetic fibers, or are visited by hot, dry winds, you are likely to suffer the premature aging effects of positive ions. To prevent or reduce the damage, the Age Reduction System recommends that you:

- Install an air ionizer in your home, car, and workplace. (Do educate yourself by reading the manufacturer's test data about ionizers before purchasing one. Some of them produce harmful ozone as well as helpful negative ions.) I prefer air ionizers that use an electrostatic ion-generating system with an activated charcoal filtering system. The charcoal filter removes large particles while the ion-generating system removes very, very small ones.
- Add green plants to your home and workplace; they produce negative ions.
- Improve your air circulation by opening windows and doors whenever possible.
- Limit your use of central heating or air-conditioning.
- Replace synthetic fibers with natural fibers. When synthetic fibers rub against each other they create a static electric friction that generates positive ions.
- Minimize use of electrical appliances.
- Avoid smoke-filled environments.
- On particularly hot, dry days, take cool showers two or three times a day.
- Take walks in environments rich in negative ions, such as the seashore and forests.

LIGHT AND THE AGING PROCESS

Without light, life cannot exist. Light is the catalyst for photosynthesis, the process by which green plants produce oxygen for us to breathe. Light is also the catalyst for your neuroendocrine system. It enters your body through your eyes and stimulates the hypothalamus and pituitary glands to produce the appropriate balance of hormones (especially sexual hormones) to maintain optimal health. Sunlight also helps you to manufacture vitamin D (and thus maintain a healthy skeletal system), increases calcium absorption, improves your ability to handle stress or emotional disturbances, reduces blood cholesterol and arthritic pain, and stimulates the immune system.

Most centenarians are farmers who spend nearly every day working in the sun. Although it's true that their faces look weathered and wrinkled, it's also true that nature has endowed them with dark skin that contains an abundance of protective pigments against overexposure.

Our own culture has a more bizarre relationship with the sun. Under most circumstances we avoid it, wearing dark sunglasses and working under artificial light. Then, perversely, we expose the length of our vulnerable torsos to it for long hours without the least protection. Even worse, those of us with northern European roots are actually semi-albinos, with little or no natural protective pigments!

The appropriate formula for sunlight exposure is consistent with the entire Age Reduction System: not too little, not too much.

Too little light results in understimulation of the neuroendocrine and immune systems, underproduction of vitamin D, and reduced ability to handle stress or emotional disturbances. The wrong kind of light (i.e., artificial light) has been linked to hypertension, arthritis, cancer, depression, and hormonal imbalances. Too much light causes DNA and RNA breakdown and cross-linkage (both of which cause cellular aging), skin aging, cataracts, sunburn, and skin cancer.

For a dramatic demonstration of the aging effects of sun, wind, and other weather, simply compare the texture of the skin covering your buttocks to the texture of the skin covering your face. Even very old people have soft, supple skin where it has been protected.

Some controversy exists about which ultraviolet rays (A, B, C, or all of them) cause free radicals, cross-linkage, skin damage, and cancer. My point of view is very simple: Protect yourself from every ray as much and as often as possible. There are so many occasions when you are unexpectedly or indirectly exposed to sunlight that any exposure you can anticipate you should protect against.

Most sunscreens on the market today carry a sun protection factor (SPF) rating. The higher the number, the greater the degree of protection. You must choose your degree, but do so with this understanding: *Any* tan

TABLE 10

Sun Protectors

Supplement	Daily Amount	Effects
Beta carotene	40,000–160,000 IU*	Prevents damage from all wave-lengths of ultraviolet rays (cancer, sunburn, and aging)
PABA		Increases resistance to ultraviolet B rays (cancer, sunburn, and aging). *Caution:* Taken internally may cause diarrhea and nausea in some people. May diminish effectiveness of sulfonamide antibiotics. Safest method of use is as a topical application in a moisturizing sunscreen.
Cell aids	(See Chapter 13)	Counteract free radicals and cross-linkage caused by overexposure to sun
Skin-care cosmetics containing sunblock (SPF 8–15) with moisturizer		Prevent skin aging, cross-linkage, free radicals, skin cancer, and burning

*More than 100,000 IU of beta carotene may turn your skin yellow.

See the Age Reduction Supplement Guide (Chapter 9) for a list of supplement suppliers and complete instructions on the correct and safe use of supplements.

you now enjoy will pay off in later years in broken capillaries, wrinkles, and a leather-textured skin.

To experience the benefits of sunlight without the hazards, the Age Reduction System recommends that you:

- Spend some time, one hour if possible, outdoors every day without glasses or contact lenses, but with a sunscreen. (NOTE: Never look directly at the sun.)
- Use a sunscreen that offers maximum protection (SPF 15). Even better, use a skin moisturizer or cosmetics that include a sunscreen, so you never leave home without it. .
- As much as possible, work under natural light. If you must work under artificial light, use special full-spectrum light bulbs such as Vita Lites (brand name), which are sold in health-food stores.
- If you must tan your body, UV-A tanning beds pose considerably less risk than natural sunlight.
- Improve your body's ability to resist sun damage by taking the supplements listed in Table 10.

POLLUTION AND ENVIRONMENTAL POISONS

It is impossible to live in the United States without being exposed to some degree of air and water pollution, food contamination, and other environmental hazards. The problem is epidemic.

Air pollution has followed the automobile the way carriages followed horses. In rural areas, fully 60 percent of the air pollution is caused by cars; in urban areas the figure soars to 90 percent. The combustion of gasoline spews ozone carbon particles, nitrous oxide, and hydrocarbons into the air. Leaded gasoline is considered the primary source for the toxic amounts of lead found in 10 to 40 percent of children under the age of five. (Lead poisoning leads to permanent brain damage, kidney disease, cerebral palsy, and sterility.) Other automobile-related air pollutants include asphalt, rubber products, dust, and pollen, all thrown up in the air by turbulence created by vehicles traveling over roads.

Airplanes dump a heavy load of air pollution on the areas surrounding airports.

Industry contributes by burning gas, coal, oil, wood, and refuse. Chemical industries are particularly prolific, polluting the air with acids, alkalines, plastics, pharmaceuticals, rubber products, and other inorganic materials. The construction industry contributes paints, bricks, insulation materials, concrete, asphalt, ceramics, and plastics that poison the air. Most food-processing plants, easily recognized by their distinctive odor, pollute the air. And the agricultural use of poisons such as insecticides, rodenticides, herbicides, and fungicides contribute to air, water, and food contamination.

One final form of air pollution: cigarette smoke. Smoking is one of the most dangerous forms of air pollution because it literally fills the lungs with toxic metals and poisons such as lead, arsenic, cadmium, acetaldehyde, and nicotine. Smoking plays a role in 30 percent of all cancer deaths and has recently been linked to stiffening of the wall of the heart muscle, leading to cardiac failure.

Whether you smoke or are merely surrounded by smokers, you should know that you are risking the following fallout:

- Tars contain polynucleated aromatic hydrocarbons, which damage DNA and cause cancer and arteriosclerotic plaques.
- Acetaldehyde creates cross-linkage, which causes skin aging and wrinkling, emphysema, lung fibrosis with accompanying loss of flexibility and stamina, and difficulty breathing.
- Nicotine is a poison that raises blood pressure and cholesterol levels and increases adrenal gland secretions. Commercially, nicotine is sold as an insecticide!
- Carbon monoxide destroys the blood's oxygen-carrying capabilities, inducing cellular aging.
- Lead, arsenic, and cadmium destroy the immune system and disrupt normal chemical reactions, causing neuroendocrinological aging.
- Nitrates and nitrosamines cause cancer.
- Radon, a radioactive element found in the soil, is concentrated in tobacco leaves and produces cellular damage and cancer.

Toxic metals are another prevalent environmental hazard. Aluminum, for example, is found in food storage foil and cookware and is a common ingredient in antacids and baking powder. Aluminum causes cross-linkage (and, therefore, cellular aging) and is suspected as an underlying cause of Alzheimer's disease and senile dementia. Cook foods in white porcelain and stainless steel pots and pans and Corning-type glassware. Store foods in high-density polyethylene containers such as Tupperware.

Mercury, used in medicine, agriculture, and industry, wrecks havoc on the liver, kidneys, and brain.

Cadmium, found in refined foods, water, and cigarette smoke–filled air, promotes free radicals and cross-linkage, alters DNA and RNA functions, weakens cell repair mechanisms, and prevents cellular reproduction. Some of the diseases resulting from cadmium poisoning are hypertension (which causes heart enlargement and kidney and artery diseases), heart failure, coronary thrombosis, strokes, and hemorrhages.

Formaldehyde is a toxic chemical found in diesel engine exhaust, nail hardeners, soap, and hair-growth products. According to recent research, formaldehyde cross-links DNA and prevents cells from reproducing, and a single molecule of formaldehyde is sufficient to initiate damage within a cell.

Environmental hazards also exist in the form of pollution by radioactive substances such as X rays and microwaves, and electromagnetic phenomena such as living near high-voltage power lines. Research in the last decade has indicated that low-voltage electrical current and magnetic waves are biological stressors capable of damaging the body's hormonal balance, nervous system, and muscular conduction of electrical currents.

Isolating environmental poisons as the source of a problem is difficult because the symptoms are so many: irritation; fatigue; headaches; allergic reactions; respiratory infections; burning, red, or watery eyes; nausea; pulmonary disease; cancer. The symptoms are almost endless, and they all contribute to premature aging.

Laboratory tests and hair analysis are sometimes useful in determining toxic levels of different substances already in the body. For a preventive approach, the Age Reduction System recommends that you:

- Avoid living in high-risk areas. If your current home or workplace is located anywhere near a toxic waste dump site, high-voltage power lines, power plants of any kind, factories, food-processing plants, or mining operations, seriously consider moving to a different location. Don't wait for your child to suffer brain damage from lead poisoning or leukemia from exposure to toxic wastes. Life is too valuable to surrender it to such unnecessary hazards.
- Compensate for poor air and water quality by using an air purifier or ionizer and a good water purifier. The two best types of water purifiers are high-quality water filters and reverse-osmosis water purifiers. (In the reverse-osmosis system, water flows over a membrane full of tiny pores. Pure water molecules pass through the pores, but polluted molecules are too large and wash harmlessly down into the sink.) Make sure you match air and water cleansers to the kind and amount of pollution found in your home. You can get this information by buying your equipment from local experts who are familiar with the conditions in your area. Many air and water filter manufacturers supply independent test reports about their apparatus. I use a seven-stage water filter and prefilter available from Vital Corporation (listed among the supplement suppliers given in Chapter 9).
- Stop smoking or allowing others to smoke around you. If you don't think you can quit cold turkey, join a stop-smoking center or cut back gradually. Substitute somewhat less poisonous nicotine gum. Practice stress-reduction techniques if you believe your desire to smoke is associated with anxiety. Do whatever you have to do, but stop smoking.
- Consider detoxification procedures (explained in the next section of this chapter) to periodically rid your body of accumulated poisons and wastes.

- The cell aid supplements and strategies listed in Chapter 13 will protect you to some extent against the damage from smoking and other environmental hazards.
- If you feel you need professional assistance in identifying and eliminating environmental toxins, contact the Society for Clinical Ecology, 1750 Humbold Street, Denver, Colorado 80218.

How to Achieve Detoxification

Detoxification is the process of removing hazardous environmental toxins and metabolic wastes from your body. It is a longevity-developing process introduced by evolution to help man live longer.

Your body already has a highly effective built-in detoxification program, which includes five systems and five cellular and metabolic processes.

The systems are:

- The respiratory system (nasal passages, pharynx, larynx, trachea, bronchial tubes, and lungs)
- The digestive system (esophagus, stomach, liver, gall bladder, large and small intestines, rectum, and anus)
- The urinary system (kidneys, ureter, urinary bladder, and urethra)
- The dermal system (sweat and sebaceous glands of the skin)
- The immune system (antibodies)

The cellular and metabolic processes are:

- Cell repair and reproduction, which prevents DNA-damaged cells from reproducing and causing cellular aging
- Kupfer cells in the liver, which deactivate circulating toxins in the blood
- Naturally occurring antioxidants such as ascorbates and urates, which protect you from free radicals and foreign invaders
- Enzymes such as superoxide dismutase (SOD) and catalase, which protect your cells by deactivating free radicals
- Protein digestive enzymes that work to break down cross-linkage

In the environment for which we were designed, your natural detoxification system would be more than sufficient. Unfortunately, we breathe air, drink water, and eat food that is so poisoned that natural detoxification is not enough. In fact, most of us are exposed to so many toxins that our natural detoxification mechanisms have begun to malfunction or shut down.

When this happens, your body begins to poison itself. Polluted air penetrates your natural filters and accumulates in your lungs, causing cellular damage, infections, cancer. Poisoned food fails to be neutralized or excreted by the digestive system. Instead it becomes putrid and highly toxic, contributing to diverticular disease, constipation, diarrhea, hernias, spastic colon, depressed immune responses, cancer. Toxic metals and chemicals and other poisons overwhelm the kidneys' filtering systems and are absorbed into your body, where they are converted into deadly free radicals, destroying your DNA, depressing your cell repair rates, and fostering cellular aging. The dermal system, clogged by antiperspirants, cosmetics, perfumes, and other substances, is no longer able to pass toxins into the air. The aging liver no longer removes toxins from the blood. The immune system is overloaded by poisons and eventually fails to recognize harmful invaders; it may even attack itself. Poisons steadily accumulate, becoming more dangerous as they interact with each other.

Unlike allergic reactions, which affect only some people, toxins affect everyone. Any person exposed to them eventually shows symptoms. Whether symptoms occur depends on degree of exposure, inherited susceptibility, and the strength of your detoxification systems. These are some common reactions to exposure to toxins:*

- Headache often occurring at a particular place or time of day
- Migraine headache
- Hair loss in clumps
- Burning, tearing, or dry eyes
- Coughing, wheezing, or breathing difficulties
- Itching or bleeding nose, difficulty smelling
- Metallic taste in mouth or garlic breath
- Toothaches or swollen jaw
- Ringing ears or temporary deafness
- Skin eruptions, redness, rash, irritations, itching, bluish color, hives, cracks, dryness, numbness, bloating, or temporary tingling
- Muscle tension, weakness, or spasms
- Appetite loss or sudden weight loss
- Moodiness, restlessness, depression, thinking difficulties, hyperactivity, irritability—often occurring at a particular place or time of day
- Sexual decline
- Painful or frequent urination
- General fatigue or weakness or insomnia
- Stomach pain, nausea, or vomiting
- Rapid, slow, or irregular heartbeat
- Bloating or excess perspiration

It's interesting to note how many toxic reactions mimic disease symptoms. People and health professionals commonly mistake sickness for toxicity and vice versa.

The Age Reduction System minimizes internal pollution and mitigates the damage. Cleaning up your home and work environment reduces your exposure to environmental hazards. Installing air ionizers in your home,

---

* Adapted from Saifer, P., and M. Zellerbach. *Detox*. Los Angeles: Jeremy P. Tarcher, Inc., 1984. © 1984 by Merea Zellerbach and Phyllis Saifer.

car, and work environment limits the amount of air pollution your lungs have to filter. By eating the natural foods for longevity and a calorie-restricted diet you minimize the amount of poisoned food your digestive system has to detoxify. So just by following the Age Reduction System's general recommendations you can provide powerful assistance to your natural detoxification systems.

However, if you scored from 0 to 265 on the Environmental Aging Factors checklist, you may need something more.

The Age Reduction System's two-week detoxification program provides a kind of spring cleaning for your inner environment. Like spring cleaning, you probably won't want to do it more than two to three times a year, but you're going to love having done it. You'll feel lighter, more energetic. You may smell better, too.

Some doctors recommend a seven-day juice fast. Comfrey tea, pineapple juice, lemon and water, carrot juice, beet juice, green vegetable juice, and distilled water are drunk on each of the seven days. This method, while effective, is dangerous unless supervised by professionals.

A *word of caution:* The Age Reduction System's detoxification program is safe but *not suitable for everyone.* If you are substantially underweight or malnourished, are currently taking prescribed medication, or are pregnant, *do not undertake this program.* Anyone contemplating it should consult with a physician about the advisability of undergoing the detoxification program, especially if you have diabetes, heart disease, cancer, or another serious disorder.

During the fourteen days of detoxification you will be eating a modified version of the Age Reduction Diet, as described in Chapter 10.

If you prefer not to follow the Age Reduction Diet, you can achieve similar results over a longer period of time. Restrict your calories to a lesser degree, eat the natural foods for longevity listed on page 121 and ingest the recommended detoxification fibers and supplements.

Detoxification Supplements

For the next fourteen days, you will be consuming a carefully balanced mixture of fibers, herbs, activated charcoal, vitamins, and other supplements.

Begin by determining the level at which you should start, which varies according to your weight.

Weight in Pounds	Beginning Level	Maximum Level
Less than 99	1	3
100–149	1	4
150–199	2	5
200 or more	3	6

The next step is to determine the amount of detoxification mixture you should take each day, based on your level. Starting at Day 2, increase the amount one level each day until you reach your maximum level, which you will then consume until the end of the program. (NOTE: It is normal to feel fullness or experience abdominal swelling from consuming the detoxification mixture. The psyllium husks and guar gum fiber absorb water and swell. However, if you experience actual abdominal pains, you should discontinue the program. Some people are allergic to psyllium husks.)

Level	Detoxification Mixture Amount (mix with 8 ounces of juice)
1	1 level teaspoon twice daily
2	1 level teaspoon four times daily
3	1 rounded teaspoon four times daily
4	1 heaping teaspoon four times daily
5	1½ heaping teaspoons four times daily
6	2 heaping teaspoons four times daily

Detoxification Mixture Recipe

This recipe makes approximately one pound of detoxification mixture. Raw ingredients and combinations of these ingredients are available from the supplement suppliers listed in Chapter 9 and in most health food stores.

Ingredients	Amounts
Fibers	
Psyllium husks (100% pure)	160 grams
Bran fiber (oat, rice, or wheat)	60 grams
Guar gum	40 grams
Apple pectin	30 grams
Sodium alginate	25 grams
Irish moss	10 grams
Herbs	
Deodorized garlic	40 grams
Cloves	10 grams
Blessed thistle	10 grams
Corn silk	10 grams
Red clover	10 grams
Plantain	10 grams
Echinancea	10 grams
Miscellaneous	
Lactobacilli cultures	30 grams total

While you are detoxifying, you should take the basic fat-soluble, water-soluble, and mineral nutrients identified in Chapter 9. Vitamin C and sulfhydryl amino acids such as cysteine are very important.

The final supplement of the program is activated charcoal. This gritty black powder effectively removes toxins from the intestines as well as the blood and has extended life, according to recent Russian research. Mix one teaspoon of activated charcoal with a cup of juice, water, or other beverage. Drink one cup in the morning and one at night on each day of the program.

NOTE: Activated charcoal does cause one unfortunate side effect: constipation. Since the detoxification program is more effective with activated charcoal, I recommend that you compensate for constipation by taking 100 to 200 milligrams a day of cascara sagrada extract, a gentle herbal laxative.

Simplified Supplement Program

If formulating your own detoxification supplements appears too time-consuming or complicated, use my simplified supplement program.

Twice a day (in the morning and at night) drink 8 ounces of water or pure juice with the following ingredients:

Psyllium husks	1 teaspoon
Activated charcoal	1 teaspoon
Lactobacilli	1 teaspoon
Apple pectin	¼ teaspoon
Sodium alginate	¼ teaspoon

In addition take 2 grams of aged, deodorized garlic, the basic nutrient supplements suggested in Chapter 9, and the digestive aids described in Chapter 13. Relieve constipation with cascara sagrada extract, if needed.

The Detoxification Diet

The best diet while detoxifying is a modified version of the Age Reduction Diet described in Chapter 10. Men should eat the recommended portions of food in their target zone, between 1600 and 2000 calories a day. Women should eat the portions in their target zone, between 1400 and 1800 calories a day.

For maximum detoxification benefits, follow these additional guidelines:

• Do not eat any meat protein while detoxifying. Eat only vegetables, dairy products, fresh fish, or poultry without any skin. Poultry should be organically raised if possible. Try to keep your intake of animal protein as low as possible.

• Increase your consumption of fresh fruit juice and pure vegetable juice in place of solid complex carbohydrate foods. Carefully clean all vegetables and fruits. If you can purchase genuine organic produce, do so.

- Do not consume foods in the dessert, dairy, sweet, or alcoholic beverage exchange groups. (See the Age Reduction Diet food groups listed in Chapter 10.)
- Drink at least one quart of pure water on each day of the program.
- Limit your use of spices and condiments. Do not use vinegar while detoxifying.

While detoxifying you should also avoid sugar, salt, coffee, harmful chemicals, foods containing preservatives, alcohol, cocaine, marijuana, and drugs unless prescribed by your doctor. Limit your contact with cleansers, toiletries, soaps, and detergents. Many of these products are highly toxic.

Exercise and Detoxification

Exercising aerobically (see Chapter 11) and sweating enhance detoxification. Exercise increases your circulation, perspiration, metabolic rate, and fat metabolism. More toxins are excreted via your sweat, urine, liver bile, lungs, and fat metabolization (fat stores toxins such as DDT). Sustained aerobic exercise creates lactic acid, a moderately powerful chelating agent that removes toxic metals.

Checking Your Progress

You may notice during the course of this program that your feces change shape, color, and smell. This is a sign that the procedure is working. Activated charcoal causes grayish black feces. By the end of the program, your feces should be long and thick, float instead of sink, and be without odor. When activated charcoal leaves your system in a day or two, your feces will be a lighter color than they were before detoxifying.

The Detoxification Maintenance Program

I suggest daily use of the detoxification formula (two to five teaspoons a day) especially if your diet is deficient in dietary fibers (see Chapter 8). It contains a good mixture of fiber and other beneficial ingredients. Activated charcoal should be used two days a week to prevent cellular damage. Mix it in beverages along with psyllium seed husks and other fibers.

Detoxification Symptoms and Withdrawal Reactions

Detoxification, especially from addictive substances (nicotine, sugar, alcohol, caffeine, cocaine, medications, and chemicals), causes withdrawal

TABLE 11

Detoxification Withdrawal Symptoms

Toxin

Symptoms	Alcohol	Caffeine	Chemicals and pollutants	Cocaine	Food	Marijuana	Medicine and drugs	Nicotine	Refined sugar
Brain									
Anxiety and tension	X	X	X	X	X	X	X	X	X
Craving addicted substances and depression	X	X	X	X	X	X	X	X	X
Insomnia	X	X		X		X	X	X	
Dizziness	X	X	X		X		X		X
Drowsiness		X		X				X	
Hyperactivity	X		X		X	X	X		X
Fatigue	X				X		X		
Concentration loss	X	X	X	X				X	X
Headaches			X		X		X	X	X
Migraines		X							
Ears									
Ear-ringing		X							
Earaches							X		
Eyes									
Blurriness					X		X		X
Dilated pupils	X						X		
Wateriness							X		
Digestion									
Diarrhea		X			X		X	X	
Constipation							X	X	
Nausea	X	X			X		X	X	
Mouth									
Bad taste							X		
Dryness	X								
Gum or tongue soreness								X	
Muscles									
Weakness	X	X	X	X			X		X
Aches		X		X			X	X	
Nose									
Dripping		X		X			X		
Irritated				X					
Bad smells							X		
Skin									
Chills	X	X			X		X		
Goose bumps							X		
Flushing		X							
Rash					X		X		
Itching			X		X				
Sweating	X	X			X		X		

Adapted from Saifer, P., and M. Zellerbach. *Detox*. Los Angeles: Jeremy P. Tarcher, Inc., 1984. © 1984 by Merla Zellerbach and Phyllis Saifer.

signs. Withdrawal signs are metabolic and psychological adjustments when your body is deprived of the addictive substance. The release of stored toxins from your fat and cells also causes symptoms. High toxicity and rapid detoxification increase the incidence of withdrawal symptoms. For example, if you're a chronic drinker who inhales cocaine and abuses other drugs regularly, a sudden stoppage of your addictive substances will cause withdrawal symptoms. The Age Reduction System of detoxification has been designed to decrease the severity of withdrawal symptoms. Table 11 shows typical detoxification symptoms from common substances.

If you suffer from any of these symptoms for more than half a day or are uneasy about the discomfort, call your physician. If you suffer from any of these more serious symptoms: hallucinations, panic, irregular heartbeat, severe diarrhea, intense constipation, vomiting, seizures, double vision, twitching, uncontrolled eye movement, or fever, call your physician immediately.

Most people only have minor discomfort. Still, it's a good idea to alert your family and discuss with your doctor beforehand what you are going to do and where he can be reached.

To minimize toxic reactions, go for long walks in fresh air, use meditation or hypnosis to calm your mind, and remember that part of getting better may involve withdrawal symptoms.

SECTION II

Age Reduction Through Optimal Nutrition and Exercise

8

Optimal Nutrition for Age Reduction

Improving your eating habits is probably the fastest and easiest change you can make to reduce your biological age.

Food is the fuel that nourishes individual cells, helps maintain biochemical processes, determines your blood sugar level, and produces the energy to maintain life.

Both genetic and non-genetic cellular aging theories revolve primarily around the over- and undernutrition your cells receive. DNA and RNA damage, the accumulation of toxic wastes, lipofuscin deposits, free radicals, and cross-linkage damage may all be traced at least partly to diet. Your diet can also induce neuroendocrinological aging by damaging the immune system.

By eating the right food in the right amount at the right time (and by taking the right supplements), you can:

- Provide your cells with the kind of food, water, and oxygen they require to reproduce correctly, properly transmit information to other systems, and effectively repair any damage
- Improve your emotional stability and energy level by supplying a continuous source of usable fuel
- Help your body purge itself of dangerous toxins and waste materials which, left to accumulate, could cause cancer or other degenerative diseases
- Decrease your risk of developing cancer, arteriosclerosis, hypertension, heart disease, osteoporosis, senility, and depression
- Help synchronize your body rhythms
- Add years to your life by returning to the dietary habits dictated by evolution.

OPTIMAL NUTRITION
VERSUS THE AMERICAN DIET

To discover the "optimal" diet, we must understand the eating habits we had for the first several thousand years of our existence, when evolution was perfecting our digestion.

In those days we were divided into two primary groups: nomadic tribes who wandered wherever fresh food was available and farming communities where the art of agriculture was born.

Since fire wasn't discovered for some time, the diet of our earliest ancestors consisted primarily of raw fruits and vegetables, nuts, and seeds. There is strong evidence to suggest that man was not initially carnivorous. One rule of thumb for determining dietary preferences is to examine the way a species drinks water. Carnivorous species, such as cats, dogs, bears, and wolves, lap water. Herbivorous species, such as cows, horses, elephants, chickens—and man—suck water. For man, meat eating is an acquired taste. Unfortunately, our ability to digest it was not so easily acquired.

The optimal diet is nontoxic, provides the correct amount of nutrients and fuel, and is fast and easy to digest and eliminate. Fruits, especially the sweeter ones such as dates, figs, and raisins, should be consumed in moderate amounts only throughout the day. They are high in calories, rapidly digested and converted into energy, then eliminated quickly from your body. Complex carbohydrates such as starchy vegetables and grains are also easily digested. They provide a gradual sustained release of energy, furnish protein, and offer bulk and fiber to aid in elimination. While meats provide protein, they are an inefficient source of fuel for readily usable energy, unlike high-protein vegetarian foods. Moreover, due to their lack of fiber, meats pass sluggishly through the intestines and are eliminated slowly. Daily consumption of meat increases your risk of developing pancreatic and colon cancer.

Natural Foods Promote Longevity

The diets of most centenarian cultures mimic our ancestral diet. They drink pure mountain water, moderate amounts of alcohol distilled from local fruits and vegetables, or dairy products. They eat fresh produce grown on their own unpolluted soil. Since food processing procedures are primitive, they don't consume chemical additives, preservatives, food colorings, hormones, or antibiotics common to "civilized" cultures. They bake their own bread from whole grains. They consume very little fat, salt, or sugar. Perhaps most important, their eating habits are determined by the historical cycle of feast and famine. When food is plentiful, they eat plenty and store what they don't need for energy as fat. When food is scarce, they convert their fat deposits to energy, just as evolution intended. When both feast and famine are accounted for, most centenarians consume between 1200 and 2000 calories per day.

To create your own long-life diet in twentieth-century America, most of your meals should be made up of these foods:

- Raw or lightly cooked whole grains and breakfast cereals
- Raw or lightly steamed fresh vegetables and sprouts
- Raw fresh fruit (in the skin, whenever possible)
- Lightly cooked legumes (dried beans, lentils, or peas)
- Nonhomogenized dairy products, especially yogurt and other cultured dairy products
- Raw nuts and seeds (be sure they are unsalted and fresh, not rancid)
- Fresh, unadulterated meat, fish, and poultry (preferably skinless), no more than twice a week.

See Table 12 for the appropriate amount of each food group.

The Age Reduction System also recommends that you take the basic vitamin, mineral, and nutrient supplements described in Chapter 9. Since there is no way to avoid food contamination completely, you should at least compensate for it.

Plan your meals so that you consume most of your protein in the morning and most of your complex carbohydrates later in the day. As noted in Chapter 6, protein stimulates your dopamine cycle while carbohydrates stimulate your serotonin cycle. The correct balance of these cycles helps you maintain balanced body rhythms and delay aging.

My final advice is to avoid becoming a fanatic. As you read the succeeding pages you may be so repelled by the state of food affairs in America that you believe drastic measures are required. I agree, but it's important to realize that the price of outrage over every little agricultural insult is negative stress that may be more debilitating than the bad food.

TABLE 12

Proper Balance of Nutrients

Nutrient	Typical American Diet	Proper Nutrient Amount
Fat	40–45%	10–20%
Protein	15–20%	10–20%
Carbohydrate		
Refined or simple sugars	20–25%	0–5%
Complex (whole grains and cereals, vegetables, fruits)	20–25%	65% or more

The Price of Progress

To say the American diet is less than ideal is an understatement. It isn't just that we don't always eat what's best for us; we rarely eat what's genuinely edible.

Most Americans (and particularly Baby Boomers) were raised on food that came out of a package or a can. Forty-five percent of the average American's total calories comes from totally or partially prepared "convenience foods."

After World War II, American ingenuity turned its attention to agriculture. We wanted to raise more food faster and on fewer acres than any other country in the world.

We invented pesticides, insecticides, herbicides, and fertilizers to increase the yield of our crops. We developed chemical additives, colorings, and preservatives to improve the taste, smell, color, and shelf life of our food products. We built processing mills to convert fresh foods into prepackaged meals any busy homemaker could serve. We developed growth hormones and antibiotics to produce more meat at less cost.

In the process we also poisoned our soil, contaminated our food, and stripped fruits, vegetables, and grains of their abundant natural nutritional value.

At the risk of standing on a (prepackaged) soap box, I want to share with you just a few examples of how little your food dollars are buying.

Packaged, canned, frozen, or prepared foods provide less nutritional value. Frozen vegetables contain 25 percent less common vitamins (vitamin A, vitamin C, vitamin B-1, vitamin B-2, and vitamin B-3) in comparison with cooked fresh vegetables. Frozen fruit contains 20 percent less common vitamins in comparison with fresh fruit. Canned fruits and vegetables contain two to three times less of the common vitamins in comparison with frozen vegetables. Canned peas, for example, have lost 96 percent of their vitamin C by the time they are spooned onto your plate. Potatoes that are peeled, cut, soaked in water for two hours, and baked are missing 76 percent of their vitamin C. Meats that are frozen and then cooked lose from 15 to 40 percent of their vitamin B-1 and from 5 to 15 percent of their niacin.

Not everybody has the luxury of being able to obtain fresh produce and food, however. How does the nutrient content of frozen foods and packaged items compare with fresh fruit that has traveled long distances and spent days sitting in trucks and eventually in the supermarkets that most urban dwellers rely on? Under the worst conditions, fresh foods may become entirely inedible after delivery to urban centers before reaching your mouth unless they are properly packaged and preserved by techniques such as freezing.

The kinetics of food degeneration is very complex. The shelf life of each nutrient in a food varies with the degree of exposure to oxygen, carbon dioxide, temperature, moisture, and light, as well as to any physical damage that disrupts cells. For example, spinach becomes unusable thirteen times as rapidly when stored at room temperature than when refrigerated near freezing temperature.

The potential degree of loss in fresh food from harvest time until it reaches your mouth is highly variable in comparison to the fixed degree of loss described above for frozen foods. If you live in an urban center or rely on supermarket produce left out on open shelves that may have been inadequately refrigerated or improperly protected for considerable periods of time, eating frozen foods is often the better option.

The only definite conclusion one can reach is the need for supplemental nutrients to compensate for nutrition lost in the processes used in our modern agricultural system.

Cattle are kept in small pens because exercise builds strong muscles, which translates into tough meat. They are overfed on grain laced with growth hormones to produce the maximum amount of fat-marbled meat in the minimum time. And then they are deluged with antibiotics to encourage growth and stave off disease until slaughter. Recent research at the Center for Disease Control in Atlanta, Georgia, has found a connection between antibiotics fed to animals and the development of drug-resistant infectious bacteria in people.

In the post-slaughter stage, beef is tenderized by aging (which is simply decomposition) and injected with chemicals to disguise the smell of decaying flesh and improve the color. All this you can purchase for $1.50 to $9.00 per pound.

And finally, there are chickens, those little creatures that used to scratch around barnyards and lay eggs in strange places. Today chickens are cooped up in tiny cages and stacked one atop the other in hen houses where artificial lights glare twenty-four hours a day in hopes of tricking them into laying more eggs. (Talk about disrupting circadian rhythms!) They're fed a diet loaded with hormones and antibiotics to encourage growth and keep them from developing unprofitable diseases. When they do get sick—cancer is epidemic among chickens—farmers simply cut off cancerous wings or legs and sell what remains as higher-priced chicken parts in your local grocery store.

Before I direct too much of my indignation toward farmers, I must admit that our economy has placed them firmly between a rock and a hard place. Farmers are compelled to extract every last ounce of yield from crops and livestock, and still many of them are forced into bankruptcy.

Once food enters our kitchens, we, too, play a role doing ourselves nutritional damage. We douse our food with salt or sugar, cook it at high temperatures or for long periods, and eat much more of it than we need for optimal health.

It's no wonder that more than half the American population suffers from some degree of malnutrition.

Here are just a few of the items we choose to call food that you will avoid if you wish to grow younger instead of older:
- Presweetened cereals
- Canned vegetables or fruits
- Luncheon meats
- Desserts containing refined sugar
- TV dinners
- Refined flour or cereal products
- Soft drinks and sweetened fruit drinks
- Prepackaged, instant, or artificial foods
- Fast or snack foods
- Salted and fried potato or corn chips
- Sugar products
- Roasted, salted nuts and seeds
- Fried foods
- Food products containing caffeine
- Excessive alcohol

To compensate for the deficiencies of the American diet and achieve optimal nutrition, you'll have to eliminate your bad eating habits and develop some good ones.

In terms of negative impact on health and longevity, these are the six worst eating habits:
- Consuming too many calories
- Eating too much salt
- Overindulging in sugar
- Consuming excess fats of the wrong kinds
- Eating insufficient fiber
- Eating excess protein

OVEREATING: THE GREAT ESCAPE

Most Americans do not eat simply to satisfy hunger or provide needed nourishment. We eat to satisfy subtle psychological needs—to assuage loneliness or frustration, to stave off boredom. In America, eating is the illusory antidote for whatever ails us. It's no wonder that more than 30 percent of Americans are overweight. (The many causes and solutions for this problem are discussed extensively in Chapter 10.)

Regardless of the cause of excess weight, the results remain the same: increased incidence of hypertension, heart disease, stroke, diabetes, respiratory disease, gall bladder disease, arteriosclerosis, osteoarthritis, and cancer. Excess weight has also been linked to immune system dysfunction, free radical damage, sugar intolerance, free fatty acids, cross-linkage, cell and tissue damage.

TAKING IT WITH A GRAIN OF SALT

There's good news and there's bad news about salt. The good news is that you actually do need some salt in your diet. About 200 milligrams per day of sodium, one of salt's two components, is needed for many different physiological functions, including energy production. A sodium deficiency causes depression, fatigue, and weakness. Sodium deficiency occurs primarily as a result of hot weather and excessive sweating during heavy work. Chloride, the other component, is required to digest food in your stomach.

The bad news is that most of us consume about twenty times as much salt as we need, about 8 pounds per year. The result is increased blood pressure and water retention, higher incidence of premenstrual tension, prostate disorders, and likelihood of heart attack and stroke.

It is possible, however, for one element to displace another. Salt is displaced by calcium, potassium, and magnesium. Increasing your intake of these minerals while reducing your intake of salt may add years to your life. Table 13 lists the salty foods you should avoid. In addition, you should season foods with herbs instead of salt. If you must use salt, use:

- Sea salt, which contains 75 percent sodium chloride and 25 percent trace minerals
- Kelp, which contains only 18 percent sodium chloride and is rich in trace minerals

TABLE 13

Sodium-Rich Foods

Beverages	Commercial buttermilk, tomato juice, V8 juice
Fats	Gravy, regular peanut butter, commercial salad dressings
Protein foods	Cured meats (ham, bacon, luncheon meats), hot dogs, regular canned salmon and tuna, frozen dinners, cheese, caviar
Snacks	Salted pretzels, potato chips, popcorn, pizza, salted crackers (and many, many more!)
Vegetables	Sauerkraut, most canned vegetables, olives, pickles
Soups	Commercial soups, bouillon, broth
Condiments	Catsups, meat sauces, soy sauce, chili sauce, prepared mustard, seasoned salt, MSG (monosodium glutamate), meat tenderizers, steak sauce

• Miso, which contains only 12 percent sodium chloride, 15 to 20 percent protein, 5 to 8 percent fat, and 12 to 22 percent carbohydrates. (Kelp and miso as you can see are superior to sea salt.)

See the Age Reduction Supplement Guide in Chapter 9 for a list of supplement suppliers and complete instructions on the correct and safe use of supplements.

THE SWEETEST ENEMY

Do you suppose that Eve was really trying to satisfy a craving for sweets rather than a thirst for knowledge when she plucked that fateful apple? If you are addicted to sugar, you know how irrational you can become in pursuit of sweet-tooth satisfaction. The first symptoms are fatigue and irritability, followed by inability to concentrate, a queasy stomach, tremors, possibly a headache, and an insatiable urge for sugar. But then, sweet relief. Within ten minutes of consuming candy or anything like it you experience a wonderful lift. Energy, power, enthusiasm return. For the next thirty to forty-five minutes you are operating at peak efficiency. Then you notice a vague feeling of fatigue, irritability . . . And so on, and so on, and so on.

Sugar, whether it's called sucrose, glucose, dextrose, brown sugar, raw sugar, or turbinado sugar, is a carbohydrate that provides instant energy. When consumed in diluted form, such as in fresh fruits, it won't overload your blood sugar system. If you're eating pure, refined sugar, however, you might as well inject it directly into your veins. So much of it enters your blood system so quickly that your pancreas glands are forced to release massive doses of insulin to restabilize your blood sugar level. (Insulin is antagonistic to glucose.) Unfortunately, just about the time you have produced enough insulin to restabilize your blood sugar level, the energy fix you've given yourself fails, so your blood sugar level now plummets far below normal. You reexperience the symptoms already described and find yourself on the vicious treadmill of sugar addiction.

Sugar comprises 22 percent of most Americans' daily calories. Some experts believe that chronically high sugar intake (more than 16 percent of daily calories) contributes not only toward dental cavities but also to vitamin deficiencies (sugar contains no nutrients and still people substitute it for food), fat gain, muscular degeneration, immune system dysfunction due to the repression of growth hormone, cardiovascular problems, arteriosclerosis, high blood sugar (diabetes), and low blood sugar (hypoglycemia). Recent evidence uncovered by researcher Richard Bucola at Rockefeller University indicates that excess glucose is a crosslinking agent that binds collagen and other cell tissues so that DNA is damaged and cells cannot reproduce properly.

Approximately 35 percent of Americans suffer from some degree of hypoglycemia—abnormally low blood sugar. It is sometimes called the "divorce disease" because of the emotional instability, insecurity, and irritability it produces. Other symptoms include fatigue, trembling, rapid heartbeat, and loss of coordination and sexual drive. Both hypoglycemia and diabetes are more likely to occur with age, as the body develops an intolerance to carbohydrates.

The first step you should take to cut sugar consumption is to read food labels. Since food manufacturers are required by law to list ingredients in descending order of amount, you can quickly determine if sugar is one of the first ingredients. Beware, though, of manufacturers who try to conceal the fact that sugar is the primary ingredient by breaking it down into sucrose, glucose, and corn sugar. If you see several kinds of sugar listed, don't buy the product.

The next phase of your sugar strategy is substitution. Table 14 contains a complete list of substitutes and supplements. Increasing your intake of complex carbohydrates such as whole grains and sugar-free cereals will also reduce your craving for sugar.

Finally, if you suspect you may be hypoglycemic or diabetic, take a glucose tolerance test at a local clinic. If the results are positive for blood

TABLE 14

Sugar Regulators

Supplements	Daily Amount	Effect
Cysteine	500–1000 mg.	Modulate your release of insulin and stabilize blood
Vitamin C	1–2 gm	sugar levels
Vitamin B-1	10–60 mg.	
Zinc	30–50 mg.	
GTF chromium	200–300 mcg.	
Dietary fibers (before meals)	2–3 gm	Slow down the absorption of sugar and the release of
Guar gum	500–1000 mg.	insulin
High methoxy pectin		
NutraSweet	Minimal	Sugar substitute that does not stimulate release of
		insulin
Bupleurum	6.0 gm	Traditional Chinese formula—"Bupleurum
Ginger	4.0 gm	Combination plus Rehmannia"—that controls
Rhubarb	1.0 gm	blood sugar and treats diabetes
Scute	3.0 gm	
Chih-shih	2.0 gm	
Jejube	3.0 gm	
Pinellia	3.0 gm	
Peony	3.0 gm	
Rehmannia	3.0 gm	

See the Age Reduction Supplement Guide in Chapter 9 for a list of supplement suppliers and complete instructions on the correct and safe use of supplements.

sugar intolerance, the Age Reduction System recommends that you eat a diet rich in complex carbohydrates (see pages 199–201) in several small meals throughout the day. The high-protein mini-meal diet traditionally recommended by doctors negatively influences longevity due to its excessive protein and fat and insufficient fiber. (We'll review each of these factors in succeeding sections of this chapter.)

The need to sweeten foods is a common dietary crutch. Even though I don't recommend using artificial sweeteners or eating refined sugar, I recognize that people with an acquired sweet tooth have a hard time doing without sweets. Given the choice between using refined sugar, which alters the blood sugar level, elevates blood lipids, cross-links, and is addictive, and using either aspartame (commonly known as NutraSweet) or saccharin, I believe NutraSweet is safest. NutraSweet is a protein 200 times sweeter than sugar and contains two amino acids, aspartic acid and phenylalanine, and methanol. Because it is metabolized as a protein it does not cause a release of insulin. It tastes better than saccharin and does not cause tumors in animals, as saccharin does.

Critics have attacked NutraSweet's safety on different fronts. Some critics feel that the phenylalanine it contains interferes with the absorption of neutral amino acids such as tryptophan by competing with their protein carriers. Impeded absorption of tryptophan would mean a decrease of serotonin in the brain. These critics maintain that phenylalanine will also increase dopamine levels. According to their scenario, aspartame alters brain chemistry and behavior.

Studies have shown that high amounts of aspartame fed to rats along with glucose decreased the amount of serotonin in their tiny brains. In human dosages, however, aspartame does not alter emotions, behavior, and neurochemistry. Besides, the potential effect of phenylalanine, an anti-aging nutrient, on neurochemistry may be beneficial, not harmful. Experimental research suggests that raising dopamine and lowering serotonin extends life.

The second area of criticism concerns methanol toxicity. But the amount of methanol in an amount of NutraSweet equivalent to one teaspoon of sugar is one-twentieth of the amount of methanol contained in eight ounces of tomato juice.

It is true that a small segment of the population suffering from PKU (phenylketonuria) cannot metabolize phenylalanine or use aspartame. If you suffer from PKU, I recommend using foods sweetened with sorbitol, a slow metabolizing sugar-derived alcohol that does not increase insulin.

A DIET OVERSATURATED WITH FAT

Our diet has the paradoxical distinction of containing excessive fat (40 to 45 percent of daily calories) while simultaneously offering an inadequate supply of the essential fatty acids required to maintain health.

Fat contains twice as many calories as protein or carbohydrates. If you reduce your fat intake to less than 20 percent of your daily calories by substituting the same quantity of complex carbohydrates and reduced-fat foods, you could cut more than 1000 calories a day out of your diet. And by doing so, you could also appreciably extend your life expectancy.

Table 15 (see pages 130–131) provides an example of a person removing 1460 calories by eliminating foods containing 49 percent fat and 3100 calories and substituting for them foods containing only 17 percent fat and 1640 calories.

Some fat in the diet is essential. Natural fats are needed to:
• Provide a concentrated form of energy
• Improve the taste of food
• Create the correct environment to digest fat-soluble vitamins
• Provide the essential fatty acids, which maintain cellular structure and function through regulators such as prostaglandin, prostacyclins, and thromboxanes

Natural fats include saturated fats—solid fats formed from dairy, meat, and fish products—and unsaturated fats—liquid fats extracted from vegetable and fish oils.

Cod liver oil and evening primrose oil are two excellent natural sources of essential fatty acids. (Both oils are part of my basic fat-soluble nutrients listed in Chapter 9.) Cod liver oil contains essential fatty acids that convert to EPA and DHA, two well-documented heart protectors. The circulation-smoothing effect of EPA and DHA may explain why Eskimos and Japanese, both of whom consume an abundance of fat, have a low incidence of heart attack.

The essential fatty acid gamma linolenic, found in evening primrose oil, is also beneficial to the heart. It has been shown to lower cholesterol, lower blood pressure, heal eczema, alleviate hangovers, relieve premenstrual tension, and control weight in the obese without dieting.

Olive oil is a monounsaturated fat used since biblical times. Recent research shows it increases your HDL to LDL cholesterol ratio by lowering LDL cholesterol without affecting HDL cholesterol. In contrast, polyunsaturated fats such as sesame seed oil and sunflower seed oil lower both HDL and LDL cholesterol. Polyunsaturated fats are also more susceptible to auto-oxidation (turning rancid) and may suppress your immune system and damage your cells. Use extra-virgin olive oil pressed manually. Hydraulic pressing may generate heat that damages the oil.

Lecithin is another form of natural fat found in almost every plant and animal cell. Lecithin contains glycerol, fatty acids, phosphorus, and a nitrogen-based choline. (Choline converts into the neurotransmitter acetylcholine, which can improve memory and intellectual abilities, as well as alleviate signs of senility.) Lecithin has been clinically proven to lower total blood cholesterol. It also controls blood fat levels, prevents

TABLE 15

A Sample Fat-Substitution Menu

Old Diet	New Diet Substitution
BREAKFAST:	
3 scrambled eggs made with whole milk and butter or oil	Scrambled eggs made with the whites of 3 eggs, 1 egg yolk, and skim milk in a nonstick pan
2 English muffins with 2 pats of butter	2 whole wheat English muffins with 2 teaspoons of whipped butter
1 cup of coffee with 2 teaspoons of cream	1 cup of decaffeinated coffee with 2 teaspoons of low-fat milk
740 calories **36 grams of fat**	**480 calories** **11 grams of fat**
LUNCH:	
1 cup cream of celery soup	1 cup vegetable soup
Tunafish sandwich with 1 teaspoon of mayonnaise	Tunafish sandwich with 1 tablespoon of low-calorie mayonnaise
Apple pie	Large apple
Tea	Herbal tea
860 calories **36 grams of fat**	**410 calories** **3 grams of fat**

liver degeneration, improves blood circulation, and aids the nervous system. Soybeans provide a superior form of lecithin. (See the "Age Reduction Supplement Guide" in Chapter 9 for complete instructions on the correct use of lecithin.)

While consuming a moderate amount of natural fats is both useful and necessary, consuming any amount of unnatural fats is harmful. Hydrogenated fats, such as margarine and shortening, are the most common unnatural fats. The hydrogenation process converts a liquid (unsaturated) fat to a solid (saturated) fat by exposing the fat molecules to hydrogen. Hydrogenated fats create unwieldy molecules that prevent the production of prostaglandins, hormonelike substances that are a prerequisite for healthy cells and tissues. Since margarine contains less cholesterol and

Old Diet	New Diet Substitution
DINNER:	
Fried chicken	Roasted chicken
¾ cup hash brown potatoes	Baked potato
Dinner salad with 1 tablespoon of blue cheese dressing	Dinner salad with 1 tablespoon of low-calorie blue cheese dressing
1 biscuit with 1 pat of butter	1 whole wheat roll with 1 teaspoon of whipped butter
Coffee with 1 tablespoon of cream	Decaffeinated coffee with 1 tablespoon of low-fat milk
1 scoop of ice cream with 4 tablespoons of whipped cream	1 scoop of orange sherbet with 4 tablespoons of whipped, chilled skim evaporated milk

**1500 calories
96 grams of fat**

**750 calories
17 grams of fat**

Totals:
  3100 calories
  49% fat

Totals:
  1640 calories
  17% fat

You saved 1460 calories

saturated fat than butter, some nutritionists and doctors recommend substituting margarine for butter to control cholesterol in your blood. This is wrong. Studies indicate that the unnatural molecules in margarine actually raise blood cholesterol rather than lower it. Moreover, hydrogenated fats increase free radicals and provide an unwelcome lining for your arteries—fat deposits that inhibit blood circulation. Some of the most common results of eating a diet high in unnatural fats are cardiovascular disease, heart attack, stroke, arteriosclerosis, and cancer.

How Fats Become the Body's Enemy

Both natural and unnatural fats can become health hazards through a process called auto-oxidation. Oxidants, primarily oxygen and hydrogen peroxide, combine with molecules to form free radicals, those unstable and destructive aging forces described in Chapter 2. Free radicals are so reactive they are willing to attack anything in sight, but polyunsaturated fats are especially vulnerable because of unfilled bonds between their atoms.

The situation is akin to the childhood game "Red Rover," in which two lines of children stand facing each other, each line holding hands. One team calls out, "Red Rover, Red Rover, send Sally over." Sally, a free radical in our analogy, sizes up the opposite line for its weakest point. If the chemical chain is an unsaturated fat, Sally quickly perceives that there are holes in the chain—places where children (atoms) are not holding hands (linked), obviously the ideal place to attack. If the chemical chain is a saturated fat, Sally can still comfort herself with the knowledge that none of these kids (atoms) have strong arms (bonds). She races over,

TABLE 16

How to Prevent Auto-Oxidation

Factors Encouraging Fat Oxidation	Methods Preventing Fat Oxidation
Using unsaturated fats instead of saturated ones.	Use saturated fats such as butter.
	If you do use liquid unsaturated fats, make sure the label states the addition of antioxidants (nutrients or food additives that prevent the auto-oxidation process from taking place). The most common antioxidants are BHA (butylated hydroxyanisole), BHT (butylated hydroxytoluene), PG (propyl gallate), TGPA (thiodiopropionic acid), NDGA (nordihydroguaiaretic acid), TBHQ (2-tertiary butylhydroquinone), and AP (ascorbyl palmitate). If the oils you prefer do not contain antioxidants, you can add them yourself—250 mg. of BHT will preserve 47 fluid ounces of nonoxidized cooking oil for more than 100 days. Some antioxidants are available from suppliers by mail; others are sold in health food stores.
Exposure to oxygen	Purchase small bottles of fats and refrigerate them in tightly sealed bottles with narrow necks to limit oxygen exposure. Use quickly (even those with antioxidants) and discard after two months.
Being heated to high temperatures or for long periods; being reheated	Purchase cold-pressed oils so that fats will not have been preheated.
	Use butter instead of oils for slow-cooking meals. Butter is more resistant to oxygenation.
	Heat fats to moderate temperatures (no more than 300° F while cooking.
	Do not reheat fats. Discard after one use.

bursts through the line, breaks the chain, and destroys her opponent. Free radicals have won the day.

Table 16 lists other factors that encourage oxidation and tells you how to prevent it.

One final comment about fats. For years, high-fat diets have been associated with high blood cholesterol levels. And high blood cholesterol (a fatlike alcohol) has been associated with increased risk of heart disease, cancer, immune system failure, atherosclerosis, and hypertension.

THE TRUTH ABOUT CHOLESTEROL

On December 13, 1984, the *New York Times* carried a front-page story detailing the latest developments on cholesterol and disease. In one of the most sweeping statements yet made on the subject, a panel of experts convened by the National Institute of Health found that elevated blood cholesterol is a *direct cause* of heart disease and not just a "risk factor," as was previously supposed. *More than half the American population dies of heart disease.*

The panel also found that blood cholesterol levels previously considered normal were actually too high. (Typical middle-aged Americans have cholesterol readings of 220 to 260 milligrams.) The panel recommended reducing cholesterol levels to less than 180 milligrams for adults in their twenties and less than 200 milligrams for those thirty and older.

The panel's recommendations for reducing blood cholesterol included restricting calorie consumption in general and dietary fat in particular (no more than 30 percent of total calories), maintaining normal body weight, avoiding cigarette smoking, maintaining a normal blood pressure, and engaging in a regular and moderate exercise program. In essence, the panel advised a watered-down version of the Age Reduction System.

Not addressed in the article were these very salient points:

- More than 90 percent of your blood cholesterol is *produced by your own body*. So simply reducing dietary cholesterol is unlikely to affect your total blood cholesterol level significantly. However, reducing dietary cholesterol will decrease cortisol. Excess amounts of cortisol help produce degenerative aging diseases, including heart disease (see Chapter 5).
- Your total blood cholesterol level is as critical to health and longevity as the ratio of LDL to HDL cholesterol. LDL (low-density lipoprotein) cholesterol carries cholesterol to the tissues; HDL (high-density lipoprotein) cholesterol removes cholesterol from the tissues and flushes it out of the body. The average man's LDL to HDL ratio is 3.5; the average woman's is 3.2. A preferred value for a man is less than 1; for a woman it is less than 1.5.

Excess cholesterol and triglycerides damage your immune system.

There is some evidence that excess cholesterol may indicate the presence of tumors.

If your cholesterol level is too high, it's not because your body produces too much of it but because your body excretes too little of it. Some of the factors influencing this process are:

- Carrying too much body fat
- Exercising too little
- Consuming too much fat (especially saturated fats), calories, and sugar
- Excessive stress and depression
- Smoking
- High blood pressure
- Liver problems
- Genetic predisposition toward overproduction of cholesterol
- Consuming too little of the essential fatty acids that regulate blood fat
- Ingesting too few lipid-control agents (e.g., lecithin), which act as detergents to remove blood fats
- Consuming too little fiber. (Fiber helps to blot up excess fats.)
- Eating meat instead of vegetable protein. Vegetable proteins contain sterols, which block the absorption of cholesterol from the intestines into the blood. Amino acid ratios in vegetable proteins also seem to tell your liver how much cholesterol to manufacture.

TABLE 17
Blood Fat Regulators

Supplement	Daily Amount	Effect
Evening primrose oil	1.5–3 gm	Lowers total cholesterol, maintains proper blood slipperiness
Cod liver oil	1–2 tsp.	Lowers LDL cholesterol, total cholesterol, and triglycerides; maintains proper blood slipperiness
Olive oil	1–2 tsp. as needed for salad dressings	Reduces LDL and total cholesterol
Lecithin	5–15 gm	Reduces LDL and total cholesterol
L-carnitine	300–1500 mg.	Reduces triglycerides
Vitamin C	1–2 gm	Lowers high cholesterol in some people
Vitamin E	100–200 IU	Increases HDL cholesterol, maintains proper blood slipperiness
Dietary fibers Oat bran	4–6 tsp.	Lower total cholesterol and increase HDL cholesterol
Deodorized garlic	1–2 gm	Lowers total cholesterol, LDL cholesterol, and triglycerides; increases HDL cholesterol

To counter excessive blood cholesterol you should (in addition to steps already recommended):

- Eat more fiber
- Substitute vegetable for animal protein. Your best sources are legumes (dried beans, soybeans, lentils, and peas), fermented soybeans (tofu and tempeh), tricolate (high-protein wheat), soybean sprouts, and vegetables (especially mushrooms, brussels sprouts, and broccoli).
- Use fat-free dairy products as a protein source (cottage cheese, skim milk, and yogurt)
- Control your insulin. (See Chapter 14.)
- Take the basic fat-soluble nutrients described in Chapter 9 and the supplements in Table 17.

A word of warning: Be moderate and use common sense about lowering your cholesterol, since recent research has shown that when cholesterol falls below 150 milligrams the incidence of tumors gradually rises.

INSUFFICIENT FIBER: NOW MORE DEADLY THAN INFECTIOUS DISEASE

In centuries past, death's favorite agent was a virus, bacteria, or parasite. In this century, however, infectious diseases have been replaced by degenerative diseases, the current common killer. Insufficient fiber is a primary factor in developing degenerative diseases.

Fiber is the structural material in plant walls of fruits, vegetables, grains, cereals, nuts, seeds, legumes. Fiber is also a nonstructural material used as a food additive.

The primary function of fiber is to prevent the formation of carcinogenic substances from bile acids and digestants and to absorb excess fat and calories. Fiber increases the speed with which food passes through the intestines and thus reduces exposure to carcinogens. Fiber assists in weight control by providing a feeling of fullness without excessive calories. Fiber has also been found to increase glucose tolerance and decrease abnormal insulin response, thereby forestalling metabolic shifts that could lead to premature aging and degenerative disease.

By consuming too little fiber (the U.S. average is less than 25 grams daily), we corrupt the digestive process. Our food lacks the volume naturally provided by fiber and is therefore more difficult to digest. It moves slowly through the intestines, clogging up the little filia that are trying to absorb nutrients and giving harmful bacteria too much time to multiply. Lack of fiber also makes elimination a strain, irritating the colon and bowels. Constipation is the most obvious short-term effect of insufficient fiber. Possible long-term results include:

- Diverticular disease
- Large bowel cancer
- Appendicitis
- Hemorrhoids
- Hiatus hernia

- Varicose veins
- Gall stones
- Diabetes
- Arteriosclerosis
- Colitis

Now before you begin to douse your diet with your favorite form of fiber, there are three other facts you should know.

First, shifting your normal diet to include more of the natural foods for longevity will automatically increase your fiber intake. However, you may still choose to supplement your daily diet with 10 to 35 grams of the fiber supplements listed in Table 18. These can be mixed with juices or other

TABLE 18

Fiber Sources

Type	Sources	Function
Cellulose— principal cell wall component and the only true fiber	Vegetables such as broccoli, green beans, and lettuce; psyllium husk	Swells to increase weight, reduces colonic pressure, accelerates passage of food through intestines, decreases breeding time for harmful bacteria
Hemicellulose— also a component of cell walls of many plants	Cereals, bran, whole grains, psyllium husk	Increases fecal bulk, reduces colonic pressure, helps prevent gall stones, decreases transit time and harmful bacteria and carcinogens, decreases cholesterol, has an antitoxic effect
Gums—plant secretions	Guar gum (sold in health food stores as galactomannan), gum acacia	Decrease absorption of sugars, elevate blood glucose levels, lower cholesterol, swell to cause fullness and control excess eating
Pectins—plant cement	Rinds of citrus fruit, apple peel, onion skin, carrots	Decrease cholesterol and have antitoxic effects
Mucilages— (secretions and seeds)	Legumes (e.g., dried beans), seeds, psyllium seed	Lower cholesterol, increase transit time
Algal polysaccharides— fiber from algae and seaweed	Sodium alginate, Irish moss (carrageenin)	Antitoxic effects, binds heavy metals, lowers cholesterol, binds fats
Lignins—woody plant parts	wheat bran, apples	Antitoxic effects, bind heavy metals

beverages and consumed at any time of the day. If you take them a half hour before meals, the fibers will swell in your stomach, decreasing your appetite by creating a feeling of fullness. Remember, however, that fiber does not provide nutrients or vitamins. Do not consume excessive fiber at the expense of ingesting nutritious foods in an effort to lose weight.

Second, all fiber is *not* alike. Table 18 offers a complete description of different fibers. Try to include several different kinds in making up your 40 to 60 gram daily fiber intake for maximum life-span.

Third, when consumed in large quantities, America's favorite fiber—bran—will leach minerals such as calcium, magnesium, and zinc from your system and prevent their absorption. Be sure to protect yourself by increasing your intake of these minerals and by alternating fibers.

My favorite fiber combination is given in Table 19. (The supplement suppliers in Chapter 9 sell the different fibers separately and as combination products.)

TABLE 19

Dr. Kaufman's Favorite Fiber Combinations

Type of Fiber	Daily Amounts
Psyllium husks	3–10 gm
Oat bran	3–14 gm
Guar gum	2–6 gm
Sodium alginate	500 mg.–1 gm
Apple pectin	500 mg.–1 gm
Irish moss (or carrageenin)	1–3 gm
TOTAL	10–35 gm

PROTEIN: BOTH BUILDER AND DESTROYER

As you may have noticed throughout this section, it isn't consumption that kills us—it's *over*consumption.

Protein is no exception. Its very name—derived from the Greek word meaning "of first importance"—attests to its necessity. Overconsumption of protein, however, reduces immunity, increases blood lipids and cholesterol, causes calcium to be leached from the bones (contributing to the brittle bones of old age), promotes cancer, and overtaxes the digestive and eliminative systems.

Protein is composed of specific ratios of twenty-two amino acids, eight of which are considered essential. High-quality protein contains the ideal ratio of the eight essential amino acids, while low-quality protein tends to be deficient in one or more amino acids. Animal protein is usually of a higher quality than vegetable protein.

Protein is the principal source of building material for blood, muscles, skin, hair, nails, the internal organs, the heart, the brain, and for internal secretions and enzymes.

Your daily protein requirements are principally based on your lean body weight. Your age, physical activities, and medical problems are also factors. Teenagers require more protein than the elderly. Exercising to increase muscle mass; hard-endurance training; harmful stress; recovery from broken bones, serious illness, and muscle wasting diseases increase your protein requirement.

American standards for the quantity and quality of protein you need are inflated. For example, a 154-pound man is expected to consume 54 grams of high-quality protein each day, according to the RDA. A 120-pound woman is supposed to consume 46 grams of high-quality protein. These standards are calculated to include an extra 30 percent to account for individual metabolisms, plus another 25 percent to account for less-than-perfect protein.

If American standards for protein requirements are inflated, American consumption of protein is even more so. The average American male eats 100 grams of protein every day—nearly twice the already inflated "daily requirement." Since his primary protein source is animal flesh, he simultaneously consumes more saturated fat than he needs.

Most centenarians are lightweights when it comes to protein consumption, eating between 35 and 50 grams of vegetable protein each day. They live longer and experience substantially less heart, liver, and kidney failure than do Americans on the average. Ideally, protein should account for no more than 10 to 20 percent of your daily calories. My "Permanent Weight Loss for Age Reduction" plan, detailed in the next chapter, tells you how to evaluate vegetable proteins and combine them so as to obtain high-quality protein without the excess saturated fat and calories of animal products.

Trying to satisfy your daily protein requirement by depending on the protein values given in food tables is misleading. Foods containing the same protein totals often contain different amounts of *usable* protein calories. Only certain ratios of the eight essential amino acids build new tissues, support growth, and repair cell damage. The ideal ratio is found in the amino acid composition of the white of chicken eggs. Many foods lack one or two essential amino acids and thus contain protein the body cannot use.

Table 20 shows the amount of usable protein found in different foods. It indicates how many calories you would have to eat of a particular food in order to ingest one gram of usable protein.

Overall, fish has the most usable protein, while nuts and seeds contain the least. They are very high in fats.

Correctly combining different foods increases the total usable protein. The amino acid ratios of one food can complement another food. For

TABLE 20

Usable Protein in Food

Food Class	High-Protein Foods		Low-Protein Foods	
	Calories per Usable Protein Gram			
Fish	Cod	5	Perch	13
Poultry	Chicken	7	Turkey	10
Eggs	Dried egg white	6	Whole egg	14
Dairy	Cottage cheese	7	Regular yogurt	27
Meat	Lean lamb	10	Fatty lamb	32
Vegetables	Soybean sprouts	12	White potato	60
Legume	Tofu	15	Lentils	47
Grains	Wheat germ	19	Brown rice	69
Nuts and seeds	Pumpkin seeds	32	Brazil nuts	88

example, if you eat beans with rice, you consume 40 percent more usable protein than if you ate them separately on different days. As a general rule, milk products complement grains, legumes complement grains, legumes complement seeds.

9

Supplementing
the Age Reduction
System

The notion of supplementing the American diet with vitamins, minerals, and other nutrients is little more than two decades old. Until then it was assumed that eating a "balanced" diet was sufficient to supply needed nutrients. And for many years this was probably true.

When agricultural methods were more primitive, most Americans ate fresh foods in season, grown with natural fertilizers and subjected to minimal processing methods. As I pointed out in Chapter 8, this is no longer the case.

Today the soils that produce our primary sources of vitamins and minerals are depleted and contaminated. A fresh ear of corn plucked from the stalk today doesn't contain as much natural goodness as it once did. By the time it has been cooked, canned, frozen, or creamed, its nutrient content is a shadow of its former self.

The impact of this nutrient loss has yet to be clearly defined, because most scientific efforts have focused on the *minimum* nutrients required to prevent disease and death rather than the *optimal* amount needed to maintain health and extend life. The Recommended Daily Allowance (RDA) standards cited on most ingredient labels are based on minimal requirements. Yet many Americans do not even meet RDA standards. For example, nearly 60 percent of American women age thirty to sixty consume less than two-thirds of the RDA for calcium; 45 percent of American women consume less than two-thirds of the RDA for vitamin A, according to studies by Dr. Agnes Fay Morgan, professor of nutrition in biochemistry at the California Agricultural Experimental Station, University of California.

Other studies indicate that there is no such thing as a standard requirement for a given nutrient. For example, sodium chloride requirements can vary between individuals by as much as 15,000 percent. Calcium needs may vary within 4500 percent. Even the same individual may have drastically different nutritional needs at various times, depending on current health, environment, exposure to stress, drug consumption, and myriad other factors.

In addition to helping maintain health, nutrients and other supplements have lately been shown to extend life in research animals. In 1946, researcher Thomas S. Gardener reported at a meeting of the American Chemical Society that he had been able to extend the average life of fruit flies by 46 percent through a supplementary combination of vitamin B-5 and B-6, biotin, and RNA extracts.

Vitamin B-6 also proved useful in reducing body weight, improving metabolic function, and extending the life-span of mice by an average of 11 percent in a study by scientists at NASA's Ames Research Center.

Richard Hochschild, a researcher at the Department of Medicine, University of California, Irvine, extended the life-span of mice by almost 50 percent when he fed them DMAE (dimethylaminoethanol), an alkyl-amino alcohol that converts into the neurotransmitter acetylcholine in the brain.

The supplements DHEA, coenzyme Q-10, selenium, thymus, L-cysteine, organ-specific RNA, BHA, BHT, activated charcoal, and ginseng also have been shown to extend life in research animals.

Supplemental nutrients—vitamins, minerals, herbs, essential fatty acids, amino acids, artificial antioxidants, etc.—slow aging by delaying the metabolic shifts that signal aging's onset. Still others reverse cellular aging by helping to purge accumulated toxins, maintain the integrity of cell structure, and increase the rate of cell reproduction and repair.

Special supplements for specific aging patterns are listed in the appropriate sections of the book. This chapter tells you:

- How to use herbs
- What to look for—and what to avoid—when buying supplements
- How to determine your unique nutrient requirements
- Which supplemental side effects are to be expected and which are a cause for concern
- How to use each Age Reduction System supplement
- Where you can buy safe, effective supplements

Take careful note: The information in this chapter is intended for educational purposes only. It is *not* a prescription. Any supplements you take— or any program you adopt as a result of reading this book—should be carried out under your physician's supervision. Above all, do not exceed the recommended amounts of any supplement unless you are under a doctor's supervision.

HERBS AND AGE REDUCTION

Herbal supplements and therapies, traditionally viewed as the province of folk medicine or witch doctors, are now earning serious scientific scrutiny by medical research institutes around the world.

It may be some time before the scientific data catches up to thousands of years of field work. Of the 600,000 plant species used for nutritional or therapeutic purposes, only 5 percent have been chemically or pharmacologically investigated to date! One fact, however, has already become clear. Many herbs contain pharmaceutical properties similar to those we spend untold millions on to duplicate in laboratories.

In Brazil, Pau D'Arco is used to treat cancer—its bark has been reported to contain quinoline, a substance with anti-tumor properties—but it has not been proven effective by leading research experts.

In China the traditional herbs Ligustrum and Astragalus have been documented as immune system restorers, according to the *Journal of Cancer*. The breakdown of the immune system is a primary aging factor. Scientists are now attempting to isolate the active pharmacological ingredients of these two herbs.

Ginseng, an oriental herb, has been found to contain hormonelike regulatory substances that balance the neuroendocrine system and improve stress responses. It improves memory and accelerates learning without disturbing brain cellular processes. In studies conducted between 1963 and 1978 by Dr. V. Petkov, director of the Institute of Physiology at the Bulgarian Academy of Science, ginseng appeared to slow or prevent neuroendocrinological aging by increasing levels of dopamine in the brain while simultaneously decreasing serotonin in the brainstem. Other European studies indicate that ginseng increases protein synthesis and RNA activity in rats, thereby slowing cellular aging.

In southeast Asia and China doctors prescribe herbal formulations in place of synthetic drugs to treat disease. When a patient enters an Asian hospital he may be assigned to a ward for treatment by Western medicine or by traditional Eastern measures—herbology, acupuncture, diet, and exercise.

Herbal pharmaceutics is a precise science. Herbal formulations generally contain eight to twelve ingredients in specific ratios according to four categories of herbs. The type of herbs, their ratio amounts, and their preparation determine the formula's pharmacological properties. Some formulations in use today have been used for more than 1800 years.

According to Chinese medical literature, certain recalcitrant diseases respond better to herbal therapies than to synthetic drug treatments. Aplastic anemia, polycythemia, viral hepatitis, and hemolytic anemia are just a few such diseases. The Chinese doctor selects the herbal formulation that best conforms to the patient's entire being, as confirmed through an extensive diagnostic procedure that takes into account both internal and external factors. External factors include weather, geography, environment, and life-style. The patient's internal constitution, physique, emotional makeup, and symptomatology are analyzed. The patient is also extensively questioned and palpated for vital pulses before the Chinese doctor reaches a diagnosis. The standard herbal formulation that most closely fits the patient's health conformation is modified to meet his or her specific needs and then prescribed.

The side effects from herbs are significantly less than from synthetic drugs. Only 10 percent of the herbal formulations used by Chinese doctors have a potential for side effects. The percentage of side effects from different commonly used Western drugs may range as high as 62 percent according to the United States Joint Pharmaceutical Monitoring Center in Boston. And if you receive five Western drugs instead of one, the risk of side effects is multiplied by a factor of five.

A note of caution is in order, however: Westerners seduced by the curative mystique of herbs sometimes fall victim to their misuse. For example, many Americans taking or considering taking ginseng should not. They do not fit the profile of a person for whom ginseng is suitable. Ginseng is a tonic prescribed for the elderly, weak, or chronically sick and debilitated. Young, strong, and healthy people with fiery temperaments generally should not use ginseng.

Scientific evidence indicates that ingesting 3 grams of ginseng a day for two or more years may lead to Ginseng Abuse Syndrome. Its symptoms include high blood pressure, morning diarrhea, insomnia, skin eruptions, and nervousness. Ginseng and other herbs are powerful. They deserve respect and proper guidance in use.

Other herbs may be hazardous in high dosages when used by themselves or in amateurishly concocted formulations. Table 21 (next page) lists some herbs that you should not take unless prescribed and in combinations specifically measured to counteract any toxic potential.

I seriously doubt the safety and benefits of many common herbal formulations found in health food stores. Their dosages are too low to do any good and the formulations are not designed to conform specifically to the profile of each potential user. In addition, some formulations include one or two toxic herbs in high amounts. For example, Ephedra (Ma Huang) is sold as an energy potion in health food stores along with other toxic herbs.

Keep these guidelines in mind relative to the use of herbs:

• Store herbs in your refrigerator to prevent bacterial degradation.
• Do not use herbs at the same time you are using synthetic drugs.
• Pregnant or lactating women should *never* use herbs without consulting their medical doctor.

TABLE 21

Hazards of Herbs

Herb	Effect
Sassafras Comfrey	Liver cancer in animals
Buckthorn Senna Dock Aluti Rhubarb	Strong evacuation from bowels
Burdock Catnip Juniper Hydrangea Lobelia Jimson weed Wormweed Mandrake Ephedra	Autonomic nervous system imbalance, euphoria or depression, disturbed behavior
St. John's Wort tea	Oversensitivity of skin to light
Pokeweed or ink berry	Stomach and intestinal inflammation
Juniper berries Aconite Shave grass Horsetail	Potent diuretics

CHOOSING DIETARY SUPPLEMENTS YOUR BODY CAN USE

Taking a supplement does not ensure that your body can use it. Have you ever taken a 500 milligram vitamin C tablet only to discover that it emerged whole and undigested in your next bowel movement? That's because the manufacturing process (not to mention your own digestion and assimilation processes) is filled with pitfalls for the average supplement.

As a consultant to several supplement manufacturers and distributors, I have analyzed the active ingredients, as well as the excipients (fillers) that make up as much as 50 percent of each tablet. I have frequently witnessed inconsistent manufacturing standards and processes. And I have researched the effect of these formulas and processes on the bioavailability (ultimate usefulness) of the supplements.

When it comes to buying supplements, a little knowledge is a dangerous thing.

Manufacturers have the legal right to be quite selective about the information you read on product labels. For example, they don't have to list the source of the binders, fillers, colorings, flavorings (including sugar), and coatings that make up as much as 50 percent of the product. More than 850 inactive ingredients can be added to the supplement without being added to the label!

Some of these additives cause allergic reactions that may be wrongly attributed to the supplement itself. Others may actually prevent the supplement from being digested, assimilated, and used by your body.

Dicalcium phosphate is a commonly used filling agent that is rarely listed on product labels. Unfortunately, dicalcium phosphate is practically insoluble in water or alcohol, so it's very difficult for your body to break it down to get to the actual supplement. As dicalcium phosphate ages, it becomes even harder, so it may pass through the system undigested. Its presence in the digestive tract inhibits mineral absorption and creates a negative calcium balance that may lead to osteoporosis and arteriosclerotic diseases.

Fortunately, there is a movement afoot among consumers in this country to force manufacturers to list *all* the ingredients in their supplements. Many have already willingly complied. Most supplement manufacturers listed at the end of this chapter either list ingredients or have supplied me with reassuring formulation information. (Table 22 tells you what to look for when reading labels.)

In addition to its actual content, the bioavailability of a supplement is influenced by the supplement's form: tablet, powder, capsule, or liquid. Each form has inherent advantages and disadvantages, which are indicated in Table 23. Some supplements are safer and more effective in specific forms. For example, pancreatic digestive enzymes should be taken

TABLE 22
Preferred Supplement Excipients

Type	Formulation
Binders (hold tablets together)	Hydrogenated vegetable oil, powder, alginic acid
Fillers (fill up space in tablet molds)	Cellulose
Coating (maintains tablet potency, prevents moisture absorption)	Natural food glaze or protein
Lubricants (prevent tablet from sticking to machine)	Magnesium stearate or vegetable stearate
Drying agents (remove moisture)	Silica gel
Disintegration aid (controls breakdown of tablets in body)	Actasol (microcrystalline cellulose)

TABLE 23

Forms of Supplements

	Advantages	*Disadvantages*
Tablets	Inexpensive to manufacture Convenient to carry Measured dosages Compacted size Control of ingredient release Protection of ingredients	Contain excipients Some manufacturers' tableting machines generate heat that damage ingredients
Capsules	Few excipients Convenient to carry Measured dosages Relatively compact size Protection of ingredients	Expensive to manufacture Fatty liquids in capsules may oxidize and form free radicals
Powders	Inexpensive to manufacture No excipients Easy to swallow Easy to make a "master mixture" with different supplements	Inconvenient to carry and use Must measure dosage Caustic substances may irritate mouth Can't control release Exposure to air may spoil ingredients Bad taste of ingredients

Liquids	Easy to swallow
	Best absorption for fat soluble nutrients
		Expensive to manufacture
		Difficult to regulate dosage
		Inconvenient to carry
		May taste bad
		Fatty liquids may oxidize and form free
		   radicals
		May contain extracts from chemicals to
		   manufactured product

in tablets or capsules, as the powder form will damage your gums. Fat-soluble supplements have greater bioavailability when taken in water–liquid fat emulsions. Where appropriate, the preferred form of a supplement is listed in the Age Reduction Supplement Guide, later in this chapter.

The final factor influencing the usefulness of supplements is your own body. If you eat a lot of bran fiber, for example, you may have difficulty absorbing and using minerals. If, as a result of aging or digestive problems, you produce too little digestive bile, you could have difficulty breaking supplements down into usable forms. (See Table 43 in Chapter 13 for possible ways to improve bile production.) If you are taking any medications, you may be interfering with your body's ability to metabolize certain supplements. (See Table 7 in Chapter 6 to determine any nutrients significantly affected by drugs you normally use.)

DETERMINING
YOUR SUPPLEMENT REQUIREMENTS

Your supplement requirements change constantly to reflect changes in your environment, state of mind, physical activity, state of health, and countless other subtle and elegant interactions.

If you are like most people, you will be able to address your supplement needs simply by taking the basic water-soluble and fat-soluble vitamins and minerals recommended in the Age Reduction Supplement Guide.

You may, however, be one of those individuals who need to take supplements specifically designed to address your particular aging patterns. As you read the *Age Reduction System,* make a note of supplements suggested in the sections that apply to you. For example, if you suffer from chronic stress, you should consider taking the supplements listed in that section. The proper use of every supplement recommended in this book is described in the Age Reduction Supplement Guide.

Other ways to determine your supplement needs include blood tests and urine or computerized diet analyses such as I use with my clients. Table 24 also lists some common situations that may require additional supplementation when not due to a medical problem or toxic reaction.

TABLE 24
Individual Metabolic Requirements

Situation	Suggested Adjustment
Women before menopause	Increase iron, folic acid, vitamin B-12, vitamin E
Women after menopause	Increase calcium, magnesium, vitamin D, vitamin C, zinc
Elderly men	Increase calcium, magnesium, vitamin D, vitamin C, zinc, vitamin E
Athletes and others who perspire from heat or physical activities	Increase water-soluble nutrients, minerals (to some degree), and fluid intake
Low tolerance to alcohol	Increase B vitamins, zinc, magnesium
Sensitive to monosodium glutamate	Double vitamin B-6
Sunburn easily*	Increase vitamin B-6, vitamin B-3, beta carotene
Low stress tolerance	Increase vitamin C, vitamin B-5, B complex, magnesium
Light hair color or from northern European descent	Increase protein
Sweet tooth	Increase B complex, zinc

*Consult your physician immediately. This condition *may* indicate serious disease.

Situation	Suggested Adjustment
Insomnia or nightmares	Increase B complex
Chronic cracks at corner of nose, eyes, or lips, chapped lips	Increase vitamin B-1, vitamin B-2, vitamin B-3, B complex
Dry, scaly skin on back of arms	Increase vitamin A and beta carotene
Persistent redness of eyeball	Increase vitamin E, zinc, vitamin C complex and B complex
Can't bend fingers at second joint*	Increase vitamin B-6
Lack of ear wax or hard dark ear wax	Increase essential fatty acids (evening primrose oil, cod liver oil, soya lecithin)
Gums bleed easily	Increase folic acid, vitamin E, bioflavanoids
Poor night vision	Increase vitamin A, zinc, beta carotene
Hair loss, hair breakage	Increase B vitamins, amino acid cysteine
White spots under fingernails or ridges on fingernails	Increase iron (if low), zinc, calcium, and magnesium
Burning hands and feet	Increase vitamin B-1 and vitamin B-2
Poor taste and smell	Increase zinc and B complex
Night leg cramps	Increase calcium and magnesium
Electric shock feeling when bending neck*	Increase vitamin B-12
Oily skin with big pores or red skin areas	Increase vitamin B-2 and vitamin B-6
Hyperactive personality	Increase iron, vitamin C, copper, vitamin B-2, vitamin B-3
Emotional disturbances	Increase B complex (particularly vitamin B-1, vitamin B-6, vitamin B-12, biotin, folic acid) and vitamin C.
Low body temperature in morning, constipation, slow wound healing, heart irregularities	Increase iodine, copper, zinc, tyrosine
Red tongue	Increase B complex, especially vitamin B-2
Inflamed, red gums*	Increase vitamin E, folic acid, B-12, calcium, magnesium, vitamin B-6, and phosphorus
Chronic eczema or dermatitis	Increase zinc, B-6, essential fatty acids
Kidney stones or periodontal disease	Balance calcium, phosphorus, and magnesium; increase vitamin C
Don't remember dreams	Increase vitamin B-6

*Consult your physician immediately. This condition *may* indicate serious disease.

Situation	Suggested Adjustment
Rapid or missed heartbeat	Increase vitamin B-1, calcium, potassium, and magnesium
Nonmedical recurring back pain	Increase vitamin B-12, calcium, and manganese
Painful bones*	Increase vitamin D, calcium, and magnesium
Muscle weakness, burning lips, and tingling hands	Increase vitamin B-1 and vitamin B-2
Pink urine after eating*	Increase iron
Sore tongue or tongue sensitive to hot food and beverages	Increase folic acid, iron, vitamin B-2 or vitamin B-3
Slow wound healing	Increase protein, vitamin C, bioflavanoids, zinc, chromium, iron, copper, selenium, folic acid, and vitamin B-12
Premature, abnormal hair loss	Increase protein, cysteine, zinc, selenium, B complex, and cod liver oil
Depressed personality	Increase vitamin B-12, folic acid, vitamin B-6, and zinc
Food allergies, arthritis-like signs, migraine headaches	Increase fiber and protein-digesting enzymes

*Consult your physician immediately. This condition *may* indicate serious disease.

SIDE EFFECTS OF DIETARY SUPPLEMENTS

Each of us has an optimal range for a particular Age Reduction System supplement to produce maximum effect. Some supplements, when taken in optimal range dosages, do have a "side effect zone." Typical side effects for each supplement are described when applicable in the Age Reduction Supplement Guide. Side effects may be either annoying but harmless temporary symptoms or significant symptoms affecting overall health.

Your vulnerability to side effects is determined by:

• Your overall sensitivity to food or drugs. You may experience an allergic reaction to the basic ingredients of a specific supplement. If you do, discontinue all supplements you are taking, wait a week for your system to return to normal, then gradually reintroduce supplements one at a time, in small quantities, to discover which supplement you are allergic to. Since it may be the excipient rather than the active ingredients that is provoking the allergic reaction, you may want to try different manufacturers before abandoning the supplement.

- How you introduce your body to supplements. Side effects may result from taking a new supplement in excessive amounts without giving your body time to adjust, or from introducing too many different supplements simultaneously.
- Whether you have exceeded the recommended amount of a supplement. Some supplements are toxic in high doses.

If you experience side effects other than those described here, discontinue supplements and consult a physician.

THE AGE REDUCTION SUPPLEMENT GUIDE

This guide provides the following information, when applicable, about the Age Reduction supplements:

- Preferred sources
- Suggested daily amounts
- Intended effects
- Potential side effects
- Preferred combinations of supplements
- Whether a supplement should be taken with meals or at specific times during the day
- Which supplements work against each other
- Potential supplement/drug interactions
- Other necessary cautionary information

The suggested amounts for each supplement are given as ranges. I suggest that you begin by taking the lower amount and gradually work up to the maximum recommended amount.

The suggested amounts are based on the average needs of men and women eating a typical American diet. However, you should consider any peculiarities of your own diet. For example, if you eat a lot of dairy products, you are probably consuming as much calcium as you need. If you eat a lot of fresh, raw vegetables, you won't need as much vitamin A and C supplementation as most Americans. If you have any doubts about the nutritional quality of your diet, you may want to invest in an inexpensive computerized diet analysis by a professional nutritionist.

Perhaps most important, don't allow yourself to be overwhelmed by the length of these lists.

Taking many different types of supplements throughout the day need not be confusing and stressful if you have the correct attitude. Your individual supplement requirements are unique. But some supplements are best taken at a particular time of day under specific conditions, for example, in the morning on an empty stomach. You can put yourself under unnecessary stress trying to obey every rule governing correct supplement use and worry needlessly about the consequences from making a mistake.

The whole topic is overemphasized by nutritionists. Too many individ-

TABLE 25

Supplement Menu

Time of Day and Condition	Age Reduction Supplements
Morning (on empty stomach)	Arginine L-arginine L-ornithine DMAE (dimethylaminoethanol) L-tyrosine L-phenylalanine
Before meals	Guar gum Glycerol
Mealtime (divided dosages throughout the day)	Water-soluble nutrients: B complex Vitamin C RNA Digestive enzymes Hydrochloric acid
Mealtime (high fat content meals)	Fat-soluble nutrient supplements: Vitamins A, D Essential fatty acids Cod liver oil Evening primrose oil Beta carotene Ascorbyl palmitate Vitamin E Artificial antioxidants Coenzyme Q-10
Mealtime (protein meals)	Mineral supplements
On empty stomach (between meals)	Herbs Homeopathic medicines Detoxification fiber Activated charcoal Amino acids
Before exercising	DMG (dimethylglycine) Octacosanol L-carnitine Krebs Cycle intermediaries L-tyrosine Vitamin B-5 Ginseng Inosine Cytochrome C
Before sleep	L-tryptophan Sleep herbs L-arginine L-ornithine L-glycine Inositol

ual variables and a lack of hardcore research prevents establishment of standard laws that work for everybody taking supplements. For example, some people just can't take supplements on an empty stomach. They feel nauseated or regurgitate. To provide some reasonable order for taking your supplements, I suggest that you follow these procedures:
- Use common sense and follow the simple guidelines in the Supplement Menu given in Table 25.
- If a particular Age Reduction supplement's correct use is not stated in this menu or elsewhere in the Age Reduction System, use it according to your convenience.

Basic Fat-Soluble Nutrients

The nutrients included in this section are absorbed only in the presence of fat. Therefore, it's best to take all these nutrients at once immediately after eating a meal containing fat.

You can also increase your absorption of fat-soluble nutrients by taking them in an emulsified miscellized or liquid form. The emulsion miscellization process breaks down the fat molecules to tiny bundles that can be absorbed two to five times more effectively. It also supplies the liquid and fat needed for absorption, whereas the dry tablet and powder forms require you to supply stomach bile and water for proper absorption.

Many elderly people have difficulty digesting fat-soluble nutrients (as well as other foods) because they produce too little stomach bile and digestive enzymes. If you feel you have this problem, see Table 43 in Chapter 13 for supplements that may improve your digestive abilities.

One caution: Fatty nutrient oils oxidize rapidly to form free radicals. Maintain them in air-tight refrigerated storage. You may also protect them by adding 75 milligrams of BHT to each 16 fluid ounces of oil.

One final caution about fat-soluble nutrients: Vitamins A and D are toxic when ingested in high amounts. Do not exceed recommended amounts.

TABLE 26

Basic Fat-Soluble Nutrients

Supplement and Source	Daily Amount	Comments
Essential fatty acids, vitamins D and A		Essential fatty acids decrease risk of cardiovascular disease, prevent abnormal blood clots, lower cholesterol and triglycerides, reduce rheumatoid arthritic inflammation, enhance brain and nerve function.
		Vitamin D is essential for the absorption and utilization of calcium for strong bones and teeth. Prevents loss of calcium from bones and calcium deposits in soft tissue that lead to sclerotic diseases.

Supplement and Source	Daily Amount	Comments
		Vitamin A protects tissues against cancer and cell and pollution damage. Strengthens the immune system and thymus gland. Is necessary for night vision. Antioxidant properties fight free radicals. Decreases cancer risk.
Pure unconcentrated Norwegian cod liver oil	2 teaspoons	Provides about 500 mg. of the essential fatty acid EPA (eicosapenatenoic acid), 500 mg. of DHA (docosahexanoic acid), 900 mg. of vitamin D, and 10,000 IU of vitamin A.
or Emulsified version of above	2 tablespoons	Emulsified version (oil and water mixture) actually tastes good.
		Pregnant women should take only 1 teaspoon of cod liver oil.
and also take Beta carotene	25–100 mg. (40,000–160,000 IU)	Optional supplement that converts to vitamin A as needed by your body. Provides a nontoxic source of vitamin A for additional protection from sun damage and cancer.
		Large amounts of beta carotene may color your skin yellow.
		More than 900 IU a day of vitamin E may interfere with beta carotene absorption.
Vitamin E (dl alpha-tocopherol)	100–200 IU	The most important antioxidant fat-soluble nutrient. Reduces fat oxidation and free radical damage. Protects against abnormal blood clots, ozone, and pollution. Increases immunity, aids athletic prowess, and protects against neurological problems.
		Take several hours before or after oral contraceptives and anticoagulation drugs.
		Works synergistically when taken with organic selenium.
		Treats cuts, burns, and other skin disorders when applied topically.
		Potential side effect is the temporary increase in blood pressure, which returns to normal over time.
Fat-soluble vitamin C		Powerful antioxidant that protects fatty tissues from free radical damage. Action is synergistic with vitamin E.
Ascorbyl palmitate	1–2 gm	Available as powder or capsules. May be added to liquid fats or oils to prevent oxidation.

Supplement and Source	Daily Amount	Comments
Phosphatidyl choline/lecithin		Natural high potency source of choline. An important precursor to the neurotransmitter acetylcholine for memory and learning.
Soya lecithin concentrate that contains at least 90% phosphatidyl choline	5–15 gm	Lecithin lowers cholesterol and contains the B vitamin factor phosphatidyl-inositol. When taking high amounts of lecithin, increase your intake of calcium and magnesium. It counteracts an increase in phosphorus from lecithin.
Evening primrose oil With 8% gamma linolenic acid	1.5–3 gm 120–240 mcg.	The only source other than mother's milk of linolenic acid and gamma linolenic acid. Gamma linolenic acid manufactures a prostaglandin that lowers high blood pressure, decreases cholesterol, helps relieve PMS (premenstrual syndrome), and helps rheumatoid arthritis.

Basic Water-Soluble Nutrients

The basic water-soluble nutrients include B vitamins and related factors, vitamin C–complex nutrients, and sulfhydryl (sulfur-containing amino acids). These supplements work best when taken together three times daily.

If you smoke, take medication, exercise strenuously, have difficulty perspiring, live in a stressful or abusive manner, or are exposed to substantial environmental hazards, you have a special need for these nutrients.

Except for vitamin B-3 and vitamin B-6, current research has shown that water-soluble nutrients have little or no toxicity when taken correctly in higher doses than my general recommendations. In fact, my personal formula, which I discuss at the end of this section, contains substantially greater amounts of most water-soluble nutrients and several other Age Reduction Supplements.

Avoid taking B vitamins in time-release capsule form. Most water-soluble vitamins are absorbed primarily in the upper part of the small intestines; time-release preparations often do not release their vitamin content until well into the small intenstines. As much as 90 percent of vitamin B-1, for example, is lost through this form. Vitamin C complex, on the other hand, benefits greatly from the steady supply of time-release capsules if you don't ingest vitamin C every few hours.

TABLE 27

Basic Water-Soluble Nutrients

Supplement and Source	Daily Amount	Comments
B Vitamins and relatives		
Vitamin B-1 Thiamine hydrochloride	10–60 mg.	This sulfur-containing antioxidant fights free radical damage and protects against cross-linkage. It also helps protect you against damage from smoking, pollution, and alcohol drinking.
Vitamin B-2 Riboflavin	10–35 mg.	An antioxidant cofactor that regulates the oxidation of foods to create energy for life. Also increases immunity.
Vitamin B-3 Nicotinic acid	20–50 mg.	A powerful essential antioxidant. Megadosages of niacin, usually 1000 mg. to 3000 mg. a day administered by doctors in experimental and clinical trials have lowered cholesterol 22 percent, lowered triglycerides 52 percent, reduced recurrence of heart attack, aided sufferers of arthritis, improved immunity, and treated senility.
		Niacin (nicotinic acid) may cause temporary flushing, itching, and warming of the skin in sensitive individuals. This may occur from amounts as small as 30 to 40 mg. (I personally take 1000 mg. a day with no ill effect.) To counteract, start with small amounts and gradually increase. Taking niacin with food, in beverages, or as a time-release form diminishes this effect.
		Sufferers of heartbeat irregularities should consult their physician before use.
		Nausea, cramps, and headache may occur on very rare occasions from high dosages.
Vitamin B-5 Calcium pantothenate	40–100 mg.	An antistress vitamin that increases stamina and chemical brain signals (acetylcholine) between neurons. Has extended life and relieved arthritis in experimental research. High amounts should not be used by manic depressives during the depressive phase of illness.
Vitamin B-6 Pyridoxine hydrochloride	20–30 mg.	An antioxidant enzyme cofactor that supports the immune system, increases immunity, protects against cancer, and helps control diabetes. Vitamin B-6 deficiency may lead to atherosclerotic plaques. Clinical research

Supplement and Source	Daily Amount	Comments
		suggests that large amounts given under a doctor's supervision may relieve premenstrual syndrome (PMS).
		Do not use with the drug L-Dopa.
Vitamin B-12 Sublingual release	10–50 mcg.	Needed to form blood cells, prevent anemia, and maintain healthy brain and nervous systems. Increases the synthesis of RNA. Necessary for protein synthesis and proper mental function.
Biotin	200–600 mcg.	Assists in making fatty acids and oxidizing nutrients for energy. Stimulates proper hair growth. Biotin deficiency has been linked to *Candida albicans* yeast infection.

Folic acid
    Folacin
	400 mcg.;
	800 mcg. for
	    pregnant women;
	500 mcg. for
	    lactating women
		This is essential for red blood cell formation, growth, and healthy cell functions.

Choline
    Choline bitartrate
        or
    Phosphatidyl
        choline/lecithin
        (*See* Fat-Soluble
        Nutrients)
	200 mg.–3 gm
	
	5–15 gm
		Forms acetylocholine in the brain, a neurotransmitter necessary for memory, learning, and clear thinking. Regulates and improves the functioning of liver and gall bladder and prevents fat from accumulating in the liver. Choline bitartrate may produce stiff muscles, headaches, and a fishy body odor in high dosages; phosphatidyl choline in lecithin does not.

Inositol Myo-inositol	500–1500 mg.	Associated in nature with choline in lecithin. Found in other foods (cantaloupes, oranges, grapefruit, whole wheat bread, nuts). Slows sugar metabolism, protects against diabetes, stabilizes cell membranes, and supports growing muscles.
		Diabetics should take only under their doctor's supervision.
		Only myo-inositol is active.

Vitamin C Complex

Vitamin C
    Magnesium ascorbate
        or
    Ascorbic acid
	1–2 gm
	
	1–2 gm
		So important to your health that you should use a separate product for maximum benefits. Increases immunity, improves tissue strength, increases wound healing, combats cancer, improves stress handling, helps alleviate male infertility, lowers cholesterol, deactivates free radicals.

Supplement and Source	Daily Amount	Comments
		Time-release capsules maintain higher levels in your blood for longer periods of time. Nonacidic ascorbate forms of vitamin C offer greater bioavailability than standard vitamin C and do not upset the intestinal tract. I suggest using magnesium ascorbates, since magnesium helps maintain the correct magnesium-calcium ratio.
		Diabetics should use large doses of vitamin C only under a doctor's supervision.
		Megadoses of vitamin C often cause diarrhea.
Bioflavonoids Hesperidin *and* Rutin	100–1000 mg. 100–1000 mg.	Bioflavonoids are synergistic with vitamin C. They keep vitamin C acting longer in your body. Also fight free radicals, strengthen capillaries, and stabilize membranes. I recommend using a combination of different types of bioflavonoids.
Sulfhydryl Amino Acids		Sulfur-containing amino acids are important antioxidants that protect you against damage from smoke and alcohol drinking.
L-cysteine HCl *and*	500–1000 mg.	Increases absorption in iron-deficiency anemia, maintains flexible skin by controlling cross-linkage, and increases red and white blood cell reproduction.
L-methionine *and*	100–200 mg.	Prevents fat deposits in the liver, helps synthesize choline.
Reduced glutathione	50–150 mg.	Effective in treating allergies and controlling hypoglycemia and tumors.
		Be sure to take two to three times as much vitamin C as L-cysteine and plenty of fluids. This prevents the oxidation of water-soluble L-cysteine into insoluble L-cystine, which leads to cystine kidney or bladder stones.
		Be sure to supplement vitamin B-6 with methionine to prevent homocystine, which leads to the formation of arteriosclerotic plaques.
		Make sure that you are using the supplement L-cysteine, and not L-cystine.
		Diabetics should take L-cysteine only under a doctor's supervision.

Basic Mineral Nutrients

Minerals act as essential catalysts for many of the biological and chemical reactions that keep your cells functioning properly and slow cellular aging.

Proper mineral supplementation requires striking a delicate balance between the correct amount of *each* mineral and the correct ratio among *all* of them. Some minerals need to be consumed in relatively large amounts. They are called macro-minerals and are measured in milligrams (mg.). Minerals needed in relatively small amounts are called trace elements; they are measured in micrograms (mcg.).

Please follow these guidelines to receive maximum benefits:

- Every mineral product contains a different percentage of the actual mineral or elemental amount. For example: Magnesium oxide contains 60 percent magnesium, and magnesium orotate contains 11 percent magnesium. Most product labels and recommended amounts in literature for minerals are worthless because they don't specify the elemental amount and source. In the tables that follow I specify the recommended elemental amount after the name of each mineral and the amount of products containing the mineral to supply the elemental amount.
- Mineral products vary in bioavailability, price, and function. Mineral aspartates and orotates are expensive, low in elemental mineral content, high in bioavailability and natural chelators. Other products are cost effective, high in elemental mineral content, and high in bioavailability. I recommend a combination of orotates, aspartates, and standard products for different minerals so you get the maximum benefits. Do not purchase expensive chelated minerals. Most chelates are not genuine.
- Take all of your mineral nutrients at once and with meals. Inorganic minerals are absorbed and used more easily when combined with foods. However, avoid consuming mineral nutrients at the same time as high-bran foods such as whole wheat bread. Bran types of fiber inhibit the absorption of many minerals, including calcium, zinc, iron, and magnesium.
- Minerals with low oxidative states (the oxidative state describes the amount of electrical charges in an atom) have greater bioavailability than those with high oxidative states. The key to determining oxidative states is to examine the suffix of the mineral. Those with lower (preferable) oxidative states generally end with *-ous;* those with higher oxidation generally end with *-ic;* therefore, ferrous iron and chromous chromium are preferable to ferric iron and chromic chromium.
- Do not take phosphorus as a supplement unless blood analysis ticularly selenium, chromium, manganese, and copper, are toxic in high doses.

- Make sure you maintain the proper ratio among minerals. Taking one mineral without its opposite may do more harm than good. Calcium and magnesium, for example, should be supplemented in a ratio of 1:1. If less magnesium than calcium is consumed, you run the risk that calcium may become lodged in soft tissues, potentially causing sclerotic or heart disease. Where supplement ratios are especially important, that is noted in the text.
- Do not take phosphorus as a supplement unless blood analysis reveals a deficiency. Most people consume too much phosphorus in their diet, which is detrimental to bone metabolism.
- Do not supplement your diet with iron unless you are a pre-menopausal woman, consume less than 1500 calories daily, eat an unbalanced diet, or have discovered a deficiency through clinical testing. Iron is toxic in high amounts and difficult to remove from the body.

TABLE 28

Basic Mineral Nutrients

Supplement and Source	Daily Amount	Comments
Macrominerals		
Calcium*	600–1000 mg.	Strengthens bones, fingernails, and
Calcium orotate	500–1000 mg.	teeth. Needed for healthy blood,
and	No more than	heart, muscles, and nerve
Calcium lactate	3100–5000 mg. per day	transmissions. Protects against high blood pressure, muscle cramping, and the development of osteoporosis.
		Post-menopausal women use higher amount.
Magnesium*	600–1000 mg.	Works with calcium to strengthen bones
Orotate	1200–2000 mg.	and teeth and prevent a negative
and		calcium balance that may cause
Aspartate	600–1200 mg.	osteoporosis and arteriosclerosis.
and		Necessary for proper neuromuscular
Oxide	770–1280 mg.	contractions and a strong thymus gland for increasing immunity. Magnesium orotate helps remove age pigments and lipofuscins.
Potassium	4000–6000 mg.	Counteracts sodium's tendency to raise
Orotate	70–140 mg.	blood pressure, and helps lower blood pressure. Works with sodium for proper heartbeat, nerve transmission, and muscular function. Most potassium is obtained from food. Foods rich in potassium are green leafy vegetables, whole grains, sunflower seeds, kelp, raisins, yams, and bananas.

*Calcium and magnesium should be consumed in a 1:1 ratio.

Supplement and Source	Daily Amount	Comments

Zinc
    Orotate
    or
    Oxide
	30–50 mg.
	190–315 mg.
	
	54–90 mg.
		Required for healing and growth. Fights free radicals, stabilizes lymph and cell membranes. A powerful immune system stimulant. Prevents bone loss, reduces tissue inflammation, treats rheumatoid arthritis, helps diabetics. In men, it nourishes the prostate and prevents infertility. In women, it helps prevent premenstrual tension.

Iron Ferrous fumarate	10 mg. 30 mg.	Needed to make hemoglobin to transport oxygen to your cells. Should be used only by women between puberty and menopause and men who have a diagnosed clinical iron deficiency. Best absorbed on an empty stomach one hour before meals.
Copper Copper sulfate	1.5–2.5 mg. 5.8–9.7 mg.	Essential for proper heart function, bone and blood formation, nerve function, immunity, and reproduction. Helps fight free radicals. Deficiency causes anemia. Excess copper is quite toxic and causes free radical damage and cross-linkage. Some elderly people may need 5 mg. a day for bone formation and proper blood and heart activity. Best to take copper supplement only with professional advice.
Manganese Manganese Sulfate	10–20 mg. 32–64 mg.	Activates many essential life processes, including fighting free radicals associated with improved immune system, prevention of cancer, and improvement of glucose tolerance.
Molybdenum Molybdenum Trioxide	100–200 mcg. 150–350 mcg.	Fights free radicals, protects against cancer, and prevents anemia. Gout sufferers, consult your physician before use.

Silicon
    Horsetail herb
    or
    Colloidal silica
	100–200 mg.
	
	230–465 mg.
		Forms healthy connective tissue and flexible blood vessels. Decreases risk of heart attack.

Sulfur
    Elemental sulfur
    flowers (USP, the grade
    of quality for human
    consumption
	50–100 mg.	Part of amino acids needed for forming body tissues and collagen.

Supplement and Source	Daily Amount	Comments
Trace Elements		

Chromium
    Yeast
    or
Chromium nitrate
 	
    or
	200–300 mcg.	Stimulates enzymes to metabolize sugar and synthesize fatty acids. Helps improve control of blood sugar. Essential for weight loss and preventing diabetes and hypoglycemia. Has been found to lower cholesterol and reduce risk of heart disease.

Kelp	210–280 mg.	I recommend chromium derived from a special kelp. Also supplies organic selenium, iodine, and other trace minerals.
Iodine Kelp	280–390 mcg. 210–280 mg.	Needed for the proper function of the thyroid gland and regulation of energy production.
Selenium	200–300 mcg.	Important antioxidant fights free radicals; protects against pollution, heavy metals, and toxic chemicals. Increases male fertility, protects against heart and circulatory disorders, aids arthritic inflammations. In research, selenium inhibits cancers and strengthens the immune system. Take a combination of organic and inorganic selenium.
Sodium selenate *or*	400–600 mcg.	Sodium selenate is an organic form of lower toxicity than sodium selenite that has extended life, but it should *not* be taken at the same time as vitamin C. Selenocystine from yeast is an organic compound that works longer than sodium selenate.
Kelp	210–280 mg.	I prefer kelp-derived organic selenium. (Kelp also provides chromium and other trace minerals.) Selenium works better in combination with vitamin E and the amino acids cysteine and methionine.
Vanadium Pentaoxide	100–200 mcg. 220–440 mcg.	Inhibits cholesterol formation in blood vessels.

Additional Age Reduction Supplements

This section includes an alphabetical listing of all the supplements recommended throughout the Age Reduction System, other than the basic nutrients already described. Some of the accessory supplements recommended for specific aging patterns are amino acids, artificial antioxidants, enzymes, fungi, herbs, hormones, mucopolysaccharides, and RNA extracts.

While each supplement interacts individually with other supplements, foods, and your body rhythms and metabolism, all will produce results if you are eating a basically healthy diet and taking at least minimal amounts of the basic nutrients. Exceptional interactions are noted under the individual supplement.

I do caution you against taking only accessory supplements *without* providing your body with the basic nutrients. Taken alone, some could produce side effects.

If you experience any side effects other than the harmless ones described in the text, discontinue use. If you have any questions, are taking any medications, or have any diagnosed disorders, consult your physician before beginning a supplement program.

These supplements are not intended to treat illness or disease. The information given here is provided for educational purposes only and is not a prescription designed to replace or enhance medication you are taking or to substitute for any program of treatment your doctor has devised for you.

TABLE 29

Additional Supplements

Supplements	Daily Amount	Comments
Acidophilus		*See* Lactobacilli.
Activated charcoal (derived from peach pits and walnut shells)	¾ to 1½ teaspoons twice a day	Draws out heavy metals, toxins, and drugs from the gastrointestinal tract. Recent research shows walnut also effectively clears your blood to prevent cellular damage and extend life.
		Use as part of detoxification program on one or two consecutive days each week for continual cleansing benefits.
		Mix with 8 ounces of beverage. Brush your teeth and rinse mouth after using; otherwise it will turn the teeth dark.
		May cause constipation, which can be relieved by taking 100–200 mg. of cascara segrada or the detoxification fiber mixture (see Chapter 7).

Supplements	Daily Amount	Comments
Algin		*See* Fiber.
Amino acids		Essential protein building blocks
GABA (gamma amino butyric acid)	100–500 mg.	Inhibitory neurotransmitter, counteracts overexcited brain signals to relax the body and induce sleep. Small amounts (100 mg.) may help men increase sex drive and reduce prostate inflammation. Equally effective whether taken as powder, capsules, or tablets. May be used during the day and before bedtime.
Glycine	4–8 gm	Inexpensive amino acid which, when combined with large amounts of L-arginine and L-ornithine, induces sleep and triggers the release of growth hormone. Also used to treat degenerative muscular diseases such as multiple sclerosis. Take in powder form one-half hour before bedtime.
L-arginine	5–10 gm with L-ornithine, 10–20 gm without L-ornithine	When taken with glycine and L-ornithine, triggers the release of growth hormone. Also increases sperm count, stimulates immunity, speeds wound healing, inhibits cancer, improves male fertility, and prevents the formation of dangerous hydrocarbons. For maximum benefits take on an empty stomach, before exercise, and right before sleep. Should not be used by schizophrenics, young people, and juvenile diabetics.
L-carnitine	300–1500 mg.	Helps transfer fatty acids into mitochondria and release energy from fat metabolism. An antioxidant that fights free radicals and reduces triglycerides. Low dosages (300–800 mg.) may help male infertility. Protects against muscle weakening diseases, helps dieting. Protects against cardiovascular disease. The presently marketed DL-carnitine may cause myasthenia—a progressive muscle weakening disease.
L-ornithine	4–10 gm with L-arginine, 6–15 gm without L-arginine	When taken in combination with glycine and L-arginine, triggers the release of growth hormone. Also stimulates immunity and helps detoxify ammonia.

Supplements	Daily Amount	Comments
		For maximum benefit take on an empty stomach, before exercise, and right before sleep.
		Should not be used by young people, schizophrenics, and juvenile diabetics.
L-phenylalanine	200–1000 mg.	Controls appetite, enhances neurofunction, and acts as an antidepressant.
		Begin with low dosages and gradually increase amounts. Monitor blood pressure to see if it rises, a common side effect. If it does, revert to lower dosages.
		Do not use this supplement if you are hypertensive, are taking MAO inhibitor drugs, or suffer from PKU (phenylketonuria).
L-tryptophan	400–800 mg.	Is converted by the brain into serotonin, a sleep-inducing hormone. May be used sparingly and infrequently to treat insomnia or depression.
		Because high levels of serotonin are associated with premature aging, you should maintain critical ratios of serotonin to dopamine (its hormonal opposite) by combining supplemental L-tryptophan with supplemental L-tyrosine, a dopamine precursor. (See Table 3 in Chapter 6 for a complete discussion of serotonin/dopamine supplementation.)
		For maximum results take L-tryptophan in the evening with vitamin B-6 (100 mg.).
L-tyrosine	500–1500 mg.	Increases dopamine that stimulates daytime metabolic processes, releases growth hormone, and delays sexual decline.
		Begin with low dosages and gradually increase amounts. L-tyrosine should stabilize blood pressure, but monitor it anyway.
		Insomnia is a potential side effect that indicates a dopamine/serotonin hormonal imbalance. If you suffer from it, reduce L-tyrosine amounts, or take small amounts of L-tryptophan, a serotonin precursor, to counteract effect.
		Obtain maximum results by taking L-tyrosine early in the day and separate from other amino acids or protein foods.

Supplements	Daily Amount	Comments
Artificial antioxidants		Help prevent and destroy free radical formation and lipid oxidation. Reduce risk of cancer.
BHT (butylated hydroxytoluene)	125–300 mg.	BHT has extended life in experimental research with animals.
BHA (butylated hydroxyanisole)	125–300 mg.	May be consumed directly or added to foods and oils. If consumed directly, maximum benefits and minimum side effects are achieved by using a *variety* of antioxidants. If added to oils, 50 mg. of BHA or BHT will protect 10 fluid ounces of vegetable oil from oxidizing and forming free radicals.
Thiodipropionic acid	25–75 mg.	
		Pregnant and lactating women or individuals with kidney or liver ailments should not use artificial antioxidants.
Aspergillum		Fungal-derived digestant predigests food in your stomach before the secretion of stomach acid. Stomach acid temporarily deactivates aspergillum. Reactivated by pH rise in intestines. May be taken in capsules or tablets and sprinkled on food. Recommend using aspergillum along with pancreatin for maximum digestive benefits.
Protease	10–20 mg.	
Amylase	26–52 mg.	
Lipase	5–10 mg.	
Cellulase	4–8 mg.	
Betain HCl		*See* Hydrochloric acid.
BHA		*See* Artificial antioxidants.
BHT		*See* Artificial antioxidants.
Bran		*See* Fiber.
Bromelain		*See* Protein-digesting enzymes.
Catalase		*See* Enzymes.
Chlorella	2–6 gm	Unicellular micro algae containing protein, vitamins, minerals, and chlorophyll. Japanese studies indicate chlorella increases immunity, fights viral infections, treats peptic ulcers, lowers cholesterol, fights tumors, aids weight loss, and eliminates constipation. Start with small amounts and gradually increase.
Chondroitan sulfate A		*See* Mucopolysaccharides.
Chymotrypsin		*See* Protein-digesting enzymes.
Coenzyme Q-10	15–30 mg.	Used by over 6 million Japanese to treat cardiovascular disorders. Significantly increases physical energy and has extended life in laboratory animals.

Supplements	Daily Amount	Comments
Cytochrome C	500–1000 mg.	Increases oxygen use in the mitochondria, the cell's powerhouse.
		Should be taken in powder form one-half hour before exercise to increase stamina.
DHEA (dehydroepiandrosterone)	(undetermined)	An anti-obesity, anti-cancer, anti-aging hormone produced by the adrenal gland. Inhibits weight gain without suppressing appetite.
Mexican wild yam		Available in low concentration tablets derived from wild Mexican yams. It's currently difficult to project the amount needed in people based on the high amounts used in original animal studies.
DMAE (dimethylaminethanol) Bitartrate salts	100–300 mg.	Precursor of the neurotransmitter acetylcholine, which is necessary for brain function, memory, and nerve transmission. Removes lipofuscin deposits.
DMG (dimethylglycine)	50–200 mg.	Increases stamina by controlling lactic acid buildup from exercise.
		Best taken in the sublingual form for quick absorption.
		Recommend using the sublingual form one-half hour before exercising, along with the other energy supplements.
Enzymes		Superior free radical scavengers and anti-aging cell aids.
SOD (superoxide dismutase)	6000 IU or more	Deactivates dangerous super oxide radicals. High levels of SOD enzymes are associated with maximum life-span in some species. However, increasing overall SOD levels by supplementation is futile due to high levels already present in the body and destruction by stomach acid. However, tablets absorbed under the tongue prevent destruction of SOD by stomach acid.
Catalase	100,000 IU or more	Deactivates free radicals.
Glutathionine peroxidase	12,000 IU or more	Deactivates free radicals.
Fiber		Daily fiber requirement depends on fiber content of your food. I suggest a combination of fibers; some nutritionists recommend single fibers.

Supplements	Daily Amount	Comments
		Take fibers in divided daily dosages. Blend with 8 ounces of beverage in each session.
		Not for individuals with intestinal adhesions or narrowing. Individuals with gross intestinal pathology may suffer an impaction from fiber.
Algin	500–1000 mg.	A fiber derivative of algae that binds and removes radioactive substances and heavy metals such as cadmium and lead.
		Should be taken with meals that do not include supplemental minerals.
Bran	3–14 gm	Contains lignin, which absorbs heavy metals and toxins and reduces cholesterol. Reduces triglycerides and excess blood sugar levels. Has been used to treat constipation, diverticulosis, varicose veins, and colon tumors.
		2 to 3 tablespoons of bran by itself helps constipation but binds minerals.
		Use oat or rice bran if allergic to wheat.
Guar gum	2–6 gm	Improves glucose tolerance and lowers triglyceride levels. 2 grams are taken with 8 ounces of liquids one-half hour before meals. Guar gum depresses the appetite by swelling in the stomach to create a feeling of fullness. Aids diabetes and hypoglycemia.
		Sold commercially under the name Galactomannan.
Pectin (high methoxy)	500 mg.–1 gm	A fiber which, when taken one-half hour before meals, helps prevent excessive blood sugar levels. Aids diabetics and hypoglycemics. Lowers serum cholesterol and triglycerides. Eliminates heavy metals from the body.
Psyllium husk	3–10 gm	Excellent bowel regulator; doesn't bind minerals. Increases transit time, eliminates waste and mucus buildup.
		Up to 30 grams of psyllium husk in daily divided dosages used by itself treats constipation.

Supplements	Daily Amount	Comments

Garlic
    Deodorized aged
      garlic extract
      (social garlic)
	800–1600 mg.	Reduces blood pressure, cholesterol, and excess blood sugar levels. Is a strong antibiotic and detoxifier of heavy metals. Guards against atherosclerosis and coronary artery disorders. Also contains selenium, a powerful antioxidant. Available in powder or capsules.

Glycerol Glycerine USP	1 tsp. 15–30 min. before each meal	Weight-loss aid. This is the substance in all fat that signals your appetite-control center to decrease appetite and food intake.
Glutamic acid HCl		*See* Hydrochloric acid.
Glutathionine peroxidase		*See* Enzymes.
L-glycine		*See* Amino acids.
Guar gum		*See* Fiber.
Hydrochloric acid		Lowers pH to help initiate digestion. Should not be used by individuals with ulcers.
Glutamic acid HCl	100–150 mg.	
Betaine HCl	300–450 mg.	
Inosine	300–600 mg.	Metabolic product improves oxygen-carrying capacity of blood to muscles. Reduces fatigue. Use powder form one-half hour before exercise, along with other muscular aids. May be helpful in treating angina, senility, and a weak heart.

Krebs Cycle
  intermediaries
    Succinic acid
    Fumaric acid
    Malic acid
    L-aspartic acid
    L-glutamic acid
    L-valine
	
	1–2 gm
	1–2 gm
	1–2 gm
	1–2 gm
	1–2 gm
	1–2 gm
		Stimulate oxidation of carbohydrates, fats, and proteins to produce the universal energy molecule ATP (adenosine triphosphate). Succinic acid also increases hypothalamic sensitivity.
		
		Use one-half hour before exercise to increase endurance.
		
		Current recommended amounts are provisional pending further experimental data.
		
		Use with an aluminum-free antacid if upsetting to stomach.

Lactobacilli		Improve intestinal functions, enhance immunity, lower cholesterol, and decrease risk of cancer.

Supplements	Daily Amount	Comments
Acidophilus	1–2 teaspoons dry culture	Lactobacilli acidophilus and bulgaricus are natural antibiotics that kill pathogenic substances and deactivate toxins. DDS-1 is the most potent strain of acidophilus.
Bulgaricus		
or		
Bifidus	1 tablespoon liquid	Bifidus enhances liver function.
or		
Cancasicus	10 billion IU	For best results, consume a mixture of these lactobacilli cultures.
L-arginine		*See* Amino acids.
L-carnitine		*See* Amino acids.
L-glutamine		*See* Amino acids.
L-ornithine		*See* Amino acids.
L-phenylalanine		*See* Amino acids.
L-tryptophan		*See* Amino acids.
L-tyrosine		*See* Amino acids.
Lecithin		*See* Table 26, Basic Fat-Soluble Nutrients— Phosphatidyl choline
Mucopolysaccharides		A combination of carbohydrates and proteins that are good defense against arterial damage. Maintain flexibility of blood vessels. Lower serum cholesterol and triglycerides.
Chondroitan sulfate A	2–6 gm	Most often recommended by medical professionals. (Available without prescription but extremely expensive.)
or		
Extracts of trachea and aorta	2–6 gm	When correctly extracted, may be as powerful as chondroitan sulfate A, but less expensive.
or possibly		
Compound plant extract of *Chondrus crispus*	2–6 gm	Some researchers believe that different factions of *Chondrus crispus* (carrageenin) work like chondroitan sulfate A at a fraction of its cost.
Lipase	500–1400 IU	Fat-digesting enzyme attacks cholesterol, triglycerides, and atherosclerotic lesions.

Use with protein-digesting enzymes and other chelating agents. |

Supplements	Daily Amount	Comments

Octacosanol
  Viobin brand,
    derived from
      wheat germ oil
	500–2000 mcg.	Improves endurance and reaction time while eliminating excess cholesterol.
		
		Use one-half hour before exercising.
		
		Those sensitive or allergic to wheat should not use this supplement.

Organ-specific RNA	5 cc./6 mg. vials of each type	Increases protein synthesis in the particular organ from which it was extracted. Imported from Europe and available through selected physicians. Over 40 types of organ-specific RNA are available for injection treatments. A three-week series of treatments costs around $600. Homeopathically prepared organ-specific RNA may produce similar results for a fraction of the cost.
Pancreatin (4×)	400–1000 mg.	Contains all of the enzymes necessary to digest food in the intestines. Available in different concentrations. An 8× concentration requires one-half the amount as in 4×. Do not use enteric-coated pancreatin, as testing indicates this coating substance is mildly toxic and reduces the potency of the supplement.
Papain		*See* Protein-digesting enzymes.
Pectin		*See* Fiber.

Pineal gland
  Epithalamin
 	
    or
	(Currently
	unknown)
		Increases immunity, improves hypothalamic regulation, and fights cancer in experimental research.

Crude extract		Crude extracts are available but expensive. Their degree of activity and required daily amount are unknown.

Protein-digesting
  enzymes
    Bromelain
 	
    or
	240–900 GDU
	(gelatin-
	digesting
	units)
		Uses are determined by dosage. In low dosages, protein-digesting enzymes help to digest proteins and relieve food allergies resulting from incomplete protein digestion. In moderate amounts, enzymes help heal bruises and contusions. In high doses, enzymes attack cross-linkage, dissolve blood clots, and chelate your body.

Supplements	Daily Amount	Comments
Papain	300–1200 MCU (milk, clotting units)	Ranges indicated here are moderate to high dosages.
and		*Enzyme activity rating* is just as important as the number of milligrams consumed.
Chymotrypsin	1–10 mg. concentrated	Similar amounts may vary in potency by 20–30 times. Determine activity rating by questioning the manufacturer, buying a product from a supplier that labels activity, or consulting a nutritionist.
RNA (ribonucleic acid)	1–3 gm	Necessary for memory and learning, protein acid formation, and cellular activities. An antioxidant that attacks free radicals.
		Caution: RNA increases uric acid. Gout sufferers and yeast-sensitive individuals should not use it.
		Raw thymus gland provides an excellent source of RNA.
SOD (superoxide dismutase)		*See* Enzymes.
Thiodipropionic acid		*See* Artificial antioxidants.
Thymus Thymosin *or*	(Currently unknown)	Limited research shows thymus gland peptides improve immunity and stress-handling capabilities, while reducing risk of autoimmune disorders.
Crude extract		Product quality and quantity vary dramatically both in manufacturing and experimental use.
		Recommended amount is uncertain pending further research.

A Personal Difference

My personal supplement program—designed for my environment, lifestyle, and body—differs slightly from my general recommendations for your body. I ingest the substantially higher amounts below of vitamin E and of certain basic water-soluble nutrients. You should not attempt to follow my personal program but, with the help of your physician, who knows your health profile, tailor one to your own unique needs.

Vitamin E—800–1000 IU daily

Extra vitamin E helps protect me against the pollutants and toxins of Los Angeles. I'm not 100 percent sure that vitamin E increases my endurance while exercising (although it probably does), but it definitely diminishes free radical damage from overexercise. Vitamin E decreases the potential for blood clots, brain damage from lipid peroxidation in neurons, precarcinogenic conditions, and immunodeficiency.

> **Vitamin B-1 (thiamine)—250 mg. daily;**
> **400 mg. daily during stress**

Thiamine helps convert the supplement choline, which I ingest daily, into the neurotransmitter acetylcholine for continued brain power. Thiamine guards me against thiamine destruction from stress and bisulfites added to foods in restaurants to prevent spoilage. As a bachelor, I frequently eat in restaurants with salad bars and other foods that may occasionally contain unhealthy bisulfites.

> **Vitamin B-3 (niacin)—1000 mg. daily**

I follow the advice about niacin from Dr. Abram Hoffer, a pioneer in orthomolecular medicine and president of the Huxley Institute for Bio-social Research. Among other things, I believe that vitamin B-3 prevents my blood from sludging (abnormal stickiness), lowers my cholesterol, and stimulates my brain.

> **Vitamin B-5 (pantothenic acid)—1500 mg. daily**

Megadosage of vitamin B-5 controls the arthritic pain remaining from my Belgian motorcycle accident, increases my resistance to stress, aids my endurance, and forms acetylcholine for nerve transmission.

> **Vitamin B-6 (pyridoxine)—500 mg. daily**

I believe that vitamin B-6 decreases my risk of developing cancer and atherosclerosis.

> **Vitamin B-12—1500–2000 mg. daily**

My current intake level of B-12 is extrapolated from an obscure animal study. According to that study, supplemental vitamin B-12 increased learning in RNA (ribonucleic acid) synthesis in brain cells. Decreased RNA activity contributes towards senility and aging throughout the body.

> **PABA (para-aminobenzoic acid—1000 mg. daily**

PABA reduces the toxicity of the picturesque ozone-rich smog layer in Los Angeles.

Vitamin C—5–7 grams daily

I follow the research findings about vitamin C reported by the world's foremost authority, two-time Nobel Prize laureate Linus Pauling, and the 1937 Nobel laureate, Albert Szent-Gyorgyi, the man who first identified and synthesized vitamin C.

Within the next several years I will chelate my body to remove deleterious minerals that contribute towards pathology and premature aging. I believe that chelating my body by exercise will accumulate lactic acid and infuse the man-made amino acid EDTA (ethylene diamine tetra-acetic acid) into my veins as recommended by Johan Byorksten, the originator of the cross-linkage theory of aging, to extend life.

Finally, I will undergo Regeneresen (organ-specific RNA) therapy. Intramuscular injections of RNA (ribonucleic acid) extracted from different animal organs will have an affinity for the same organ in my body and increase protein synthesis in the target organs. The systemic decrease of protein synthesis is a major cause of cellular aging.

SUPPLEMENT SUPPLIERS

Various companies sell anti-aging combination products. Others sell the raw ingredients. Below is a list of companies that specialize in selling these products and raw ingredients. The list is intended as a guide only and does not constitute a recommendation or guarantee of any product. The fact that a supplier is not included in this listing does not indicate criticism of that supplier's products; I have listed only those with whom I am familiar. As a careful consumer, you should study the products described in the suppliers' catalogues, compare prices if possible, and make an informed choice of products you wish to use in your Age Reduction Program.

Age Reduction, Inc.
P.O. Box 85152
Department MB159
San Diego, CA 92138
1-800-621-0852, ext. 585

Sells a complete series of supplemental and skin care products based on my combinations of Age Reduction System supplements, nutrients, and herbs. Sells water purifiers, homeopathic first aid kits, age reduction programs, and other anti-aging tools.

John A. Borneman & Sons
1208 Amosland Road
Norwood, PA 19074
215-532-2035

Sells homeopathic remedies.

Brion Corporation
12020 B Centralia
Hawaiian Gardens, CA 90716
213-924-8875

Sells scientifically prepared herbal formulas.

Connex Enterprises
1626 West Temple Street
Los Angeles, CA 90026
213-617-1586

also

151 Mott St.
New York, N.Y. 10013
212-925-7466

Sells over 1000 different Chinese herbs.

General Research Labs
8900 Winnetka Avenue
Northridge, CA 91324
1-800-421-1856

Sells high quality enzyme combinations, raw supplements, and combination products.

Life Extension Foundation
2835 Hollywood Boulevard
Hollywood, FL 33020
1-800-327-6110

Sells high quality nutrient formulas, raw ingredients, books, and other products to control aging.

The Longevity Institute
Avenida Federico Boyd y Calle 51
P.O. Box 2689 Balboa
Panama, Republic of Panama

Sells organ-specific RNA and anti-aging drugs.

Natures Herb Company
281 Ellis Street
San Francisco, CA 94102
415-474-2756

Sells powdered herbs.

Star and Crescent
8561 Thys Court
Sacramento, CA 95828
916-381-7025
Sells powdered herbs.

Sun Ten Pharmaceutical Works Co. Ltd.
114 Chung-Ching South Road Section 3
Taipei, Taiwan
Sells scientifically prepared Chinese herbal formulas.

Twin Laboratories
Ronkonkoma, NY 11779
Sells anti-aging nutrients through health food stores.

Vitamin Research Products
2044-A Old Middlefield Way
Mountain View, CA 94043
415-967-7775
Sells bulk anti-aging nutrients and combination products. I recommend only their raw ingredients.

Whole Herb Company
P.O. Box 1085
Mill Valley, CA 94941
415-383-6485
Sells powdered herbs and Chinese herbal combinations.

10
The Age
Reduction Diet

Restricting calories and manipulating nutrients is the single most power-ful age reduction tool at your disposal today. If recent experiments with rats (which closely mimic human biological responses) are any indication, you may potentially add more than fifty years to your life by following the Age Reduction Diet described in this chapter.

To understand why manipulating your consumption of calories and nutrients can have such a dramatic effect on your life-span, reconsider the evolutionary model discussed in Chapter 8. Your body was designed not just to survive feast and famine but *to thrive* on it.

AN EVOLUTIONARY APPROACH TO EATING

The sophisticated system by which you consume food, digest it, turn it into heat or energy, store it as fat, detoxify and eliminate it was created in response to firmly established eating habits. Or, perhaps more accurately, in response to non-eating habits.

In the beginning, food availability was best described as feast or famine. When times were good, people ate everything in sight. (Of course, refined sugar, excess salt and fats, and other goodies were then unknown.) The bodies of our early ancestors stored calories the way a chipmunk stores nuts, each saving something for a rainy day. When that fateful rainy day or week or month arrived, their bodies were ready to switch to Plan B: the conversion of fat to fuel or heat. It was, and is, an excellent system.

There's only one problem: We changed our eating habits without in-forming evolution. For at least the last century, Americans have taken a lopsided approach to this historic pattern. We love to feast but hate to be famished. Consequently, our bodies cheerfully continue to store calories against a fateful day that never arrives. The result is obesity, cell damage, breakdown of the digestion and elimination systems, premature aging, development of degenerative disease, and early death.

Restricting calories balances the yin/yang of the evolutionary eating equation by reintroducing a form of famine.

The famine phase allows your body to purge itself of accumulated wastes and toxins (reducing the formation of free radicals and cross-linkage), rest the digestion and elimination systems, refortify the immune system, and divert energy normally devoted to digestion to cell repair and reproduction.

RESTRICTING CALORIES EXTENDS LIFE

In experiments with white rats, caloric restriction has yielded astonishing life extension results.

For example, researcher Morris H. Ross, at the Institute for Cancer Research, Philadelphia, Pennsylvania, restricted the food intake of rats to 30 percent of normal. At twenty-one days of age, these rats had a life expectancy of 1100 days. Rats in the control group, who were fed a normal amount of the same diet, had life expectancies of 600 days.

A number of the nutrient-restricted rats survived more than 1800 days, a life-span far beyond any previously recorded. In human terms this is equivalent to 180 years. In contrast, the last of the control rats died some 700 days earlier.

In many scientific studies conducted around the world equally astounding results have been reported. Many of these studies are listed in my bibliography and reference section.

WHAT MAKES
THE AGE REDUCTION DIET DIFFERENT?

The Age Reduction System's calorie-restriction program, the Age Reduction Diet, is a highly advanced life extension technique. Its primary goals are to reduce body fat while maintaining lean muscle mass, to slow down your metabolism so your body lasts longer, and to delay the metabolic shifts of aging. This calorie-restricted diet also has a beneficial effect on the degenerative diseases of aging: adult-onset diabetes, cancer, hypertension, obesity, atherosclerosis, immune system depression, and autoimmune disorders.

Most weight-loss programs measure success by the amount of weight you lose, regardless of the consequences to your health. Their methods attempt to provoke your metabolism into burning calories the way a race car engine burns fuel—and with the same short-lived results! Maximum life-span, on the other hand, is achieved by *gradually* eliminating excess weight while pampering the metabolism and delaying its inevitable breakdown, not by forcing the metabolism to run at open throttle.

In addition to overtaxing the metabolism, many weight-loss programs shorten life-span by selectively restricting or overindulging in particular food groups or nutrients. Some diets rely heavily on artificial powders and liquids that have caused death in humans and laboratory animals. Other diets recommend excessive protein consumption, whose life-shortening effects were discussed in Chapter 8. Even the American Diabetic Association's Exchange Diet (the parent of many weight-loss programs) allows you to eat refined carbohydrates and recommends (on its 2000-calories-a-day plan) that you consume 104 grams of protein. That is two times the normal protein requirement for a person weighing 150 pounds!

Reduces Weight and Biological Age at the Same Time

The Age Reduction Diet is a nutritionally balanced program that allows your body to naturally shed excess weight, delay the metabolic shifts of aging, and reduce your biological age. It incorporates the principles discussed in Chapter 8, and takes them one step farther into the future of optimal weight, health, and longevity.

You will find the Age Reduction Diet's recommendations easy to follow, requiring few sacrifices and offering many rewards. You can take it anywhere—into restaurants and friends' homes, even on vacations. Since I follow the Age Reduction Diet myself, I had to make it simple, flexible, and practical enough to accommodate my ever-changing needs.

Although the Age Reduction Diet is based on natural eating patterns, it is not appropriate for everyone. Pregnant and lactating women, hypoglycemics, diabetics, and those recovering from serious illnesses should not use the program. If you have to eat much more than most people you know to maintain a moderate weight, do not use this program. As with any other calorie-restricted diet, this one is best conducted under a health professional's supervision.

I have supervised the use of the Age Reduction Diet for myself and my clients for more than six years with excellent results. Although I have never needed to lose weight (except perhaps in college, when I attempted a single-handed survey of every Belgian waffle in Brussels), I restrict myself to 1500 calories per day, consumed in one and one-half meals. I keep my total body fat at about 6 percent. From my own experience, as well as that of my clients, I can assure you that long-term caloric restriction is not only healthy, it's immediately rewarding. I have more energy, stamina, and emotional stability than I did as a teenage athlete.

The only real conflict I've experienced as a result of my unusual eating habits has been during social or business meals. Reactions range from raised eyebrows to outright hostility. It is amazing how threatening people sometimes find change, even in others. I find that laughing at my own peculiarities generally makes it easier for myself and others.

Address Every Aspect
of Weight Gain/Loss and Longevity

The Age Reduction Diet addresses each factor influencing body weight and longevity in five easy phases:

Phase 1: Getting to Know You. In this phase we'll determine your ideal weight, as compared to your current weight, and explore the reasons why you might be overweight.

Phase 2: Designing Your Own Diet. The Age Reduction Diet is as individual as your fingerprints. To design the diet that is right for you, we will first determine how many calories you are consuming on average each day and how efficient your metabolism is at converting those calories into fuel. Then I will explain the Age Reduction Diet levels, the nutrient exchange system, and help you pinpoint your target calorie zones.

Phase 3: Creating Your Age Reduction Exercise Program. Exercise does more than just burn up calories. In this phase I'll explain how exercise alters your metabolism to burn more calories even when you aren't exercising and how it delays metabolic shifts that cause aging.

Phase 4: Supporting the Diet with Stress Reduction. Chronic negative stress is a key ingredient in fat gain. In this phase, I'll tell you why and what you can do about it.

Phase 5: Supplementing Your Diet. This final phase explains how you can use vitamins, amino acids, special oils, fibers, and other nutrients to make your Age Reduction Diet an almost effortless success.

PHASE I: GETTING TO KNOW YOU

The true measure of your degree of fitness for longevity is body fat, not body weight.

Body fat can be measured by hydrostatic (underwater) weighing, skinfold (pinch) measuring, circumference measurements, and a new system involving computer analysis of electrical resistance between fat and muscle. If you have access to any of these measuring systems, I strongly urge you to use them instead of the less accurate but more common body weight scales. If weight scales are the only available method, however, the following tables indicating ideal weights for men and women will help you to approximate your ideal weight.

The values are extrapolated from the lifelong research of Albert Behnke, one of the world's foremost experts in anthropometry—the measurement of size, weight, and proportions—who has measured thousands of subjects.

Your lifelong ideal weight range for Age Reduction falls between the standard weight and minimum weight of healthy young people. In my opinion, the current tables of the Metropolitan Life Insurance Company are too permissive. To control aging, maintain your muscles at the level of a twenty-five-year-old. If your muscles are hypertrophied, that is, if you lift weights or have large muscles, height and weight tables are less accurate than for people with normal musculature.

The long-life goal of men should be to keep total body fat less than 15 percent; women should keep theirs at less than 22 percent. Since some body fat is essential to cushion organs and supply energy, water, and nutrients in periods of deprivation, men should not allow body fat to fall below 3 percent; women must retain at least 12 to 14 percent to remain healthy.

If your body fat content is up to 5 percent above the maximum levels suggested or if your body weight is up to 15 pounds more than the maximum levels suggested by Table 30, you are probably accelerating the aging process. Your body is forced to create miles of new blood vessels to feed the fat, putting an unnecessary strain on the cardiopulmonary system. Moreover, fat accumulates inside the blood vessels, making the heart work harder to move the same amount of blood.

If your body fat content is *more than* 5 percent above maximum suggested levels or if your body weight is *more than* 15 pounds above the maximum levels suggested, you are obese.

Obesity is a disease that both accelerates and results from the aging process. Excess fat *accelerates* aging by provoking the metabolic shift in which your body switches from using carbohydrates to fats as its primary energy source. As we have already discussed in Chapter 2, this metabolic shift leads to immune system and growth hormone depression, excessive insulin response, and the malfunction of the neuroendocrine system charged with regulating energy production. Some of the degenerative diseases associated with this metabolic shift include adult-onset diabetes, hypertension, heart attack, and cancer.

Obesity may also *result* from the natural aging process. As you grow older your energy metabolism gradually deteriorates. The RAS and the hypothalamus are less sensitive to information; the cells become less tolerant of glucose as the primary fuel source; the thyroid gland (which determines whether food will be converted into fat or fuel) becomes less active. The neuroendocrine system becomes deregulated, releasing the wrong amounts of chemicals and hormones at the wrong time. The outcome of obesity, whether it occurs from aging, overeating, or metabolic abberations, is the same. Alteration in your metabolic apparatus from aging is similar to gaining fat from overeating, lack of exercise, and metabolic defects. Growth hormone and the immune system are depressed. (Since growth hormone is responsible for building lean muscle

TABLE 30

Ideal Weights

For Men

Height*	Standard Weight* (lb.) (12% fat)	Minimum Weight* (lb.) (3% essential fat)
6'6"	192 or less	174
6'4"	184 or less	167
6'3"	180 or less	163
6'2"	176 or less	159
6'1"	172 or less	155
6'0"	168 or less	151
5'11"	164 or less	148
5'10"	160 or less	145
5'9"	156 or less	141
5'8"	152 or less	137
5'7"	148 or less	134
5'6"	144 or less	131
5'5"	141 or less	128
5'4"	137 or less	124
5'3"	134 or less	121
5'2"	130 or less	118

For Women

Height*	Standard Weight* (lb.) (22% or less body fat)	Minimum Weight* (lb.) (14% Fat)
6'3"	150 or less	138
6'2"	146 or less	134
6'1"	143 or less	131
6'0"	140 or less	128
5'11"	136 or less	125
5'10"	133 or less	122
5'9"	130 or less	119
5'8"	127 or less	116
5'7"	123 or less	114
5'6"	120 or less	111
5'5"	117 or less	109
5'4"	114 or less	105
5'3"	111 or less	102
5'2"	108 or less	100
5'1"	106 or less	97
5'0"	103 or less	94

*Without shoes and clothes

mass, its depression causes muscle wasting and fat gain.) Excessive insulin causes fat to be stored rather than burned as fuel. Low thyroid activity encourages calories to be stored as fat.

The accumulation of fat leads to further breakdown in energy metabolism, leading to accumulating even more fat and the degenerative diseases already described.

The only way to break the vicious cycle is by caloric restriction, adequate exercise, and supplemental nutrients. If you become obese during childhood, adolescence, or the maturity phase of life you will *significantly accelerate* the aging process. If you become obese during the physiological decline stage of life, as a *result* of aging, you will still accelerate decline and death, but not to the same degree.

It is important to eliminate excess fat as early as possible, before it has a chance to provoke premature metabolic shifts.

Why You Gain Fat

I once saw a cartoon in which an overweight, middle-aged woman had puffed her way to the top of a Himalayan peak to visit a guru. Upon her arrival, she sat down heavily and inquired of the guru, "Please tell me, what is the secret of the universe?" The guru stared at her silently for a few minutes, then replied, "Burn more calories than you eat."

While this simple axiom is mainly true, it is not entirely true. In addition to overeating, you may be overweight because:

- One (or both) of your parents was overweight. If one parent was overweight, there is a 40 percent chance that you will be, too. Two overweight parents increase your risk of being overweight to 80 percent.
- You possess too many fat cells. Either through heredity or overfeeding at critical periods of development, you have overproduced fat cells, which increase your tendency to convert food to fat instead of fuel.
- Your metabolism helps your body to store calories the way a camel stores water.
- Your brown fat—a special type of fat containing blood vessels and found around the internal organs and the heart's blood vessels—is sluggish about converting calories into heat.
- You suffer from hypothalamus, thyroid, adrenal, or pancreas gland dysfunction. These are the primary glands governing the release of at least eleven hormones influencing the conversion of food into fuel or fat.
- Your sodium pump, a mechanism that controls the passage of minerals across cell membranes, may be sluggish. In order to operate, it must consume considerable caloric energy.

The Dynamics of Calorie Conversion

The Law of Thermodynamics takes a simple mathematical approach to weight gain and loss. It assumes that:

- Food contains potential energy in the form of calories. (Calories are a

unit for measuring energy. One calorie is the amount of energy required to raise the temperature of one kilogram of water one degree.)
- Your body uses food calories as an energy source for internal and external physical activity.
- If you consume exactly as many food calories as you need to perform these activities, you will maintain a stable weight. Consume more and you will gain weight. Consume less and you will lose it.

According to mathematical calculations based on ideal thermodynamic principles, 3500 calories equal one pound of body weight. In real life, some sedentary people could eat 7000 calories per day and never gain an ounce, while others may consume less than 1000 calories a day and never lose an ounce. I have never met a perfect 3500-calorie client in my life.

Why? Because the Law of Thermodynamics does not account for individual idiosyncrasies. Your age, body type, and state of health influence your conversion of calories. If you exercise (especially aerobically), you increase your metabolic rate (the rate at which you burn calories) not just while you are exercising, but for up to *six hours* afterward. If you eat a high-fiber diet or have digestive problems, you will absorb fewer of the calories you consume than most people do. In this chapter we'll explore these and other factors affecting weight gain and loss. The Age Reduction System offers techniques for coping with each of them and will help you strike the balance between weight gain and loss that's right for you.

Finding Your Metabolic Type

There are several physical factors that predispose you toward having either a fast metabolism, which tends to burn calories as energy, or a slow metabolism, which tends to store calories as fat. Your metabolic rate decreases rapidly until the age of twenty and then more gradually until death. Other primary factors determining your basal metabolic rate (BMR) are listed below.

Your BMR and caloric requirements increase if you are:	Your BMR and caloric requirements decrease if you are:
Tall	Short
Thin	Fat
Muscular	Nonmuscular
Male	Female
Above normal body temperature	Below normal body temperature
Pregnant or lactating	
Living in tropical climate	

Another factor determining weight gain or loss is how much and what kind of food you eat. The American diet is high in calories not just because we eat more but also because of the kind of food we eat. Fats and refined sugars make up over 55 percent of the calories most Americans consume each day.

Excessive chronic sugar consumption will also cause you to gain weight for another reason: It creates an abnormal and excessive insulin response. *Insulin is the most powerful fat-promoting hormone in the body.* It binds fat to cell membranes, fights the release of fat from cells, and increases your conversion of sugar into fat. An abnormally high insulin secretion from the pancreas will cause you to gain fat and stay fat. The aging process increases both insulin and fat.

A high-fat diet will also cause you to gain weight, not only because of its high caloric content but because fat is a secondary fuel source. Your body prefers to convert carbohydrates to energy and will store fat for future necessity.

Many people find that they lose weight permanently and without dieting simply by following the principles set forth in Chapter 8. This high-carbohydrate, low-protein, low-fat diet is automatically low in calories while providing sufficient fiber to move food quickly through the intestines, thus slightly reducing calorie absorption.

The Brown Fat Blues

Brown fat is an infrequently discussed aspect of calorie conversion. Brown fat, as I have explained, is a special type of fat surrounding and cushioning the internal organs. It converts calories into heat. Cold weather stimulates the adrenal glands to produce adrenaline, which in turn stimulates brown fat metabolism to create heat that protects essential organs from freezing. Constant moving from a warm to a cold climate increases energy and stimulates brown fat to warm your body and lose weight. Other catalysts for brown fat metabolism include eating, which increases brown fat activity by 10 to 20 percent for up to six hours, and exercise, which increases brown fat activity for four to six hours. Maximum exertion in a short time period (e.g., sprinting or weight lifting) is a powerful brown fat stimulator.

Factors that tend to decrease brown fat metabolism are: living in an excessively warm or constant temperature climate, chronically overeating (as compared to eating frequent small meals), physical inactivity, having an underactive thyroid gland, being dominated by the parasympathetic nervous system, and growing old.

The amount of caffeine contained in two cups of mildly brewed coffee (200 milligrams) has also been found to increase brown fat activity by about 10 percent for three hours following consumption.

Under the Influence of Hormones

Your neuroendocrine system, through the autonomic nervous system, governs the more than eleven hormones known to influence the formation of fat. When the autonomic nervous system is balanced, it releases the appropriate amount of hormones to maintain a balanced weight. When the autonomic nervous system is unbalanced, it releases hormones that cause weight gain or loss and induces neuroendocrinological aging. Insulin, as I've already mentioned, is the primary fat-producing hormone.

Raising blood sugar levels, especially by eating sweets, triggers an insulin response. Insulin travels to your brain and stimulates the sympathetic nervous system, thyroid gland, and brown fat for temporary energy. Insulin also signals satiety about twenty minutes after eating.

Eating sweets before meals to control appetite is advised by some nutritionists. I don't recommend it. Artificially inducing hyper/hypoglycemia deregulates growth hormone activity, insulin control, and energy balance—all of which accelerate aging (see Chapter 14).

The thyroid gland produces hormones that control your basal metabolic rate, stimulate brown fat, and increase or decrease appetite. The thyroid gland determines your overall tendency to turn calories into fat or fuel. Overeating increases thyroid activity, and undereating decreases thyroid activity.

Thyroid response naturally diminishes with age. It is also reduced by parasympathetic nervous system dominance. The thyroid gland depends upon the sympathetic nervous system to help stimulate energy production through the hormones dopamine, adrenaline, and noradrenaline.

In spite of the popularity of "thyroid problems" as an excuse for fat gain, the truth is that hypothyroidism, a clinical deficiency of thyroid gland hormone, is quite rare. Its symptoms, in addition to fat gain, include fatigue and coarse, puffy skin.

Growth hormone is produced abundantly in adolescence to burn off fat and build muscles. With the onset of the maturity phase, growth hormone production is somewhat diminished. More importantly, self-created aging patterns such as stress; overconsumption of sugar, calories, fats, and refined foods; and lack of exercise suppress the release of growth hormone. That's an important reason why older people often have less lean muscle mass and more fat.

Adrenaline and noradrenaline, released by the sympathetic nervous system, are antifat hormones that activate brown fat metabolism. This may be why sympathetic-dominant, nervous types of people are frequently thin.

Cortisol is a fat-promoting hormone whose production is triggered by chronic negative stress and the prolonged use of corticosteroid drugs. Obesity develops from the distribution of fat in a girdle around the waist and a buffalo hump of fat pads between the shoulders. Common corticosteroids include betamethasone, cortisone acetate, hydrocortisone, prednisone, and dexamethasone. Cortisol also promotes fat gain by over-stimulating the appetite, causing you to eat more.

Sex hormones account for the differences in the percentage of body fat carried by men and women. The female hormones estrogen and pro-gesterone cause fat to be deposited on the hips, thighs, buttocks, and breasts. Progesterone production increases during the two weeks prior to menstruation. It acts as an appetite stimulant, causing women to eat more during these periods. Birth control pills contain these hormones in varying amounts and may also cause weight gain.

Endorphins and enkephalins are peptide hormones produced by the brain and distributed throughout the autonomic nervous system, digestive tract, and internal organs. They modulate nerve transmissions. Production of these natural (and powerful) pain killers is triggered by the sympathetic nervous system in response to sudden stress or pain and acupuncture. Besides killing pain, endorphins and enkephalins integrate emotions, mo-bilize fat, regulate reproduction, and increase appetite.

Cholecystokinin is a digestive hormone produced mainly in the di-gestive tract and distributed in the brain. Cholecystokinin stimulates growth hormone and numbs pain. But its primary purpose is to tell your hypothalamus whether you are hungry or full. The release of cho-lecystokin is governed by the vagus nerve and serotonin (the neu-rotransmitter discussed in Chapter 6). A stomach full of food transmits a signal that indicates satiety to the brain through the vagus nerve. Since, as we have already discussed, serotonin production decreases with age, so does production of cholecystokinin. The hypothalamus receives fewer signals that you are full, so you tend to eat more than you need. Stress also depresses cholecystokinin levels by stimulating the sympathetic nervous system to release cortisol and adrenaline, both cholecystokinin antag-onists. The more negative stress you experience, the fewer satiety signals reach your hypothalamus, and the more you eat. So stress offers chemical as well as psychological causes for overeating.

As you can see, gaining fat is a process that results from both self-created and preprogrammed patterns. The Age Reduction Diet will help you to overcome destructive habits and improve metabolic efficiency by:

- Restricting calories
- Depressing your appetite
- Stimulating both regular and brown fat metabolism
- Making use of the stress-reduction techniques discussed in Chapter 5
- Complementing the fitness program for longevity described in Chap-ter 11
- Supplementing your diet with the amino acids, enzymes, vitamins, fibers, and other nutrients necessary for optimal metabolic efficiency and longevity.

PHASE 2: YOU CAN DESIGN YOUR OWN DIET

Let me remind you at this point that this program's primary goals are not just to lose excess weight but to reduce your biological age. Most crash diets are aptly named—they cause the crash of your digestive, immune, and neuroendocrine systems by forcing them to adapt to unnatural conditions. High-protein and low-carbohydrate diets are among the worst of these. The Age Reduction Diet recommends reducing your daily intake of calories not just today or next week, but for the rest of your life.

The first step is to determine how many calories you consume on average each day. I recommend that you keep an accurate log of every mouthful you eat for at least five days spanning one weekend. Do not attempt to diet or otherwise improve your eating habits during this period. Do not forget to record the three bites of chicken curry you sampled of your friend's dinner last night or the cookie you washed down with the glass of milk just before bed. You will be amazed to discover how these little bits and pieces add up, particularly in terms of your fat consumption.

At the end of the five-day period, calculate your average calorie consumption with the help of a complete calorie-counter book (widely available in bookstores). Make a note of your average daily calorie consumption.

If your metabolic rate is very rapid, that is, you are continually eating food just to maintain your weight or prevent weight loss, or if you're very, very thin and can never gain weight even by overeating and rapidly lose weight, then the Age Reduction Diet is not suited for you.

If you're metabolically normal or if you have a sluggish metabolism, that is, you eat few calories and you have a difficult time losing weight even under those circumstances, the Age Reduction Diet will benefit your health and longevity.

Finding Your Target Zone

In Phase 1 of this program, you determined your relationship to your ideal body weight or body fat ratio.

If you are underweight or underfat, *do not* follow the Age Reduction Diet.

If you are very close to your correct body weight/body fat ratio, you may still choose to follow this diet to reap its age reduction benefits. If so, I recommend that you compare your average daily calorie consumption to the target zone shown below. If your average calorie consumption is at the maximum target level suggested for your sex, you should begin the Age Reduction Diet on the next lower level. If your average daily calorie consumption is at the bottom of the preferred target zone levels, do not further restrict your calories. Instead, manipulate the amount and type of proteins, carbohydrates, and fats you consume (as recommended by the Age Reduction Diet) to maximize life extension effects.

If you are overweight and overfat, you should treat yourself to two weeks of amazing results by limiting yourself to 1000 calories if you are a woman, 1200 calories if you are a man. After two weeks, women should consume 1200 calories, and men should consume 1400 calories. Continue at these levels until you have achieved your ideal body weight/body fat ratio. Then slowly increase your caloric consumption by 100 calories a day. Maintain this new level for one week. Then, if measurements or scales show that you have not gained weight or fat, increase it by another 100 calories. Continue until you either reach the maximum amount of calories for your target zone or begin to gain weight or fat. If necessary, revert to the next lower target zone level.

These are the ideal target zones for men and women.

Daily Calories Consumed
2000
Male target zone — 1800
1600 — Female target zone
1400
1200
1000

When choosing the target zone that's right for you, remember that less is not necessarily best. Here are some other factors you should keep in mind:

Lower Calorie Levels	Higher Calorie Levels
Small body	Large body
Sedentary	Active
Excessive body fat	Little body fat
Slow metabolic rate	Fast metabolic rate

Do not undertake any level of the Age Reduction Diet without first consulting your physician.

An Alternate Method: Feast/Famine

If you find the idea of restricting calories day in and day out, year after year, too difficult to digest, you may want to consider another approach to the Age Reduction Diet.

The feast/famine approach mimics the eating habits designed by evolution. In essence, you allow yourself to overeat one day and balance it by eating less the next. The method also helps people who occasionally overindulge and lack discipline.

If you are following the Age Reduction Diet and "binge out," these are the key guidelines when taking the feast/famine approach:

- Keep track of the extra portions you eat of protein, carbohydrates, and fats.
- Over the following day or two eliminate the same number and type of food portions you overate.
- Make sure that you drink at least six to eight glasses of pure water or vegetable or fruit juices on your low-calorie days.

If you are following the Age Reduction Diet for its life extension benefits, you can systematically use the feast/famine approach as follows:

- For five days each week, consume 30 to 35 percent more calories per day than your ideal target zone. For optimal health the additional portions should contain no more than 20 percent protein and 10 percent fat, with the remainder being composed of complex carbohydrates.
- For two days each week, drink 400 calories (eight portions) of fresh fruit and vegetable juices throughout the day. Dilute the juices in pure water at a ratio of 1:1. Also drink at least four large glasses of water throughout the day.

If you choose to use the feast/famine technique, you should be aware of the following facts:

- If you do not increase your protein consumption 40 percent on feast days, you may develop a protein deficiency.
- Some people feel nauseated, weak, and dizzy if they go through a whole day without eating solid foods.
- If you do not drink the recommended liquids on your famine days, you may become dehydrated, preventing proper cell metabolism.

Caution: If you are suffering from hypoglycemia or diabetes, you should not follow the feast/famine method.

The Six Age Reduction Diet Levels

The Age Reduction Diet offers a complete program for each of the six calorie levels listed in the target zones. Each level specifies the number of portions you should eat of each food group to provide the essential nutrients and proper balance of proteins, carbohydrates, and fats for maximum life-span. Since I have already carefully calculated the calories and composition of each food group, you won't have to count calories. For example, the number of protein portions is based on the number of usable grams of protein provided by meat, fowl, fish, dairy, vegetables, and grains and cereals. Fat portions also account for the fat contained in protein sources such as meat. Because protein requirements are based primarily on lean body weight rather than on percentage of calories, I have included a simple protein adjustment table at the bottom of each calorie level. If you are exercising to build bigger muscles or recovering from a muscle-wasting disorder, adding one or two low-fat proteins in place of carbohydrates and fat may be advantageous.

The foods in any given category—proteins, carbohydrates, fats—are freely interchangeable, and a wide variety is suggested to help you stay with the program for the rest of your lengthened life.

If you are using the Age Reduction Diet to lose weight or substantially restrict the number of calories you normally consume, you may find the following suggestions useful:

- Eat small meals throughout the day, rather than one or two large ones. Small meals provide a constant flow of energy, whereas large meals produce more energy than you immediately need, so are stored as fat.
- Do not eat refined carbohydrate foods such as candy, cookies, cakes, desserts (including most commercial desserts), typical children's breakfast cereals, waffles, and pastries; or sugar. These foods digest rapidly, create too much energy, and tend to be stored as fat.
- Avoid eating for about two hours before you go to bed. Your energy requirements are at their lowest ebb during sleep, so food eaten immediately before retiring is often stored as fat.
- "Preload" your stomach to help you eat less at mealtime. Drink five to six glasses of water. Consume the fibers recommended in Phase 4 of this diet, or eat vegetables one-half hour before meals to trigger the production of cholecystokinin, the digestive hormone that tells your hypothalamus you are full.
- Help maintain your circadian rhythms (including digestion) by eating most of your protein foods, which stimulate dopamine, in the morning and most carbohydrates, which stimulate serotonin, at night. (See Chapter 6 for a complete discussion of body rhythms.)

NOTE: If you experience chronic fatigue, weakness, or hair loss while following an Age Reduction Diet, either increase your calorie consumption to the next level or abandon the program.

The 1800-calorie diet following shows how you can distribute the required daily food portions in a typical Age Reduction Diet.

Age Reduction Diet Food Groups

Now that you've reviewed the target zone levels and found the one that's best for you, the next pages will tell you exactly how much and what kind of each food group will help you reach your target zone.

This section includes the correct portion size, nutritional information, and cooking tips for each of the following groups:

- Proteins, such as meat, fish, fowl, and dairy products
- Complex carbohydrates, such as grains and cereals, vegetables, and fruits
- Fats, such as butter and oils
- Beverages (both alcoholic and nonalcoholic)

• Optional desserts
• Condiments

As you can see, the Age Reduction Diet includes all the foods you need to live longer and enjoy it.

A Sample 1800-Calorie-Level Diet

Food	Portions
Early	
3 ounces of fish or poultry or 3 eggs*	3 proteins
1 slice of bread with 1 pat of butter	1 complex carbohydrate 1 fat
Herbal tea	
Midday	
Homemade vegetable soup—1 bowl	2 vegetables
Large fruit salad with ⅔ cup cottage cheese or 1 cup yogurt	3 fruits 2 proteins
Whole wheat English muffin with 1 pat of butter	2 complex carbohydrates 1 fat
Noncaloric beverage	
Snacks	
1 apple	1 fruit
3 whole wheat crackers of average size	1 complex carbohydrate
1 cup vegetable juice	1 vegetable
1 ounce *low-fat* cheese	1 protein
Late	
1 cup of spaghetti or pasta with tomato sauce and mushrooms	2 complex carbohydrates 1 vegetable
1 whole wheat roll with 1 pat of butter	1 complex carbohydrate 1 fat
Corn (fresh cooked, sliced off the cob, or frozen cooked), ⅔ cup	2 complex carbohydrates
Vegetable salad with 1 Tbsp. of regular dressing or 3–4 tsp. of low-calorie salad dressing	2 vegetables 1 fat
1½ cups strawberries	1 fruit
Noncaloric beverage	

*Use only one or two egg yolks and three or four egg whites.

2000-Calorie Level

Exchange Group	Daily Portion
Proteins Meat, fowl, fish, and/or dairy	6
Complex carbohydrates Grains and cereals Vegetables Fruits	11 7 6
Fats Butter and oils	5

Exchange Group Adjustments

If your ideal weight
is *more* than 215 pounds

Add:
Subtract:

2 proteins
1 fat and
1 complex carbohydrate
or
2 fats

If your ideal weight
is between 190 and 214 pounds

Add:
Subtract:

1 protein
1 fat

If your ideal weight
is between 150 and 189 pounds

No change is necessary.

If your ideal weight
is between 130 and 149 pounds

Subtract:
Add:

1 protein
1 complex carbohydrate

If your ideal weight
is *less* than 130 pounds

Subtract:
Add:

2 proteins
1 fat and
1 complex carbohydrate
or
2 complex carbohydrates

1800-Calorie Level

Exchange Group	Daily Portion
Proteins Meat, fowl, fish, and/or dairy	6
Complex carbohydrates Grains and cereals Vegetables Fruits	9 6 5
Fats Butter and oils	4

Exchange Group Adjustments

If your ideal weight is *more* than 205 pounds	Add: Subtract:	2 proteins 1 fat and 1 complex carbohydrate
If your ideal weight is between 185 and 204 pounds	Add: Subtract:	1 protein 1 fat
If your ideal weight is between 140 and 184 pounds	No change is necessary.	
If your ideal weight is between 121 and 139 pounds	Subtract: Add:	1 protein 1 fat
If your ideal weight is *less* than 120 pounds	Subtract: Add:	2 proteins 2 complex carbohydrates *or* 1 fat and 1 complex carbohydrate

1600-Calorie Level

Exchange Group	Daily Portion
Proteins Meat, fowl, fish, and/or dairy	6
Complex carbohydrates Grains and cereals Vegetables Fruits	8 6 4
Fats Butter and oils	3

Exchange Group Adjustments

If your ideal weight is *more* than 195 pounds	Add: Subtract:	2 proteins 2 complex carbohydrates
If your ideal weight is between 175 and 194 pounds	Add: Subtract:	1 protein 1 complex carbohydrate
If your ideal weight is between 135 and 174 pounds	No change is necessary.	
If your ideal weight is between 116 and 134 pounds	Subtract: Add:	1 protein 1 complex carbohydrate
If you weight *less* than 115 pounds	Subtract: Add:	2 proteins 1 fat and 1 complex carbohydrate *or* 2 complex carbohydrates

1400-Calorie Level

Exchange Group	Daily Portion
Proteins Meat, fowl, fish, and/or dairy	5
Complex carbohydrates Grains and cereals Vegetables Fruits	7 5 4
Fats Butter and oils	3

Exchange Group Adjustments

If your ideal weight is *more* than 170 pounds	Add: Subtract:	2 proteins (low fat) 1 fat and 1 complex carbohydrate
If your ideal weight is between 155 and 169 pounds	Add: Subtract:	1 protein (low fat) 1 fat (preferably) *or* 1 complex carbohydrate
If your ideal weight is between 116 and 154 pounds	No change is necessary.	
If your ideal weight is *less* than 115 pounds	Subtract: Add:	1 protein 1 complex carbohydrate

1200-Calorie Level

Exchange Group	Daily Portion
Proteins Meat, fowl, fish, and/or dairy	5
Complex carbohydrates Grains and cereals Vegetables Fruits	5 4 4
Fats Butter and oils	2–3*

Exchange Group Adjustments

If your ideal weight is *more* than 165 pounds	Add: Subtract:	2 proteins (low fat) 1 fat and 1 complex carbohydrate
If your ideal weight is between 150 and 164 pounds	Add: Subtract:	1 protein (low fat) 1 fat *or* 1 complex carbohydrate
If your ideal weight is between 111 and 149 pounds	No change is necessary.	
If your ideal weight is *less* than 110 pounds	Subtract: Add:	1 protein 1 complex carbohydrate (preferably) *or* 1 fat

---

*Less than three a day is preferable.

1000-Calorie Level

Exchange Group	Daily Portion
Proteins Meat, fowl, fish, and/or dairy	5
Complex carbohydrates Grains and cereals Vegetables Fruits	5 4 4
Fats Butter and oils	2–3*

Exchange Group Adjustments

If your ideal weight is *more* than 170 pounds	Add: Subtract:	3 proteins (low fat only) 1 fat and 2 complex carbohydrates
If your ideal weight is between 150 and 169 pounds	Add: Subtract:	2 proteins (low fat) 1 fat and 1 complex carbohydrate
If your ideal weight is between 130 and 149 pounds	Add: Subtract:	1 protein (low fat) 1 fat
If you weigh *less* than 129 pounds	No change is necessary.	

*Less than three a day is preferable

Protein Group

One protein portion equals: 65 calories
5 grams usable protein
3–4 grams fat
0 grams carbohydrate

Animal Sources

Poultry—1 ounce
    Chicken
    Cornish game hen
    Turkey
    (all without skin)

Meat—1 ounce
    Lean beef
    Organs
    Veal
    Ham (center cuts only)
    Lamb (lean only)

Fish—1 ounce
    All fresh fish except salmon
    Tuna must be canned in water

Eggs—1 small egg

Dairy—low-fat group
    Cottage cheese—⅓ cup
    Low-fat milk—¾ cup
    Skim milk or buttermilk—¾ cup
    Low-fat yogurt—½ cup
    Low-fat mozzarella—1 ounce

Dairy—high-fat group*
    Cheeses—1 ounce
    Whole milk—½ cup
    Kefir—½ cup

Vegetable Sources

Soy sprouts—1½ cups
Brussels sprouts—14 medium
Broccoli—2 cups
Mushrooms—3½ cups
Tofu or tempeh—4 ounces

---

*Because high-fat dairy products contain substantially more fat and calories than other protein sources, you should limit your consumption to four servings per week. If you are a vegetarian and must consume more, count each serving as one protein portion *and* one fat portion.

Protein Tips

- Limit your consumption of meat to eight portions per week. Meat contains a high proportion of saturated fats and carcinogenic substances and is difficult to digest. If you must eat meat, choose higher-quality grades with less fat. Also use only unsaturated fats to fulfill your fat portion requirements. Cook without oil in nonstick pans.
- Fish provides the highest-quality protein with the least calories and fat. Poultry and low-fat dairy products follow.
- If you are a vegetarian, see the Age Reduction Supplement Guide (Chapter 9) for complete instructions on the correct use of supplemental vitamin B-12. If you do not eat dairy products, review the Skeletal System Supporters in Chapter 13 for bone-building nutrients.
- Make sure you buy cheeses free of preservatives or coloring agents. Avoid "cheese foods," "processed cheese," and other fake foods.
- Be aware of the difficulty of digesting cheese and other dairy products. About 30 million people (and 60 to 80 percent of Jews, mixed Indians, blacks, and Hispanics) can't tolerate dairy products because their intestines do not produce lactase, the enzyme needed to digest

the milk sugar lactose. Common signs of lactose intolerance include bloating, gas, cramps, and diarrhea.

If you believe you might be "allergic" to cheese, check with your doctor. As a rule of thumb, if your ancestors regularly ate cheese (most northern Europeans, for example), you should be able to digest it, too. If not, you may want to add supplemental lactase (widely available in health food stores) to your dairy products.

Complex Carbohydrates Group—Grain/Cereals

One grain or cereals portion equals: 65 calories
1 gram usable protein
0 grams fat
15 grams carbohydrate

Breads	Crackers	Pancakes
Sliced bread—1 slice	Melba and white—3 crackers	4"—1
Bagel—½		
Biscuit, roll—1–2"	Flat (Akmak)—2 pieces	*Starchy Vegetables*
Cornbread—1½" cube		Corn—⅓ cup
Hamburger roll—½	*Flours*	Green beans—½ cup
Muffin (English or other)—½	All—½ cup	Parsnips—1½ cups
Pita bread—½		Peas—1½ cups
Tortilla (6")—1	*Grains*	Potatoes (with skin)—1 small
Taco shell	Millet, grits, kasha, barley, oats, wheat berries—½ cup cooked	Pumpkin—¾ cup
Cereals		Squash (acorn, winter, butternut)—½ cup
	Wheat germ—¼ cup	
Dry cereal—½ cup		Rutabaga—½ cup
Cooked cereal—½ cup	*Pasta*	Sweet potato (yams)—⅓ cup
Bran—½ cup	Rice, spaghetti, noodles, etc.—½ cup cooked	

Starch Tips

- Use only whole grain breads, pastas, cereals, and other baked goods.
- Read all labels to avoid added preservatives, sugar, and other chemicals.
- If you see an ingredient listed on the label whose name you don't understand, don't buy the product.
- The less refined your cereal products, the better. Be wary of commercial boxed cereals claiming to be "natural." They may be loaded with sugar, salt, and a host of other unnecessary elements. Check the ingredients list to be certain of what you are buying.

Vegetable Tips

- Choose a balance of vegetables from the four groups: vitamin A, vitamin C, high-mineral, and indoles. Indoles are chemicals in cru-

Complex Carbohydrates Group—Vegetables

One vegetable portion equals: 50 calories
1½ grams usable protein
0 grams fat
10 grams carbohydrate

Portion size is 1 cup for all vegetables (unless otherwise marked).

Vitamin A	*Vitamin C*	*Indoles*	*Other High-Mineral Vegetables*
Peppers	Peppers	Cauliflower	Artichoke
Dandelion greens	Kale	Brussels sprouts	Bamboo shoots (½ cup)
Carrots	Parsley (2 cups)	Broccoli	Beets
Collard leaves	Collards	Cabbage (2 cups)	Celery (1½ cups)
Kale	Turnips		Cucumber
Parsley (2 cups)	Broccoli	*Seaweeds*	Chard (1½ cups)
Spinach	Brussels sprouts	Nori	Endive (2 cups)
All greens	Mustard greens	Kombu	Eggplant
	Watercress	Wakame	Kohlrabi
	Cauliflower (2 cups)	Etc.	Lettuce (5 cups)
	Red cabbage		Mushrooms
		Vegetable Juice	Okra
			Onions
		Carrot (½ cup)	Radishes
		Other vegetable juices	Rhubarb
			Scallions
		Legumes	Sprouts
			String beans
		Lima beans	Summer squash
		Lentils	Tomatoes
		Kidney beans	Turnips
		Black beans	Water chestnuts
		Soybeans	Zucchini
		Peas	
		Chickpeas	

ciferous vegetables (broccoli, cabbage, brussels sprouts, and cauliflower) that increase enzymes to fight cancer.

· Be sure your diet contains dark green, yellow, and red vegetables. Seaweeds represent a potent source of trace minerals and other nutrients.

· Invest in a pressure cooker or vegetable steamer to prepare vegetables without oil and prevent nutrient losses from cooking. Instantly brown vegetables in your broiler without using oil.

· Vegetable juices, while high in concentrated nutrients, contain less fiber than whole vegetables. If you purchase bottled vegetable juices, be sure they contain no added salt.

· Eat most of your vegetables in their fresh, raw state to extract the maximum benefits from their vitamin, mineral, and stomach-filling fiber properties. Avoid canned and frozen vegetables, as processing

Complex Carbohydrates Group—Fruit

One portion of fruit equals: 75 calories
0 grams usable protein
0 grams fat
19 grams carbohydrate

Vitamin C Fruits	*Other Fruits*
Acerola—10 ounces	Apples—1 medium
Guava—⅗ medium	Apricots—4 medium
Strawberries—20 large	Berries—⅘ cup
Papaya—⅔ medium	Banana—1 very small
Orange—1 medium	Cranberries—¾ cup
Lemon—3 medium	Cherries—⅔ cup
Grapefruit—¾ medium	Dates—10 medium
Elderberries—3½ ounces	Figs—3 small
Cantaloupe—½ melon	Grapes—25 medium
Tangerines—3 small	Kiwi—1
Raspberries—⅔ cup	Prunes—2 medium
Loganberries—⅔ cup	Pineapple—1 cup
Honeydew melon—½ medium	Pear—⅗
Lime—3 medium	Plums—3 medium
Kumquat—5–6 medium	Peaches—2–3 medium
	Persimmon—1
	Pomegranate—1
	Pumpkin—10 ounces
	Raisins and currants—3 Tbsp.
	Watermelon—1½ cups

has robbed them of most of their vitamins, minerals, and other nutrients. It has also added unwanted sugar, sodium, and preservatives.

Fruit Tips

- Space your intake of fruit throughout the day to provide a steady source of instant energy. Eat apart from meals (not with other food).
- Concentrate your fruit choices on those that contain a lot of water and fiber (for example, strawberries, watermelon, papaya). The water and fiber dilute the fruit sugar so it doesn't enter the bloodstream too quickly, causing an excessive insulin response.
- Avoid overeating dates, figs, raisins, currants, plums, and cooked and dried fruits. They contain a concentrated dose of fruit sugar and calories.
- Dilute all fruit juices with water. (A good ratio is 1:1.) Remember, fruit juices contain a concentrated amount of sugar without the fiber found in whole fruits. Use your taste buds as a guide to the sugar content of fruit juices. For example, grape juice, currant juice, and cherry juice all taste sweet because they contain high amounts of sugar.

Fats Group

One portion of fat equals: 50 calories
0 grams usable protein
5½ grams fat
0 grams carbohydrate

Saturated	*Unsaturated*
Butter—1 tsp.	*Oils*
Cream cheese—1 Tbsp.	
Cream—1 tsp. (half and half)	Vegetable, olive, corn, wheat germ oil—1 tsp.
Lard—1 tsp.	
Sour cream—1 Tbsp.	*Fruits*
Shredded coconut—1 Tbsp.	
	Olives—5 small
	Avocado—⅛ medium
	Salad Dressing
	Regular—2 tsp.
	Low-cal—3 Tbsp.
	Mayonnaise—1 tsp.
	Nuts
	Nut butter—2 tsp.
	Almonds—10 whole
	Cashews—3–4
	Macadamia—3
	Peanuts—15 whole
	Pecans—2 large
	Walnuts—6 small
	Other nuts—6 small
	All Seeds
	Sesame, sunflower, etc.—2 tsp.

Fat Tips

- Balance your diet between saturated and unsaturated fats. If you eat dairy products and other animal protein, use only unsaturated fats.
- Use vegetable oils protected against oxidation by artificial antioxidants.
- Chill stews and soups in your refrigerator. Remove the coagulated fat and then heat and serve. Use nonstick pots and pans that don't require butter and oil in cooking. Boil, bake, and poach instead of frying in oil and butter. Sauté and season foods in water or clear stock. Use uncreamed cottage cheese in place of creamed. Use egg whites in place of whole egg. (Egg whites are pure protein. The yellow is pure fat.) Quick broil meat, fish, and poultry under the broiler instead of frying. Marinate with wine, vinegar, lemon juice, and vegetable broth in place of fats and oils. Use whipped butter instead of regular butter.

It contains one-half the calories per tablespoon. Use dietary salad dressings in place of regular ones. Combine lemon juice with basil and yogurt for a low-calorie salad dressing. Always mix mayonnaise with yogurt to cut calories and add nutrients.

Beverage Tips

- Drink six to eight glasses of pure water a day. (Mineral water or purified water are best.)
- Herbal tea and decaffeinated coffee are not acceptable as a pure water substitute.
- Drink caffeinated beverages between 3 and 4 P.M. to avoid disrupting body rhythms. (See Chapter 6 for more information.)
- Vegetable juices free of added salt and sugar are a good source of pure water and nutrients. Vegetables act like a sophisticated filter and nutrient additive system.
- Dry wine is better than sweet wine because it contains less sugar.
- If you are overweight, do not drink more than two alcoholic drinks per week (which count as two servings of grains and cereals each). If you are maintaining a low-calorie diet, do not consume more than seven alcoholic drinks per week.

Beverages

0-Calorie Beverages	100-Calorie Alcoholic Beverages
Mineral water Herbal tea Decaffeinated coffee Coffee and tea (no more than 2 cups daily) Consomme and clear broth	Light beer—10 ounces Regular beer—8 ounces Liquor—1½ ounces Dry wine—4 ounces Sweet wine—3 ounces

Dessert and Sweetener Tips

- Use desserts and sweeteners *sparingly*. If you are using the Age Reduction Diet to lose excess weight, do not eat any desserts or use any sweeteners during the first two weeks of the diet. Those maintaining a low-calorie diet can eat up to four dessert portions and four sweetener portions each week. Each dessert portion counts as one complex carbohydrate and one fat portion. Each sweetener serving counts as one fruit portion.
- Read the labels on "natural" goodies to make sure that sugar isn't listed as sucrose, dextrose, fructose, or honey.
- Desserts sweetened with fruit juice or fructose do not cause a quick release of insulin.

Desserts and Sweeteners

Desserts—100 calories	Sweeteners—50 calories	Sweeteners—0 calories
Tofutti—½ cup Frozen yogurt—½ cup Popcorn (minus oil and salt)—1 quart Whole grain cookies and other baked goods sweetened with fruit juices (portion size depends on calories and fat content)	Raw sorghum—1 Tbsp. Date sugar—1 Tbsp. Fructose—1 Tbsp. Raw molasses—1 Tbsp. Sugar-free jam and jelly—1 Tbsp. Carob powder—1 Tbsp. Barley malt—1 Tbsp. Dried fruit—20 grams	Aspartame (NutraSweet)

Condiment Tips

- When used in moderation to flavor foods, condiments contain few or no calories.
- Substitute these condiments for oils, mayonnaise, and other high-calorie sauces.
- Commercial soups, including consomme, stocks, and bouillon, generally contain excessive amounts of sodium. Low-sodium versions are sold in health food storers and some supermarkets.

Condiments

One condiment portion equals: 0 calories

Cornstarch (for thickening sauces and gravies) Plain gelatin Herbs and spices Horseradish (uncreamed) Hot sauce Ketchup (sugar- and honey-free) NutraSweet (aspartame)	Lemon juice Lime juice Salt substitutes—low-sodium soy sauce, Tamari sauce Kelp Sea salt (in moderation) Vegit Soups—consomme, fat-free stock, bouillon

PHASE 3: HOW TO CREATE YOUR PERSONAL AGE REDUCTION EXERCISE PROGRAM

The next phases of the Age Reduction Diet are designed to support your calorie-counting efforts. Exercise helps you lose excess weight and reduce your biological age by:

- Suppressing your appetite
- Activating brown fat and sodium pump metabolism
- Releasing growth hormones to burn fat and build muscle
- Burning stored fat during long, strenuous workouts and increasing metabolic rate for up to six hours afterward

• Preventing the muscular wasting that occurs on most weight-loss programs. Loss of lean muscle mass accelerates aging by reducing strength, physical coordination, and energy requirements.

Chapter 11 will tell you all you need to know to create the fitness program that's right for you. For the purposes of the Age Reduction Diet, the most important type of exercise is aerobic. Sustained oxygen-demanding exercises will burn up the most calories and stimulate your energy and brown fat metabolisms to peak efficiency levels. To benefit you must perform aerobic exercises at least one hour a day, three days a week. Table 31 indicates the number of pounds you can lose per month solely from exercising while eating the number of calories that would maintain a constant body weight if you were not exercising.

However, since the primary goal of the Age Reduction Diet is to reduce your biological age, I strongly urge you to develop a program that addresses each of the six fitness factors discussed in the next chapter.

One final note about exercise: If you are a professional athlete or are extremely active, exercise will enhance your appetite, not suppress it.

TABLE 31

Weight Loss from Aerobic Exercise

Hours of Aerobic Activity (Weekly)	Body Weight						
	100 lbs.	120 lbs.	150 lbs.	175 lbs.	200 lbs.	250 lbs.	
½	.3	.3	.4	.5	.5	.6	
1	.5	.7	.8	.9	1.1	1.2	
1½	.8	1.0	1.2	1.4	1.6	1.8	Weight
2½	1.4	1.6	2.0	2.4	2.7	3.0	loss in
5	2.7	3.4	4.0	5.0	5.5	6.0	pounds
10	5.1	6.0	8.0	10.0	11.0	12.0	per
15	8.0	10.0	12.0	14.0	16.0	18.0	month
20	12.0	15.0	17.0	19.0	22.0	24.0	

PHASE 4: SUPPORTING THE DIET WITH STRESS REDUCTION

Although the myriad aging effects of stress have already been reported in Chapter 5, negative stress also exerts some particular effects on fat gain. By learning to cope with negative stress, you can also:

• Eliminate the psychological need to overeat
• Prevent the release of excessive cortisol and a fat-promoting hormone discussed earlier in this chapter
• Balance the autonomic nervous system, so that the sympathetic nervous system keeps your metabolism running at peak efficiency

TABLE 32

Potential Body Fat Regulators

Supplement	Amount	Effect
Growth hormone stimulators	*See* individual supplements in the section Growth Hormone Stimulators (Chapter 13).	Release growth hormone that burns fat and builds muscles
Evening primrose oil with gamma linolenic acid	1–3 gm	Synthesizes prostaglandins that activate brown fat to burn calories as heat in overweight people
DHEA (dehydroepiandrosterone)	*See* Age Reduction Supplement Guide in Chapter 9.	Adrenal gland hormone that removes fat and increases vitality
L-phenylalanine	400–800 mg.	Decreases appetite by releasing cholecystokinin
Vitamin C Vitamin B-6	400 mg. 20–30 mg. (1 hour before eating)	Work with L-phenylalanine
L-tyrosine	500–1500 mg. (in the morning or on empty stomach)	Stimulates dopamine and increases noradrenaline to activate your brown fat
Vitamin C Vitamin B-6	400 mg. 20–30 mg.	Work with L-tyrosine
Guar gum fiber and psyllium seed husks	2–4 gm (use 1 hour before meals in beverages)	Swells in stomach to control appetite and eating; inhibits absorption of fat calories; regulates insulin response to prevent fat gain
Caffeine in beverages	2 strong cups of coffee	Stimulates brown fat to burn calories
Insulin-response improvers	*See* individual supplements in the section Insulin Response Improvers (Chapter 13)	Control excessive insulin that results in weight gain
Energy and muscle aids	*See* individual supplements in the sections Energy Aids and Muscle Aids (Chapter 13)	Increase cellular and physical energy to burn calories and lose weight
Glycerol	1 tsp. 15–30 min. before each meal	Signals satiety and reduces food intake

See the Age Reduction Supplement Guide in Chapter 9 for complete instructions on the safe and correct use of supplements.

and the parasympathetic nervous system informs your hypothalamus (through the hormone cholecystokinin and other digestive processes) that you are full.

After years of study I can unequivocally say that *stress is the number one reason for overeating.*

If you feel that excessive stress plays a role in your weight, I urge you to review Chapter 5 to find the stress-reduction technique that's best for you.

PHASE 5: SUPPLEMENTING YOUR DIET

The supplements listed in Table 32 will give your metabolism a nudge in the right direction, help your hunger pains to vanish, fortify your energy, melt away excess fat, and generally make your journey to optimal weight and longevity a happy and safe one. (See the Age Reduction Supplement Guide in Chapter 9 for complete instructions on the correct use of supplements.)

11

You Can Fight Aging with Activity and Exercise

When exercise first became fashionable in the early seventies, it was imbued with the curative powers of a bath at Lourdes.

While this concept sold a lot of running shoes and warm-up suits, it did little to prepare a sedentary population adequately for transforming inflexible, flabby bodies into fit, healthy ones.

Most of us attacked exercise with all the vengeance we usually reserve for our work. Busy executives crammed an hour of racquetball into a lunch hour. Others learned to take their own pulse while running in place to ensure they were reaching 90 percent of their maximum heart rate. Aerobics instructors exhorted sweating students, "If it doesn't hurt, it doesn't work."

Today fitness has almost outgrown its fashionable origins. Instead, it has found a place in the American consciousness as one of the basic necessities of life.

Under the right conditions, physical exercise and recreation can reduce your biological age by:

- Reducing age-related deterioration of muscle tone, lean body mass, endurance, reaction speed, work capacity, pulmonary functions, neuroendocrinological information systems, and bone mass
- Conditioning the cardiovascular system, thereby protecting the heart and blood vessels, reversing arteriosclerosis, and controlling blood pressure, diabetes, and carbohydrate intolerance
- Nourishing cells and organs (especially the brain) by improving blood circulation and increasing the supply of oxygen and nutrients
- Using free fatty acids for 80 percent of the calories needed during prolonged exercise. Excess free fatty acids are a metabolic shift of aging that depresses the immune system and contributes to the de-

velopment of atherosclerosis. So using up free fatty acids during exercise delays aging

- Increasing beneficial HDL cholesterol and lowering harmful LDL cholesterol
- Improving metabolic efficiency so that food is converted into fuel instead of fat
- Triggering the release of growth hormones, which improve the immune system, build muscles, burn off fat, and produce a sense of well-being
- Producing lactic acid, a powerful chelation agent that removes accumulated toxic metals from the body
- Improving the ability to sleep and relax, both of which are critical to repairing cells and maintaining homeostasis
- Triggering the release of endorphins and enkephalins, powerful brain chemicals that create a sense of exhilaration, relieve anxiety and depression, and improve stress responses
- Increasing adaptability to weather fluctuations, another form of stress

Pretty impressive, wouldn't you say? The supporting studies are even more so.

DOCUMENTING THE BENEFITS OF EXERCISE

In the "largest human biological study undertaken of life and death," the American Cancer Society followed the lives of more than one million American men and women for twenty years. Information was collected through 68,000 volunteer interviewers. One of the key findings is: "Physical exercise lengthens life and wards off heart disease and stroke." This was particularly true among men.

Studies of athletes conducted in 1972 by T. Khosla, of the Department of Medical Statistics, Welsh National School of Medicine, suggest that people who exercise benefit not just from the exercise itself but from its ancillary effects on smoking and obesity. Khosla found that athletes were less likely to get fat or take up smoking at an early age and that this resulted in life extension benefits.

The importance of exercise, as compared to other longevity predictors, was investigated in 1977 by Charles L. Rose and Michel L. Cohen at the Veterans Administrative Outpatient Clinic, Boston. Their conclusions are based on the study of sixty-nine specific longevity variables for 500 selected white males whose death certificates were recorded in Boston City Hall during 1965. Of the sixty-nine predictors, they ranked exercise as ninth in importance. The eight factors they consider even more influential are:

- Fewer illnesses
- Younger appearance
- Less smoking
- Less worry

- Rural residence
- Sense of humor

- Higher occupational level
- Off-the-job activity

Pay attention to these factors. Don't expect to reach maximum life-span from a healthy diet and exercise only.

Perhaps even more important than the years that exercise can add to your life is the *enjoyment* that exercise can add to your years! Older people who are physically fit and active are also more alert, energetic, and able to experience joy than their sedentary counterparts, who are more susceptible to the senility and debility so common in our society.

The Pros and Cons
of Different Kinds of Exercise

When it comes to age reduction, all exercises are not equal. Some exercises are not beneficial, and too much exercise is downright detrimental.

In 1977 Anthony P. Polednak and Albert Damon, researchers at Harvard, selected a fairly homogenous group of Harvard graduates and divided them into three categories: major athletes (men who lettered in one or more sports), minor athletes (regular participants in sports who did not receive letters), and non-athletes (men with no record of sports participation). At the time of the study, 90.9 percent of those selected had died, and the age and cause of death were obtained from death certificates.

Polednak and Damon reported a result they found "surprising": ". . . minor athletes were generally and, for the most part, significantly longer lived than major athletes and non-athletic classmates. . . . In percentages of men still alive and in percentages of men reaching ages 70 and 75, minor athletes were consistently and for the most part significantly higher."

Also noteworthy is the fact that the three groups did not differ in death rates from infections, neoplasms, suicide, or cardiovascular disease, which was the leading cause of death in all groups. This indicates that minor athletes, though equally susceptible to certain causes of death, will succumb to them at a more advanced age.

Why do minor athletes outlive their more accomplished athletic counterparts? I believe it's because the body perceives excessive, abusive, or highly competitive exercise as a form of negative stress. It reacts by triggering "fight or flight" responses such as releasing adrenaline and cortisol, raising blood pressure, diverting energy from normal maintenance processes, and flooding the muscles with lactic acid, which if it isn't used up during exercise, creates stiff, sore muscles. Competitive exercise creates chronic negative stress, with all the life-shortening fallout discussed in Chapter 6. "Brute" sports—such as football, hockey, and soccer—tend to shorten life-spans. "Endurance" sports—such as track, cross-country skiing, and swimming—tend to lengthen them.

Clearly, if your fitness goal is to earn extra years (rather than trophies), it would be unwise to approach exercise with the intensity, competitiveness, and pressure for perfection so common to our culture.

THE PRIMARY FITNESS FACTORS

There are six primary fitness factors that influence longevity. They are:
- Endurance and cardiorespiratory function
- Strength and muscular development
- Speed and reaction time
- Coordination and balance
- Flexibility
- Neuromuscular relaxation

Although each factor has an important contribution to make, very few fitness programs address more than two or three. The result is a program that is incomplete, unbalanced, and potentially self-destructive.

Skin-Deep Fitness

Sarah Fingel, a former client, offers a vivid example of fitness that is only skin deep. When Sarah first came to see me about improving her health, fitness, and overall prospects for longevity, I must admit I was a little surprised. Most of my clients showed up with some obvious ailment that had catalyzed their interest in improving health. Sarah looked fit as a fiddle. Her weight was moderate, her muscle tone well developed.

She explained that she worked out with free weights religiously three tmes a week. However, she was concerned that her resting pulse rate was 78 (it should have been less than 72). Her blood pressure was slightly elevated to 138/80, instead of the 120/70 that is ideal for a woman of her age (twenty-seven), height (five feet six inches), and weight (122 pounds).

I explained to her that strength was only one of six fitness factors and that we would need to analyze her fitness in other categories. For this I used a battery of eight simple tests for which I've developed a computer program.

On completing my computer analysis, I graded Sarah on each of the six primary fitness factors as follows:
- Endurance and cardiorespiratory function   F
- Strength   A
- Speed and reaction time   B
- Coordination and balance   C
- Flexibility   D
- Neuromuscular relaxation   D

Sarah's fitness scores could easily be predicted by the exercises she did and did not do. However, that isn't always the case. Some people are naturally fast or strong or flexible (or slow or weak or inflexible) without any corresponding physical activity. (The reasons for this will become apparent as we discuss each fitness factor in more detail.)

To improve Sarah's fitness in each of the four factors in which she had scored poorly, I recommended that she adopt some different kinds of exercises. I gave her a copy of Table 33, which follows, to outline her choices.

Sarah chose jogging and aerobics classes to improve her endurance and cardiorespiratory function. She also chose to take up yoga, since it would improve her coordination and balance, flexibility, and neuromuscular relaxation abilities all at the same time.

With very little encouragement from me, Sarah incorporated these new exercises into her regular fitness program. Within six months she not only

TABLE 33

Activities for Each Fitness Factor

Endurance and Cardiorespiratory Function	Strength and Muscular Development	Speed and Reaction Time
Aerobics classes	Acrobatics	Auto racing
Aerobic dancing	Basketball	Acrobatics
Basketball	Bicycling	Badminton
Boxing	Body building	Baseball
Bicycling	Boxing	Basketball
Brisk walking	Calisthenics	Bobsledding
Hiking	Gymnastics	Boxing
Jogging	Handball	Fencing
Jumping rope	Heavy rope	Football
Lacrosse	Heavy hands	Frisbee throwing
Mid- and long-distance running	Hockey	Gymnastics
Motorcross	Isometrics	Handball
Mountain climbing	Judo	Hockey
Nordic skiing	Martial arts	Jai alai
Rowing	Motorcross	Judo
Skating	Mountain climbing	Martial arts
Snowshoeing	Racquetball	Motorcross
Swimming	Rowing	Polo (horse)
Trampolining	Squash	Polo (water)
Water polo	Snowshoeing	Racquetball
	Sprinting	Skiing (alpine)
	Swimming	Sprinting
	Tennis	Soccer
	Track and field	Squash
	Weight-lifting	Tennis
	Wrestling	Table tennis
	Yoga	Volleyball
		Wild game hunting

looked and felt better, she had lowered her resting heart rate to 68 and her blood pressure to 119/70.

What follows is a brief description of each fitness factor and why it is important.

Endurance and Cardiorespiratory Function

Endurance is the ability to perform a physical activity for a long period of time without experiencing fatigue. Shoveling snow, carrying heavy groceries for distances, doing leg kicks in aerobics classes—all these activities increase your endurance. Cardiorespiratory function influences endurance by dictating how hard your heart and lungs have to work to keep up with energy demands.

Aerobic (high oxygen demand) exercises are best for improving endurance. Almost any exercise can become aerobic if it's sustained long

Coordination and Balance		Flexibility	Neuromuscular Relaxation
Acrobatics	Horseback riding	Flotation tank floating	Archery
Auto racing	Horseshoe throwing	Hypnosis	Camping
Archery	Judo	Dancing	Croquet
Baseball	Jumping rope	Martial arts	Fishing
Basketball	Martial arts	Meditation	Flotation tank floating
Badminton	Motorcross	Stretching	Frisbee throwing
Billiards	Racquetball	Tai Chi	Gardening
Bobsledding	Rowing	Yoga	Gliding
Body surfing	Skating		Golf
Bowling	Skiing		Hypnosis
Boxing	Sky diving		Kite flying
Croquet	Soccer		Martial arts
Curling	Shooting		Meditation
Dancing	Sailing		Tai Chi
Diving	Squash		Yoga
Fencing	Surfing		
Football	Table tennis		
Frisbee throwing	Tai Chi		
Golf	Tennis		
Gliding	Trampolining		
Gymnastics	Yoga		
Handball			
Hang gliding			
Hockey			

enough. After about one and one-half minutes of sustained activity, your heart and lungs are forced to supply increased oxygen to the muscles to produce energy. When the heart and lungs are gradually and consistently made to work harder for brief periods (about twenty minutes per session), it makes them stronger and more efficient. To experience real age-reduction benefits, however, you need a session of at least thirty minutes.

If you're overweight, over forty years old, lead a sedentary life-style, and have any of these medical problems—problems with your joints or muscles, respiratory ailments, high blood pressure, diabetes, arteriosclerosis, or heart disease—consult a physician before engaging in the Age Reduction Program. If you are allowed to exercise vigorously, do not try to reach your target heart rate zone too rapidly.

The benefits of improved endurance and cardiorespiratory function are many: It prevents heart disease; prevents or reverses arteriosclerosis; inhibits diabetes; controls blood pressure; enhances the immune system; triggers the release of growth hormone, which prevents age-related increases in fat deposition and muscle degeneration; lowers cholesterol levels; prevents lung demineralization; and actively reduces your biological age. To earn these benefits, you must perform aerobic exercises at least two or more times each week.

In addition, you must exercise strenuously enough to give your heart and lungs a workout but not cause free radical damage. See Table 34 for your ideal heart rate while exercising. (Please note that your maximum rate decreases with age.) Overexertion may produce oxygen radicals that age cells prematurely. You can take your own pulse by placing your third and fourth fingers just to one side of your Adam's apple. Count the beats for ten seconds and then multiply by six to determine your active heart rate per minute. (NOTE: If your resting pulse is higher than 85 beats per

TABLE 34

Target Heart Rates for Aerobic Exercise

Age (Years)	Target Heart Rate Zone	
	70% Minimum	85% Maximum
20	140	170
25	136	166
30	133	161
35	129	157
40	126	153
45	121	147
50	116	141
55	112	136
60	108	132
65	105	127
70	102	123
75 or more	age + 20	age + 30

minute, you may be suffering from circulatory, lung, or blood problems. Consult your doctor immediately.)

As a matter of personal preference, I don't use a mechanized Target Zone Method for improving my cardiorespiratory function. (You can bet centenarians don't measure their heart rate.) I prefer a natural method called Fartlek Interval Training.

The premise of this method is that you alternate strenuous and moderate exercise in the same session, depending on how you feel. For example, while riding a bicycle I might sprint for half a mile, then return to a more leisurely pace until I feel able to sprint again. The main difference between this and Target Zone Training is that the discipline for exertion comes from the inside out, rather than from the outside in. It works with your body instead of against it. Faratlek Interval Training is ideal for anyone who is sufficiently in tune with his or her body to tell the difference between fatigue and laziness.

A caution: If you've been sedentary up till now, don't just leap into an exercise program overnight. Remember that your body regards abusive exercise as a form of negative stress, which may be worse than no exercise at all. Rather than attacking an exercise program, begin gradually to accommodate one. Start slowly and work *with* your body rather than *against* it.

Strength

Strength is the ability to summon physical force against a source of resistance.

Anaerobic (low oxygen demand) exercises are best for developing strength. Anaerobic exercises are those of short duration (ten to ninety seconds) that rely on chemical reactions and oxygen already in the muscles to produce energy.

As with endurance, you build strength by gradually and consistently overtaxing your muscles for brief periods. Each muscle group should be worked out in a variety of overlapping ways to develop *overall* strength, as compared to *specific* strength. Lifting weights, for example, may help you to increase the specific strength of your biceps, but that may not help you to throw a baseball farther. Throwing a baseball requires the coordinated strength of your arm, wrist, back, shoulder, and stomach muscles.

If you've ever pulled a muscle, you've probably been surprised by the number of movements, seemingly unconnected, that suddenly become painful. That's because it requires the coordinated efforts of many muscles to make even the simplest movement. So it's the balanced strength of all muscles that's important. Strong stomach muscles, for example, help protect your vulnerable lower back. Strong leg, arm, and back muscles help you to lift and carry objects without undue effort or strain. Strong muscles overall help to reduce age-related muscle deterioration, loss of energy, and susceptibility to injury.

I do offer one general warning, however: Overbuilt muscles may be hazardous to your health. Those bulging, sculpted muscles you see proudly displayed in body-building magazines actually shorten life-span by inhibiting flexibility, distorting proper joint function, and creating the negative stress discussed earlier—not to mention developing an oppressive narcissism that is the opposite of the easygoing, outer-directed longevity personality described in Chapter 5.

To increase your overall strength, choose several activities that you enjoy from Table 33: "Activities for Each Fitness Factor." Try to choose exercises to strengthen the upper and lower limbs at least once a week so your entire body gets stronger.

Speed and Reaction Time

Speed is self-explanatory. Reaction time is the speed with which your nervous system receives information, processes it, and produces the appropriate response. Age-related deterioration of reaction time is responsible for many accidental deaths involving cars, stairs, slippery sidewalks, and countless other everyday hazards.

Even more important, the deterioration of reaction time is one symptom of nervous system deterioration, a primary cause of neuroendocrinological aging.

Developing speed for its own sake takes a toll on your organs and muscles that will ultimately shorten your life. However, developing the ability to move and react quickly can substantially lengthen it.

Speed requires a burst of instantaneous energy. Activities that require speed are considered anaerobic because they rely on chemical energy already present in cells and tissues rather than on an inflow of oxygen to produce energy. The ability to develop speed is partly determined by genetic predisposition. Your muscles contain three different types of fibers: fast or sprint fibers; slow or endurance fibers; and fibers that contain characteristics of both. DNA decides which fibers will make up your muscles in what proportions.

Regardless of genetic predisposition, you can increase your speed and reaction time by indulging in sports (such as tennis) that require short, fast runs and accurate and speedy reactions. See Table 33 for the exercises that appeal to you. Then integrate them into your regular fitness program at least twice a week.

Coordination and Balance

Coordination and balance, which includes hand-eye and foot-eye coordination, timing, accuracy, and agility, is controlled primarily by the neuroendocrine system.

One of the key factors in improving your coordination and balance is rhythmic, natural motion. Muscles, like the cells of which they are composed, have a memory—two memories, actually: yours and that of the human species. When you perform a natural rhythmic activity like walking, your muscles remember how to do it with a minimum of effort or strain. When you perform an unnatural, awkward activity like lifting very heavy barbells, your muscles don't know how to coordinate themselves to perform this task. The result is strained and torn muscles, hernias, and other assorted injuries.

Wood chopping offers a fine example of the pleasures of coordination and balance. Remember how it feels when you do it? The air outside is a little cool, your muscles somewhat stiff. Your first few swings are a little choppy. Once you start warming up, though, you fall right into the swing of things. Gravity pulls the axe or hatchet down in a circular motion. Centrifugal force boosts it back up again. Your strokes are smooth, even, rhythmic. You find you can place the cut exactly where you want it. The wood splits in a satisfying way. And suddenly you realize that hours have passed without your having been aware of it . . . or of any bodily fatigue.

That's coordination and balance.

Centenarians understand this without even thinking about it. Spend enough time in a field, and you learn how to work it with an economy of effort.

One of the best ways to develop coordination and balance is to choose an activity you enjoy—jazz dancing, for example. Begin to practice simple steps over and over, gradually increasing the complexity of the movements. Since your muscles have a memory, you'll eventually find that the grace and coordination you experience in one activity spills over into others. See Table 33 for a list of choices, then work with your choice at least twice a week.

Flexibility

Flexibility is the ability to move, twist, turn, and stretch without experiencing pain, strain, or injury. It is one of the most important fitness factors for longevity.

Flexibility is as much a frame of mind as it is freedom of movement. In intellectual terms, flexibility and adaptability promote longevity by reducing stress and helping to prevent hardening of the arteries. In physical terms, flexibility promotes longevity by providing a greater flow of oxygen and nutrients to the cells and by protecting the spinal discs.

Interestingly, flexibility of the mind influences flexibility of the body. In yoga, for example, one stretches to the limit of comfort, then reaches into the mind for soothing thoughts or images that relax the muscles to stretch further. Conscious deep breathing releases tension, and more meaningful and painless progress is made.

Oriental medicine has long related flexibility to longevity. The Chinese believe that flexibility positively alters the flow of vital energy and returns the body to homeostasis. Western doctors such as chiropractors and osteopaths have found a connection between deteriorating discs and spinal stiffness, as well as between joint calcification and the failure to use joints to their fullest extension.

Without a doubt, the best activity to increase flexibility is yoga. Done correctly, it is simple, complete, and perfectly balanced. Even if you choose yoga, however, I recommend that you pay close attention to your mind's role in increasing flexibility. Success in this area may be easier than you think. Table 33 on fitness factor activities includes several mental routes to flexibility.

Neuromuscular Relaxation

Neuromuscular relaxation is the process by which the mind relaxes the muscles, providing the deep-level nourishment and rest required for longevity.

The tone, or resting tension, of your voluntary and involuntary muscles is determined by electrical signals sent to the brain. Too many signals create stiff muscles; too few signals result in paralysis. Both aerobic and anaerobic exercises bombard the brain with stimulation, which it translates into signals sent to the muscles. That's why most exercises create stiff, sore, contracted muscles. What's needed is some form of compensation, a relaxation response to balance the demand for activity.

Your autonomic nervous system, through the parasympathetic nervous system, creates the relaxation response. When it does, your nervous system sharply reduces its release of the stress-related chemicals adrenaline and cortisol. It also reduces your heart rate, oxygen consumption, and blood pressure; relaxes your muscles; slows and deepens your breathing; improves your physical dexterity; clarifies your thoughts; eliminates depression and fatigue; improves reaction time, coordination, and muscle control; increases flexibility, power, and muscular force; reduces fatigue from exertion; and improves the quality of your sleep.

Unfortunately, few Americans ever experience real relaxation. We travel from tenuous sleep through tension-filled days, with nary a respite in sight—that is, until our bodies demand time out by developing some dreadful disease, such as angina, coronary heart disease, or high blood pressure. Often we escape into activities we call relaxing: reading books, watching television, visiting friends, cooking, pursuing hobbies. While these activities may provide a much needed change of pace, they do not provide neuromuscular relaxation.

So what does? Yoga, meditation, hypnosis. Much has been written about these useful relaxation techniques. I practice Tai Chi Chuan for deep relaxation, stress control, and to develop internal power that can instantly turn my body from a reposed state into an effective weapon.

And then there's another relatively recent neuromuscular relaxation technique. It's called a flotation tank, and it looks like a small closet turned onto its side. The tank is lightproof, soundproof, and filled with ten inches of heavily salted water.

It may sound claustrophobic, but it isn't. Once the cover of the tank settles into place, you lose all sense of the confines of space, time, gravity, or even of the tank. Deprived of stimulation, you experience an unprecedented sense of freedom.

Floating in an isolation tank allows your body and mind to unfold as effortlessly as a Japanese fan. Your mind, released from the necessity of processing external information, turns inward. Creative, intuitive whispers, usually drowned out by the clamor of consciousness, emerge with brilliant clarity. Released from the forces of gravity and physical demands, your body dilates its blood vessels, speeding up the flow of oxygen and nutrients into your cells and the flow of accumulated wastes out of it. It is truly an extraordinary experience.

It also produces extraordinary effects.

Several studies using an electromyograph (EMG), which measures muscular tension, have compared floaters with other groups who used meditation or progressive relaxation. In every study, floaters were more quickly and deeply relaxed than non-floaters. In addition, one study found that the significant stress reduction found in floaters persisted for up to three weeks after a single float of thirty minutes to one hour.

And you thought you could never get fit lying on your back!

DEVELOPING YOUR OWN FITNESS PROGRAM

Before designing your fitness program, take a hard look at your current priorities. Do you still consider exercise an activity to be sandwiched in between "more important" commitments like business meetings or dinner dates? If you do, you are selling your life short. In the best of all possible worlds, your time would be equally and harmoniously divided among work, physical recreation, and social interaction. All are equally important to longevity.

So don't be a Scrooge about spending time on exercise. Give yourself the time and permission to abandon yourself to physical activities you enjoy. It can only make you happier, healthier, and more productive in every other area of your life.

The Three Keys to Fitness

There are three key considerations in designing your own fitness program: pleasure, completeness, and consistency.

Pleasure is probably the most important. If you don't enjoy it, you won't do it. Choose activities you really love, and change them as needed.

Completeness means that you've addressed each of the six primary fitness factors in your choices of activities. In some cases, one exercise will serve three fitness factors, so it isn't as complicated as it seems.

Consistency means that you perform these activities for the minimum time described below:

- Endurance activities in forty-minute sessions at least three times a week
- Strength-building activities in thirty-minute sessions at least twice a week (can be done on endurance days)
- Flexibility-improving activities in twenty-minute sessions at least three times a week, preferably five times
- Neuromuscular relaxation activities in thirty-minute sessions at least three times a week, preferably after endurance activities.

In broad strokes, your fitness program should begin with a warm-up period of stretching to increase blood flow to the muscles and reduce risk of injury. This should be followed by endurance and/or strength-building activities. If you've been working in your target heart range, don't move directly into strength-building activities. Instead, give yourself a chance to cool down by walking and stretching. Excess blood trapped in the muscles may cause unnecessary stiffness, dizziness, or nausea. Once you've completed your endurance or strength-building activities, treat yourself to some form of neuromuscular relaxation. It's better than a hot Jacuzzi, but you can do that, too.

Please remember that the program I've just described is the ideal to strive for. And again, let me emphasize: If you've been sedentary up to now, I do not recommend that you tackle everything at once. Begin with one exercise and stay with it until you feel comfortable. Then add another exercise. If you are just beginning endurance activities, pace yourself at 60 percent of your target heart range, rather than 70 or 80 percent.

You should consult your physician before you adopt any exercise program. Take it easy once you begin. Eventually your exercise program should burn up about 2000 calories per week and allow your body to bend, twist, and stretch in different directions. For maximum age-reduction results, moderate exercise four or more times a week is better than overstrenuous exercise two or three times each week.

I strongly urge you to start using neuromuscular relaxation techniques today. You will not only experience immediate benefits in your everyday life; they will also make your transition from being sedentary to being fit a more effortless one.

I have included a chart of my current exercise program (Table 35). Although it isn't right for everyone, it suits me.

The key factor to my fitness program is flexibility—not just physical

TABLE 35

Dr. Kaufman's Fitness Program

	Early Morning	Afternoon	Evening
Monday	Martial arts class (1 hr.)	Bicycle or walk on local errands (when schedule permits)	Jacuzzi and optional swim (1 hr.). If I watch TV (on rare occasions), I aerobic rebound or ride a stationary bicycle or hit a punching bag.
Tuesday	Aerobic rebound or bicycle and martial arts (1–2 hr.)	(Same as Monday)	(Same as Monday)
Wednesday	Martial arts class (1 hr.)	(Same as Monday)	Martial arts class (1½ hr.)
Thursday	Aerobic rebound or bicycle and martial arts (1–2 hr.)	(Same as Monday)	(Same as Monday)
Friday	Martial arts class (1 hr.)	(Same as Monday)	(Same as Monday)
Saturday	Martial arts (1–2 hr.)	Bicycle and/or roller skate (1–3 hr.)	(Same as Monday)
Sunday	Martial arts (1–2 hr.)	Bicycle and/or roller skate (1–3 hr.)	(Same as Monday)

flexibility, but scheduling flexibility. Since my work schedule fluctuates considerably (sometimes I spend whole days writing or researching; other times I scurry from appointment to appointment; still others I fly around the country giving lectures), my exercise program has to be loose enough to accommodate anything and be performed anywhere. That's one of the main reasons—in addition to my tendency to be easily bored—I perform so many different kinds of fitness activities.

I exercise every day, but the choice of exercise and the length of time it's performed vary with my schedule and mood. These are my primary fitness activities and why they work for me:

  • Martial arts. These allow me to stretch, kick, punch; practice hard and soft movements; work out with weapons, punching bags, and other training aids. Sometimes I practice alone; other times I work with an instructor or others. Martial arts promote strength, speed and reaction time, coordination and balance, and neuromuscular relaxation.

  • Tai Chi Chuan (means "grand ultimate fighting"). Although this is a martial art, Tai Chi relies on acute sensitivity to the environment as well as refined mental control over muscles and reflexes to help your opponent defeat himself. The Chinese insist you must "keep your mind like calm water to accurately reflect your opponent's intentions." Thus I find Tai Chi very useful for creating neuromuscular relaxation, relieving stress, improving coordination, balance and flexibility, and increasing conscious control of my mind and body.

- Aerobic rebound. This mini-trampoline device helps you to work up a sweat and exercise your cardiorespiratory system without the bone-crushing after-effects of jogging. In addition, I believe the acceleration improves circulation and tissue oxygenation. I have a fold-up rebounder that I take with me on business trips.
- Bicycling. I ride my twelve-speed bicycle all over Los Angeles, both for running errands and for pure pleasure. Bicycling is one of the best exercises for improving endurance and cardiorespiratory function, as well as for increasing lower body strength.
- Stationary bicycling. I use a good German flywheel bicycle that enables me to pedal both forward and backward. I have an agreement with myself that I can watch television only while bicycling. (One of my friends has gone so far as to hook up his television to a generator that can be activated only by bicycling!) I also usually wear wrist weights so I can do arm exercises while riding my stationary bicycle.
- Roller skating. Who could live in Marina del Rey, as I do, and not roller skate? Roller skating improves coordination and balance and increases endurance. I usually skate along the ocean boardwalks while listening to my favorite music through a headset.
- Swimming. Although I find swimming somewhat boring, I usually manage to swim at least twenty laps in the 25-yard pool located where I live a few times a week. Swimming has a superior influence on endurance and strength.
- Walking. I live near the ocean and walk along it whenever time permits. While walking I often practice deep breathing or meditation techniques.

SECTION III

You Can Preserve the Life Force Longer

12

Energy, Metabolic Shifts, and Aging

Consider this idea: *You are energy.*

And so is everything else in the universe. Thought, light, sound, sun, wind, soil, water, and even apparently lifeless forms such as rocks—all are energy. Each of these energy forms vibrates at a particular frequency (cycles of activity per second) to maintain its structural and functional integrity. The more complicated the energy form, the faster the frequency. Thought, for example, vibrates so quickly that we can't yet measure it. Light energy is so fast that we can't yet match its speed, as compared to sound, whose speed barrier we've only recently broken. Physical structures operate at a much slower frequency, which gives them the appearance of solidity. Rock, for example, looks solid, but that's only because its cycles per second of activity are so slow we can't see them.

Airplane propellers offer a vivid example of energy frequency in action. When a propeller is motionless, it is clearly visible. The individual blades look rock solid. As the propeller starts to turn—to increase its cycles per second of activity—its image becomes blurred. Individual blades are no longer distinct. An airplane propeller operating at full power—its highest frequency of cycles per second—is virtually invisible to the naked eye. Also noteworthy is the fact that the propeller is most powerful at its highest frequency.

All energy is the same, regardless of its vibrational or frequency level. Therefore your health, well-being, and longevity are directly affected by your own thoughts, your environment, other people—literally by everything. Physics has begun to corroborate the ancient Oriental maxim "All is one."

SCIENCE AND PHILOSOPHY:
A MIXED MARRIAGE

The first Western breakthroughs in understanding energy came about when certain contradictions and unresolved conflicts became apparent in the laws of Newtonian physics.

For most of the past 250 years, Western industrial societies have embraced the Newtonian model. Everything in the universe is assembled from solid, indestructible particles moving about in a void. What you see, touch, and feel is reality. We are bits and pieces built like a car on an assembly line.

However, with the discovery of atomic and subatomic particles from particle accelerators that split atoms, the Newtonian paradigm cracked. It simply couldn't explain why subatomic energy particles stubbornly refused to die as expected, instead reemerging from the depths of the atom-splitting cyclotron and blasting around in more energetic and sophisticated patterns than ever before. So scientists, like chicks shedding unneeded shells, stepped out into a new universe that could be seen only through a new set of eyes.

It remained for Einstein, Heisenberg, and others to describe this new universe through the concepts known as field theory, quantum theory, and relativity theory. The combined impact of these three theories has been to create a view of reality that is much more elastic, inclusive, and holistic than previous models. In this new reality, energy and matter are interchangeable according to Einstein's classic equation $E = mc^2$.

The ancient Chinese discovered that everything in the universe arises from the proportions and combinations of two forces—yin and yang. The yin force is bright, outward, and weak, while the yang force is considered heavy, solid, and inward.

Along the same lines, Nobel laureate physicist Carlo Rubbia believes that everything in the universe is formed from three basic forces. A heavy inward force holds atoms together. A light force creates radiation and electromagnetism. Lastly there is the force of gravity. Until very recently physicists thought there were four basic forces in the universe. I believe that in the near future, with the development of more sophisticated atom-smashers, research will reduce the basic forces to two that correspond with yin and yang.

How does energy relate to biology—and to you in particular? Dr. William C. Nelson, holder of four doctorates and a clinical acupuncturist and NASA engineer, has devoted the last five years to answering this question. He found that traditional biology (which is based on chemical reactions between carbon atoms) is incomplete. According to the new biology:

- All chemical reactions in your body depend on the correct energy field.

- Enzymes that catalyze chemical reactions depend on the polarity of energy.
- Nerve impulses occur from energy transfer, not from chemical transfers across the synaptic space.
- Human consciousness can be traced to quantum energy, not to electrochemical reactions.
- Cells transmute one element into another by rearranging molecules.

According to Dr. Nelson, energy controls DNA, cellular processes, and chemical reactions in your body. It pulls your strings like a puppeteer. Control energy and you control life. Restructuring body energy with acupuncture and homeopathy is a wave of the future—and invaluable medical treatment today.

Traditionally, diseases have been believed to be caused by chemical defects or by some small identifiable object—a germ or virus. Diseases are believed to develop in discrete stages: first a single symptom, then a group of symptoms, a syndrome, and finally enough pathological aberrations to qualify as a disease. Treatment is based on a biological analysis of the body's breakdown much like the way a mechanic might analyze an automobile for repair.

Medical specialists treat individual body parts when they break. If the problem can't be traced to a bodily defect, you are sent to a psychiatrist. If he fails, you are sent to a clergyman.

In the quantum model of medicine, according to Berkeley professor Dr. Kenneth Pelletier, psychological, environmental, social, and spiritual factors are weighted *equally* with biological factors when analyzing an illness. Treatment encompasses a relative understanding of each influence, as well as the relationship between doctor and patient.

ENERGY THERAPIES

Energy travels under different names. Biologists call it bioenergy. Chemists call it electrodynamic or magnetic energy. Chinese physicians call it Chi (pronounced "chee"). Indians call it prana. Theosophists call it ether. Homeopathic physicians call it vital force.

Regardless of its name, measuring energy with bioilluminence photography and acupuncture (I'll describe each technique later) and manipulating energy with acupuncture or homeopathy slow aging by preventing, detecting, and treating pathology.

Acupuncture

Five thousand years ago the Chinese discovered that energy, or Chi systematically flows through twelve meridians or channels located in your body. Energy is transmitted between a series of 800 points located on these meridians. When the energy flow is harmonious, even, and smooth, a person is healthy. When the energy flow is disharmonious, blocked, or uneven, a person is sick.

For the last thirty years, acupuncturists and biophysicists at the Sanonxi Medical College and the Institute of Biophysics in China, the Miami Heart Clinic in the United States, and research facilities around the world have scientifically validated and discovered the mechanisms behind acupuncture. Here's what they have found:

- The acupuncture meridians and points are real, not imaginary. You can see them by injecting radioactive dye, measure them with electrical detectors, and photograph them with bioilluminance photography.
- The location of acupuncture points and meridians coincides with the descriptions found in classical Chinese texts. The acupuncture meridians transport bioelectrical information between skin points of high electrical potential and low resistance. (The electrical current passes more easily through acupuncture points and meridians than surrounding skin.)
- Sixty-four variations of acupuncture energy described 4000 years ago are equivalent to the genetic code discovered by Nobel Prize winners Watson and Crick in 1962.
- The energy flowing beneath your skin generates an energy field, or aura, above it. You can photograph your aura and acupuncture points with bioilluminence photography.

The electrical changes that occur in acupuncture points and meridians correspond with disturbances in your body.

- Illness occurs when specific acupuncture points become unbalanced.
- Your muscle, urinary, nerve, and organ functions are directly linked to certain acupuncture points and meridians.
- Exercise, stress, temperature, time of day, and climate alter the electrical characteristics of particular acupuncture points.
- Acupuncture relieves pain by producing endorphins, powerful opiatelike pain relievers that block pain signals.
- Acupuncture relaxes your mind by producing alpha brain waves.

Besides diagnosing problems, clinical researchers have used acupuncture to treat disease by inserting needles or applying electrical stimulation in specific points.

- One hundred heart patients receiving acupuncture had marked improvement in heart functions. Stimulating the same points had no effect in normal people.
- Twenty asthmatics receiving acupuncture treatments showed significant improvement over nontreated patients.
- Twenty-eight subfertile men treated with acupuncture for three weeks showed increased sperm count.

- Five hundred cardiovascular disease patients suffering from ischemic heart disease, brain bleeding, high blood pressure, and other abnormalities were treated with acupuncture. They experienced significant lowering in blood pressure and improvements in blood circulation.
- Acupuncture has successfully treated psoriasis, allergies, headaches, chronic pain, insomnia, high blood pressure, autonomic nerve disorders, hypoglycemia, muscular disturbances, and nerve disorders, according to published research.
- Acupuncture allows pain-free labor and surgical operations without anesthesia.
- The Chinese and Japanese are currently testing acupuncture as a cure for cancer.
- The World Health Organization (WHO), a United Nations group dedicated to promoting health around the world, endorses acupuncture to treat disease.

If acupuncture is such a panacea, why does the traditional medical establishment consider it little better than a placebo, useful only for treating pain? According to Dr. Ralph Allan Dale, Director of the Acupuncture Education Center, Western medicine opposes acupuncture for various reasons:

- It's unprofitable for drug companies, traditional health care facilities, and doctors.
- The entire concept is contrary to the principles of health science taught in colleges, universities, and medical schools.
- Our system is based on paying for sickness, not health. It's easier to contain acupuncture than change a system to accommodate it.

Before embarking on your first visit to an acupuncturist there are a few things you should know.

First, make sure you are satisfied with the acupuncturist's credentials and methodology. Should you have any doubts, you can query the Acupuncture Education Center, whose address is listed in the Reference and Resource Guide at the end of this book. Acupuncture still exists just within the fringes of American medicine, so its training methods are not as standardized as one might wish. It takes years to learn which points to needle for a person's problems.

In traditional Chinese training an acupuncture student may spend a decade of intense personal tutoring with a master. Even today's university-trained acupuncture students in Asia receive more in-depth training than currently available in American schools, which issue diplomas after only three years of study. In fact, the best traditional acupuncturist in the United States may be an elderly Chinese person who speaks little English.

Some American-trained acupuncturists rely on anatomical measurements to determine where to place the needles. Since acupuncture relies on the intimate relationship between patient and doctor, an acupuncturist who isn't skilled or sensitive enough to "feel" the energy change as the needle enters the acupuncture point isn't likely to be very useful. A good acupuncturist can feel the energy.

I prefer Asian-trained acupuncturists with an additional medical degree from a Western university. These doctors combine the best techniques of East and West for superior care.

Use your intuition and the doctors referral services of the acupuncture organizations listed in the reference section for locating a qualified acupuncturist in your area.

You can set your mind to rest about pain during the puncturing. You can barely feel the needles enter, and once they're in you can't feel them at all.

If you have a serious phobia about needles, you may want to explore electroacupuncture. In electroacupuncture, sensitive electronic apparatus measures and stimulates acupuncture meridian points.

Different electroacupuncture systems have developed in foreign countries but the German system called EAV (electroacupuncture according to Voll, so named after Reinhold Voll, a German physician who developed the system and published data about it in the mid–1970s) is the most comprehensive and popular in the United States. EAV measures 800 acupuncture points to diagnose the initial, advanced, and final states of degeneration. The apparatus also delivers electrical pulses to unbalanced acupuncture points as treatment. EAV is used around the world and scientifically documented to:

- Detect food and environmental allergies as effectively as standard medical tests
- Diagnose then treat energy imbalances, organ problems, and pathology
- Treat pain
- Detect problems before traditional medical tests indicate the existence of pathology
- Treat pathology

I like EAV's ability to determine dosages and anticipate reactions to drugs and supplements by measuring energy compatibility without the need to ingest them. I recommend using EAV to test the effectiveness of your Age Reduction System supplements and prescribed medications.

Finally, you should be aware that you may not recognize that the healing process has taken place until well after the fact.

A client of mine, a thirty-eight-year-old Hollywood screenwriter, played tennis for an hour each day for over a year. At some point he began to notice a pain in his left hand. (Since he is left-handed, that wasn't too surprising.) He found it difficult to keep a strong grip on his racket.

Michael went to a hand specialist who diagnosed the cause as a form of bursitis, which he treated with ultrasound and whirlpool massage therapy. The pain didn't go away. Michael went to another hand specialist who took

X rays and discovered a tiny tear in the ligament between his thumb and forefinger. It wasn't serious enough to stop him from typing or writing, but it did seriously interfere with his tennis. By now he couldn't hit a ball without experiencing real pain. The specialist gave Michael a choice: Put your hand in a cast for six weeks or give up tennis for a year.

Michael, who has unlimited faith in the power of medicine (and particularly cortisone, with which the doctor proposed to inject his hand), opted for the cast. In fairness to the physician, I must say he made no guarantees.

Six weeks later the cast was removed and, lo and behold, not only was Michael's hand not better, it was much worse! Now it hurt just to move it. Physical therapy proved useless, and the specialist was at his wit's end. He suggested Michael see an acupuncturist.

I gave him the name of a highly respected Vietnamese acupuncturist who had been associated with the University of California Pain Clinic. I asked him to report her recommendations to me.

On his first visit he learned that, instead of having a little tiny problem in his left hand, he had a big problem with the entire energy meridian running from his left fingertips all the way down to his left toes.

The acupuncturist felt the primary causes of the problem were tension and a poor diet. She believed that six to eight treatments would be necessary to realign his energy.

At first Michael was optimistic. I taught him some stress-reduction meditation techniques and devised a better nutrition program for him. He found the treatments painless and rejuvenating.

About halfway through the treatment program he began to have doubts. In spite of the acupuncturist's assurances, he didn't think his hand was getting any better. It still hurt. He still couldn't play tennis. And he was under a lot of work pressure that made his weekly trips to the acupuncturist inconvenient.

Michael grudgingly continued for a total of six treatments, then quit on the pretext of schedule conflicts. Privately, he thought the entire affair had been a waste of time.

Within two weeks of ending the treatments, however, the pain disappeared. At first Michael didn't notice the change or connect it to the acupuncture, but ultimately the notion sank in. He later said to me, "I didn't believe in it, but it worked. My body just healed itself."

The whole point of energy therapy is to help your body do just that.

Bioilluminence Photography

Bioilluminence photography visually records the electrodynamic energy field surrounding and permeating all objects by exposing film to the object in the midst of a high-intensity electromagnetic field. Scientists

Semyon and Valentina Kirlian, a Russian husband-wife team, first developed the technique in 1939.

The original technique has undergone modification by Vickor Adamenko and Victor Inyushin for use in medical clinics. Bioilluminence photography is used extensively in Eastern European countries, but is relatively new in the United States.

Acupuncturists, homeopathists, and medical doctors specializing in energy disorders routinely photograph the energy illuminence from the tips of your fingers and toes as a diagnostic screen. The procedure requires less than ten minutes and costs less than $75.

Dr. David Young is a U.S.-trained medical doctor and Chinese-trained acupuncturist who practices energetic medicine in Los Angeles. He combines East and West with traditional and modern in his practice.

According to Dr. Young, specific energy patterns on these photographs precede cellular deterioration and disease. Problems are detected while traditional medical tests still indicate good health. Bioilluminence photography is a road map for restructuring your body's energy with acupuncture, herbs, homeopathy, nutrition, drugs, and other therapies. Bioilluminence photography can also point out the need to see traditional medical doctors.

Clinical trials and experimental research indicate the value of bioilluminence photography in:

- Revealing autonomic nerve imbalances, stress, and emotional disturbances
- Measuring acupuncture meridian imbalances
- Determining organ toxicity and abnormal metabolism
- Indicating predispositions to cancer and other diseases
- Localizing pain

I strongly recommend a bioilluminence photograph before beginning the Age Reduction System and every year thereafter.

Homeopathy

Though in practice not as old as acupuncture, homeopathy was officially founded by a German physician, Dr. Samuel Hahnemann, in 1779. Its name is derived from the Greek words *homeo* and *pathos,* meaning "similar suffering." Its principle is also Greek in origin. The Greek physician Hippocrates was the first to record the idea that "like cures like."

Homeopaths use extremely diluted medicines made from substances that, in stronger doses given to healthy people, would produce symptoms similar to those of the illness being treated. Allergy treatments that involve the injection of trace amounts of the allergy-provoking substances and vaccinations that stimulate immunity work on the same principle.

At the turn of the century homeopathy was a major form of medicine in the United States. So what destroyed it? The principal reason was economics. Since you can't patent homeopathic remedies, I believe greedy drug companies pressured the American Medical Association to ruin the credibility of homeopathy in the eyes of the American public.

Today homeopathy is making a comeback in the United States. Homeopathy is practiced extensively throughout England, France, Germany, Greece, India, Pakistan, South Africa, and Brazil. France has over 6000 homeopathic doctors; India has more than 120 homeopathic medical schools.

There is some controversy about homeopathy's effectiveness. Many orthodox physicians claim that it is more art than science, as evidenced by the fact that two patients presenting similar *physical* symptoms may receive widely different treatment. Homeopaths, like most energy therapists, believe that disease results from *mental, emotional, and/or physical* imbalance, so two patients presenting the same physical symptoms may be suffering from exceedingly different causes. Homeopathy focuses on highly individualized treatments that do not lend themselves to double blind medical testing on sick people. There are nonetheless several double blind studies supporting the curative powers behind homeopathy. (In double blind tests half the subjects receive the test drug while the other half receive the placebo. Neither the subject nor administrator of drugs can identify the placebo from the drugs.)

Another criticism traditional physicians level at homeopaths is that their remedies contain virtually no active ingredients and are so diluted they can't possibly work. Actually, the beneficial effects of these medicines are derived not from chemical reactions of the active ingredients in the body but from the "energy" created by the dilution process itself. Here's how it works.

Homeopathic pharmacists begin with plant or mineral extracts in a 10 percent water-alcohol solution called "mother tincture." One drop of this tincture is added to ninety-nine drops of a water-alcohol solution, then shaken a particular number of times at a specific angle. One drop of this diluted substance is again added to another ninety-nine drops of the water-alcohol solution and shaken. This process occurs at least four times, at which point the pharmacist has created a homeopathic medicine. A drop or two of the medicine is plopped into tiny pills. Homeopathics are also sold as tinctures.

The original active substance, which may be anything from strychnine to crushed wild berries from Scotland, has been diluted to about one part per million. Many of the pills may remain untouched by a single molecule of the original substance.

Homeopaths believe their remedies work by altering your energy fields to stimulate metabolic reactions against a particular problem, with little risk of side effects. This theory is corroborated by studies in which the

EAV electroacupuncture device discussed earlier has measured differences in acupuncture meridians' energy after homeopathic remedies of different potencies have been administered.

Understanding how the dilution process actually increases energy isn't too difficult. Remember Einstein's $E = mc^2$ equation that I mentioned at the beginning of this chapter? Decreasing the amount of matter during each stage of the dilution process increases the amount of energy.

Based on feedback from EAV measurements and bioilluminence photographs, sophisticated energy doctors across the country prescribe homeopathic drugs to detoxify internal organs. After homeopathic treatments energy readings return to normal.

I do not recommend treating yourself with individual homeopathic detoxification remedies in high potencies ($30 \times$ to $200 \times$). (The $\times$ after the zero is a measurement of dilution strength.) Homeopathic detoxification should be performed for less than a month and only under the guidance of a homeopathic physician.

Combinations of homeopathic medicines in lower potencies (less than $30 \times$) are sold in first aid kits for common problems. They are safe for self-prescription in conditions that don't require a visit to your doctor's office. Medicines are available for coughs, motion sickness, nausea, sore throats, flu/cold symptoms, and other common complaints. They are an alternative to synthetic over-the-counter drugs producing side effects and toxic reactions. One remedy typically costs between $6 and $12 in health food stores, homeopathic pharmacies, and through mail order. Unfortunately, some companies sell inferior products. The supplement suppliers listed in Chapter 9 offer quality manufacturers of homeopathic remedies.

I believe that homeopathic first aid remedies are a welcome addition to any family medicine cabinet. Orthodox doctors, however, are skeptical of the time it takes to effect a homeopathic cure. In this era of immediate gratification, the value of a health therapy is often judged by its speed at eliminating symptoms. Homeopathic cures may take weeks, months, or even years to have an effect. Doctors claim that, given enough time, many untreated illnesses will disappear of their own accord. They also point out that homeopathic cures may actually result from the placebo effect, in which a patient's belief that a treatment works may help him muster his own defense systems. I wish they would explain why homeopathy works in animals without belief systems!

Perhaps a more interesting question might be: *Why* do many untreated illnesses disappear of their own accord? The reason is simple. We have our own highly developed natural repair and defense systems that, when working properly, come to our aid.

Instead of overpowering and weakening our natural defenses by learning to rely on drugs, it's worthwhile to use homeopathy, acupuncture, and the power of your mind to strengthen your defense systems. I believe that homeopathy provides a useful complement to other medical therapies.

Behavioral Kinesiology

Dr. George S. Goodheart, a chiropractic physician and researcher, advanced acupuncture by his discovery in 1964 that each major acupuncture channel is linked to a different muscle. Testing the changes of strength in key muscles determines the energy imbalances in meridians and problems in associated organs. For example, weakening of your biceps indicates problems in your stomach meridian and stomach gland.

Muscle testing is popular with chiropractic doctors, accepted by energy doctors, and viewed with skepticism by traditional physicians. Clinically speaking, muscle testing results are often unreliable. The doctor performing the muscle test must feel subtle changes in muscular strength. Some doctors, regrettably, lack enough feeling to consistently perform behavioral kinesiology. Therefore I do not recommend the use of behavioral kinesiology. Instead, rely on EAV (electroacupuncture) and bioilluminence photography to measure energy.

According to Dr. David Young your body contains two types of energy. Yin energy represents the health of your internal organs. It fluctuates very little from day to day and is like a huge water reservoir. When the level of yin energy decreases, you age and develop disease.

Yin energy is visible as inside rings on bioilluminence photographs.

Yang energy represents the state of your autonomic nervous system, emotions, stress, and response to factors influencing energy balance (see Table 36 on the next page). Yang energy fluctuates from day to day and is visible as outside flares on bioilluminence photographs.

How much energy disruption you can withstand from stress, life-style, and environment before losing yin energy depends on your genetic constitution and current state of health. The degree of damage to your health caused from each energy disruption is not a precise equation. Still, it's a good idea to eliminate energy disrupters before they help eliminate you.

METABOLIC SHIFTS

Your metabolism is an energy transformer. According to Webster's dictionary, metabolism is "the chemical changes in living cells by which energy is provided for vital processes and activities and new material is assimilated to repair the waste." As much of a mouthful as that definition is, it isn't quite complete. What Webster fails to address is what causes the chemical changes in the first place. That, too, is energy.

It is the changes in energy states, or life force, discussed earlier in this chapter that direct the chemical and enzyme processes, growth, and development. In later years this same life force disrupts the metabolism. A decrease and imbalance of energy states triggers what I call "metabolic shifts," physiological changes away from balance. Metabolic shifts are signposts that your metabolism is converting energy in different ways and

TABLE 36

Factors Influencing Energy Balance

Energy Balance Enhancers	Energy Balance Disrupters
Loving and positive emotions	Being unable to love; hate and negative emotions
Maintaining a consistent but not inflexible daily schedule	Constantly changing your daily schedule, disturbances of rhythmic balance
Having a peaceful and fairly constant home and work environment	Living in a high-stress work and home environment that frequently changes
Experiencing contentment and continuity in your relationships	Experiencing traumatic or short-lived relationships
Thinking positive thoughts	Thinking negative thoughts
Indulging in regular hypnosis, meditation, or flotation tank sessions	Consuming drugs, alcohol, cigarettes, or caffeine
Practicing yoga or Tai Chi or other systems of centering	Never experiencing neuromuscular relaxation
Exercising moderately, consistently, and enjoyably	Spending most of your waking hours in sedentary activities
Performing activities that use opposite hand and leg motions	Performing activities that use only one side of the body
Using natural light as your primary means of illumination	Using fluorescent light as your primary means of illumination
Breathing fresh, pure air with balanced ions	Breathing air polluted by poisons and filled with noxious odors
Listening to harmonious and classical music	Being frequently exposed to loud, harsh noises; listening to rock and roll music
Eating fresh, live food	Eating foods poisoned by additives and pesticides, cooked in microwave ovens, processed in factories, or containing refined sugar
Living in an unindustrialized environment	Being exposed to X rays, radio waves, microwaves, electrical currents, electronic equipment, and other electromagnetic pollutants
	Exposure to foods, medicines, or environmental hazards that provoke allergic or toxic reactions

for different purposes. Menopause is a metabolic shift that signals the end of childbearing years. The woman's metabolism stops using energy to manufacture estrogen and progesterone, the primary female sex hormones; it stops manufacturing the ovary lining intended to cradle eggs, and it stops manufacturing the eggs themselves.

The Stages of Life

From the moment of conception, metabolic shifts govern your progression from birth to death. The eight primary stages of life in this progression are conception, embryonal fetal development, birth, early growth, puberty, maturity, physiological decline (or senescence), and death. The chart that follows, "Common Metabolic Shifts," describes the important changes that often accompany each of these stages, beginning with growth. (Since we are concerned here with the metabolic shifts of aging, it would serve no purpose for you to wade through the metabolic shifts prior to birth.)

Research has shown that you can add good years to your life by delaying the onset of maturity and senescence. Remember the nutrient-restriction experiment discussed in Chapter 10? Life-spans of white rats were *tripled* by delaying metabolic shifts—from 600 days to 1800 days. Remember, too, that this translated to 180 human years.

The idea that delaying metabolic shifts will extend your life is actually based on evolution. From the moment of conception, evolution has geared your energy to prepare you for siring or bearing a child. The most primitive instincts are bent on preservation of self and species. Once you've passed the childbearing age, evolution simply loses interest. On this primitive level, you are of no further use in the eyes of eternity.

If you doubt this, just reconsider the fate of the Pacific salmon discussed in Chapter 2. As soon as it swims upstream and spawns, the salmon is battered by a series of instantaneous metabolic shifts. Its adrenal hormone blood count is multiplied by a factor of ten. Its blood glucose level doubles so the fish becomes fat. These and other metabolic changes cause the salmon to die simultaneously of heart disease, brain damage, kidney damage, and other tissue destructions.

By delaying the onset of maturity, menopause, and senescence, you *can* fool Mother Nature.

TABLE 37

Common Metabolic Shifts

Stage Four: Early Growth

Cells increase in number and size.

Body height and weight increases.

The weight of organs and tissues increases.

The skeletal system ossifies.

The hypothalamus matures and increases control over the body.

The pituitary gland increases activity.

Maximum metabolic rate is reached at one year old.

The brain/nerve control of motor activities, senses, and intellect develops, so that babies can learn to walk and talk.

Body fat content increases rapidly up to the first year of life, decreases at ages six to eight, and increases during the adolescent growth spurt.

Stage Five: Puberty

Male and female sexual systems are activated by sexual hormones.

In men the testes enlarge, sperm appears, and ejaculation occurs. Body hair appears, sweat glands activate, muscle mass increases relative to fat.

In women the ovaries enlarge, breasts develop, the menstrual cycle commences, pelvic diameter increases.

Heart size and lung size increase.

Adolescent growth spurt commences.

Stage Six: Maturity

Maximum height, skeletal ossification, peak physical performance and development are reached.

Growth hormone release is maximum.

Male and female sexual systems are at peak efficiency during these prime childbearing years.

The homeostatic systems that keep pace with growth continue changing when growth is complete. Then they destabilize your internal environment and lead to the next stage: physiological decline.

Stage Seven: Physiological Decline

Protein synthesis decreases.

Free fatty acids become primary fuel source.

Growth hormone is suppressed.

Excessive insulin is secreted.

Carbohydrate intolerance develops.

Immune system deteriorates.

Cortisol increases harmful stress reactions.

Auto-antibodies increase.

Blood pressure rises.

Cholesterol, triglyceride levels increase.

Lean muscle mass decreases.

Fat accumulates inside and over body surfaces.

Men produce less testosterone and sexual functions gradually decline.

Women pass through menopause, female sexual hormones drastically decrease, and the female sexual system gradually shuts off.

Basal metabolic rate decreases.

The autonomic nervous system loses integrity.

The dopamine/serotonin cycle is unbalanced.

The hypothalamus loses sensitivity to feedback control.

The pituitary gland overstimulates receptor organs.

Energy production and metabolic efficiency decrease.

Arteries stiffen and narrow.

Number of brain cells decreases.

Neurotransmissions decrease between cells and within cells.

Nerve cell conduction speed decreases.

Muscle strength and coordination decline.

Tissues undergo cross-linkage.

Maximum heart rate declines during exercise.

Visual acuity and/or auditory functions decline.

Lung capacity decreases.

Kidney functions decrease.

Men start losing hair.

Stage Seven (continued)

Skin loses elasticity, forms lines that lead to wrinkles.

Tissue oxygenation decreases.

Sleep disturbances occur.

Brain blood flow and oxygenation decrease.

Prostate gland often undergoes some hypertrophy (after age forty).

Speed of reactions and thinking decreases.

Blood volume, red blood count, and hemoglobin decrease.

Lipofuscin age pigments appear.

Plaques develop in neurons.

Body temperature regulation decreases.

Gums recede, jaw bone decreases in size, teeth loosen and may eventually fall out.

Cartilage deteriorates.

Less hydrochloric acid and pancreatic enzymes are secreted.

There is decreased absorption and assimilation of carbohydrates.

There is a reduction in vitamin stores (vitamins C, B-6, B-5)

The number of mutated cells increases.

Cell reproduction rate decreases.

There is a decrease in stress tolerance.

Tremors and shuffling gait may occur from the loss of dopamine.

Night and color vision decrease.

There is a gradual loss of balance.

Prolactin secretion decreases in women after menopause.

A decrease in the male sex hormone testosterone occurs.

Sleep problems become common.

The need for vitamin A and vitamin B-1 may increase.

Life, Death, and Disease

Here in the West we tend to view life and death as opposites like good and bad, black and white. Disease is viewed as death's ally and therefore life's enemy.

Fortunately, it's neither that simple nor that horrible.

Life and death are really more like book covers. One may represent the beginning of your current autobiography and the other may represent the end, but quantum physics proves that energy cannot die. If energy can't die, then neither can you. I don't presume to know what form that energy takes after life as we know it ends, but if the actions of subatomic energy are any indication, it just moves to a higher level.

Besides, if you'll bear with my analogy a moment longer, it's up to you how much adventure, romance, education, accomplishment, experience, and just plain fun you fit between your covers. The Age Reduction System is designed to help you have more of these.

But I digress. We were talking about disease as death's ally. A more realistic view would be that degeneration and disease are part of the natural continuum of life and death.

To understand why this is so, you must first accept the fact that *energy cannot stand still*. It must either create or destroy. During the early phases of your life, every aspect of your being is bent on creating a whole human being in perfect condition to reproduce. Once the prime childbearing years are over, those same metabolic forces unleash disorder, disease, and death. Even the brief moment when evolution appears to hold its breath— the maturity phase—offers only the illusion of stability. In reality, the forces striving to create order and balance are merely evenly matched between the same forces striving to destroy order.

Think of it as an arm wrestling match, in which two opponents of seemingly equal strength are exerting tremendous energy. For a while their fists remain clenched upright, almost as if no forces were at work at all, but eventually one combatant prevails, slowly forcing the other's fist to the table. So it is with the inevitable descent from maturity into physiological decline.

Of course, the real-life dance between life and death is more complicated than a fist falling to a table. Far from being a matter of linear descent, aging occurs in a gestalt fashion, with each aging factor taking its individual toll, but also with all aging factors interacting and multiplying to create metabolic shifts, disease, and death.

The *whole* of aging factors is much greater than the sum of its parts.

Disease, being a natural outcome of the aging process, is no more linear than aging itself. To attempt to correlate one metabolic shift with one disease would be erroneous. In reality, many metabolic shifts combine to create all diseases. The presence of inherited genetic weaknesses or self-created aging patterns may dictate that you accumulate more symptoms for one disease than another. Most of us die from some combination of these eight primary degenerative disease groups:

- Cancers
- Heart disease
- Atherosclerosis
- Cerebrovascular disease (stroke and hypertension)
- Diabetes mellitus
- Respiratory diseases (bronchitis, emphysema, pneumonia)
- Kidney disease
- Liver disease

Conversely, each of these diseases is created by a consortium of abuses, many of which are within our control.

Most of us prefer to ignore this fact. A fifty-two-year-old cinematographer friend of mine whose compulsive daily habits include four shots of vodka, two packs of cigarettes, a twelve-hour workday, six-day work weeks, endless schedule changes and travel across time zones, and constant separation from wife and kids recently suffered a mild heart attack. I inquired what he thought might have been the cause. He looked at me in utter seriousness and replied, "Well, I've given it a lot of thought, and I've decided that I must've smoked too much that day. My heart probably wasn't getting enough oxygen."

Fortunately for him, the denial phase passed, and he's now preparing to make some significant changes in his life.

The Age Reduction System can help you extend your life in two ways: by helping you to prevent a heart attack or degenerative disease at an early age, and by helping to *delay the onset* of disease or other age-related breakdowns. Studies have shown that people who escape disease during the maturity phase of their lives usually do not contract them until late in the physiological decline stage. Therefore, if you put the Age Reduction System into practice during maturity you may be safeguarding against a precipitous decline stage and enjoy a longer, healthier life.

If you want to achieve your maximum life-span, you must begin to use what you've learned today. If you wait to use it until you've contracted a disease—even if you cure yourself—the same imbalances that created that disease may also have been at work developing other pathologies.

The entire Age Reduction System is designed to help you delay and control the metabolic shifts that invite degenerative disease. Table 38 describes each Age Reduction System technique and its action.

TABLE 38

Delaying Metabolic Shifts

Age Reduction System Technique	Metabolic Shift Delaying Action
Coping with negative stress. (*See* chapters 5 and 6)	Maintains body rhythms; reduces excessive hypothalamus, pituitary, and adrenal gland activity. Decreases use of free fatty acids as fuel. Reduces excessive secretions of adrenaline and cortisol, supports the immune system, reduces high blood pressure.
Balancing the autonomic nervous system. (*See* Chapter 5)	Synchronizes body rhythm, maintains neuroendocrine system integrity, reduces stress-induced use of free fatty acids for fuel, normalizes blood pressure, supports the immune system, reduces secretion of adrenaline and cortisol, prevents abnormal pituitary gland and organ functions.
Synchronizing body rhythms. (*See* Chapter 6)	Regulates the hypothalamus and RAS (reticular activating system), balances the production of dopamine and serotonin, normalizes neuroendocrine system, reduces cortisol levels, supports the immune system, increases daytime and nighttime metabolic functions.
Reducing consumption of caffeine, alcohol, and drugs. (*See* Chapter 6)	Maintains body rhythms and central autonomic nervous system balance, reduces high blood pressure, balances dopamine/serotonin production, reduces cross-linkage damage, supports male and female sexual systems. Saves wear and tear on the nervous system, liver, kidneys, muscles, brain, heart, immune system, digestive system, and cells. Avoids cellular toxicity.
Reducing exposure to environmental poisons and hazards. (*See* Chapter 7)	Avoids DNA damage, cross-linkage, and free radicals; saves wear and tear on brain, heart, lungs, kidneys, liver, and other organs; spares the immune system, reduces cellular, tissue, and systemic failure; prevents unrepairable cell damage leading to mutated cells and cancer. Maintains body rhythm, hormone and nervous system balance.
Detoxifying cells and intestines. (*See* Chapter 7)	Improves digestion and absorption of food, vitamins, and minerals; protects against cellular poisoning, cross-linkage, and free radicals. Prevents liver, kidney, and tissue damage. Decreases toxic bowel syndromes and intestinal tract degeneration.
Optimal nutrition. (*See* Chapter 8)	Improves digestion; regulates insulin response; reduces cross-linkage, free radicals, and other cellular damage. Supports cell reproduction and repair, reduces cholesterol levels, prevents fat increase, and reduces blood pressure. Controls bone demineralization (osteoporosis), blood pressure, glucose intolerance, atherosclerosis, and certain cancers.
Losing excess weight. (*See* Chapter 10)	Diminishes glucose intolerance, adult-onset diabetes, osteoarthritis, high blood pressure, circulatory problems, and excess stress on the heart, lungs, and internal organs. Increases weather tolerance and metabolic efficiency.

Age Reduction System Technique	Metabolic Shift Delaying Action
Restricting nutrients. (*See* Chapter 10)	Inhibits genetic and non-genetic cellular aging and neuroendocrine aging. Delays the overall development of each metabolic shift and aging disorder. Enhances detoxification, energy and vitality, and proper hypothalamus sensitivity. Maintains a healthy immune system later in life.
Appropriate physical exercise. (*See* Chapter 11)	Stimulates sluggish brown fat metabolism, maintains body rhythms, reduces high blood pressure and cortisol levels, stretches and regenerates spinal discs, increases lean muscle mass while reducing fat, increasing carbohydrate tolerance. Supports the immune system, balances the autonomic nervous system, increases stress handling. May lower biological age.
Energy therapies. (*See* Chapter 12)	Control stress; maintain proper cell regulation, neuroendocrine balance, and internal functions. May be used to control high blood pressure, digestive disorders, glucose tolerance, sexual problems, osteoarthritis, and other specific age disorders.
Age reduction supplements. (*See* chapters 9 and 13)	Specific supplements and combinations compensate for different metabolic shifts. (These are individually described in the given sections and tables.)
Anti-aging drugs. (*See* Chapter 13)	Treat specific aging disorders. (Discussed in an independent section.)

13

What Anti-Aging Agents Can Do for You— Now and in the Future

In Chapter 9 I recommended a basic supplement program that is optimal for most people most of the time. However, whether through inherited weaknesses or self-created aging patterns such as smoking or being physically inactive, you may need special help in specific areas.

The anti-aging supplements included in the next pages are specially designed to slow or reverse the aging process of specific physiological aspects, from cells to complex control systems. Each section describes the aging factors commonly at work and recommends Age Reduction techniques and supplements to mitigate aging effects.

These supplements are not a prescription and are not intended to replace or enhance any medication or medical program on which your doctor has placed you. *Consult with your doctor before embarking on any of the supplement programs recommended in this chapter.*

If you do choose to use any of the supplements recommended in this section, refer to Chapter 9, "Supplementing the Age Reduction System," for complete instructions on the safe and correct use of supplements. *Under no circumstances should you seek to treat a condition independently without regard to supplements you may already be taking.* If you are already taking the indicated supplement for any other reason, count that as part of your intake for *all other* conditions for which it is listed. Adding further quantities may subject you to risk of toxic side effects with some substances.

ENERGY ENHANCERS

One of the key metabolic shifts that cause aging occurs when your body is no longer able to use carbohydrates (and therefore glucose) as its

primary source of raw energy during the day. Due to age-related reduction of the enzymes and other elements needed to convert carbohydrates, your metabolism is forced to rely on free fatty acids as a primary energy source. Excess free fatty acids in the bloodstream induce aging by:
- Increasing blood cholesterol and triglycerides
- Increasing blood tryptophan and brain serotonin
- Depressing the immune system and growth hormone secretion
- Triggering the overproduction of insulin, which can lead to adult-onset diabetes
- Promoting body fat gain and unbalancing the neuroendocrine system, which leads to organ failure and neuroendocrinological aging

Aging also affects energy at the cellular level. As you grow older, your cells produce less ATP (adenosine triphosphate), the universal energy molecule. Less ATP means that less physical and biochemical activity can take place in your cells. This slowdown of cell repair and reproduction rates helps cause cellular aging.

You can help delay the metabolic shifts that lead to energy breakdown by keeping your body fat low (very important), exercising regularly, restricting calories, eating the natural foods for longevity that I recommend in Chapter 8, and maintaining your sense of connectedness to life and other people. The following supplements may prove helpful.

TABLE 39

Possible Energy Enhancers

Supplement	Daily Amount	Effect
Succinic acid	1–2 gm	Stimulate ATP production and improve the sensitivity of the hypothalamus. Increase chemical and physical energy
Fumaric acid	1–2 gm	
Malic acid	1–2 gm	
Citric acid	1–2 gm	
L-aspartic acid	1–2 gm	
L-glutamic acid	1–2 gm	
L-valine	1–2 gm	
Vitamin B-5	40–100 mg.	Helps produce ATP for all energy processes in life
Muscle improvers	(*See* separate supplements)	Enhance physical energy
L-tyrosine	500–1500 mg. (in morning)	Increases dopamine for energy release
Vitamin B-6	20–30 mg.	Helps convert L-tyrosine to dopamine
Vitamin C	500 mg.	
Coenzyme Q-10	15–30 mg.	Stimulates energy production

See the Age Reduction Supplement Guide (Chapter 9) for a list of supplement suppliers and complete instructions on the correct and safe uses of supplements.

IMMUNE SYSTEM SUPPORTERS

Your immune system is your single best protection against premature aging. It prevents cellular aging by destroying foreign bodies (such as bacteria or viruses) that might attack healthy cells. It staves off troublesome metabolic shifts by policing the cells, tissues, and organs whose breakdown triggers these metabolic shifts. It also prevents degenerative disease by destroying mutant or damaged cells before they have a chance to multiply into cancer and other diseases.

As your immune system ages, it breaks down in one of two ways: It loses its ability to identify and destroy harmful and foreign bodies; it mistakes your own tissue for foreign bodies and so attacks you.

If you suffer from frequent colds, flus, or allergies, your system is, at least temporarily, unable to identify and destroy foreign bodies. Multiple sclerosis and rheumatoid arthritis are two examples of autoimmune disorders, in which your immune system mistakenly attacks healthy cells.

Many factors can depress or weaken your immune system. Genetic defects and natural genetic aging cause the gradual breakdown of the immune system. Negative stress causes the thymus gland (an integral part of the immune system) to shrink and wither; negative stress also triggers the release of corticosteroids, immune system antagonists. Excess sugar and refined foods, overexposure to environmental toxins, pollution, radiation, and lack of exercise also contribute to immune system depression. Some prescription drugs used to treat diseases actually prevent your immune system from working. Consult your physician about side effects associated with these drugs: antazoline sulfate, P-aminosalicyclic acid, chloropromazine (Thorazine), dipyrone, isonicotonic acid, penicillin (in large doses), phenytoin, phenacetin, Pyramidon, quinine, tetracycline, corticosteroids, cancer chemotherapy agents, and sulfonamide antibiotics.

One final factor influencing the deterioration of the immune system is shifts in metabolism and neuroendocrine function. When your metabolism shifts from using carbohydrates to using free fatty acids as the primary energy source, the resulting rise in cholesterol, triglycerides, insulin secretion, and glucose intolerance causes your immune system to falter and break down.

In addition to eliminating the immune system antagonists already discussed, you can protect and strengthen your immune system by keeping your body fat low and following a long-term fat- and calorie-restriction diet, increasing growth hormone, periodically following the detoxification program described in Chapter 7, and perhaps by taking the supplements listed in Table 40.

TABLE 40

Possible Immune System Supporters

Supplement	Daily Amount	Effect
Vitamin B-3	50 mg.	Water-soluble nutrients necessary for immunity. Vitamin B-3 is
Vitamin B-5	40–100 mg.	prescribed for autoimmune disorders but may cause
Vitamin B-6	20–30 mg.	temporary redness and itching in people sensitive to niacin.
Vitamin B-12	10–50 mcg.	
Folic acid	400 mcg.	
Vitamin C	1–2 gm	
Vitamin A	5000–10,000 IU	Fat-soluble nutrients necessary for immunity
Beta carotene	40,000–160,000 IU	
Vitamin E	100–200 IU	
Selenium	200–300 mcg.	Essential minerals that activate your immune system. Zinc is
Magnesium	400–600 mg.	very important.
Zinc	30–50 mg.	
L-arginine*	5–10 gm	Amino acids that stimulate/support your immune system
L-ornithine*	5–10 gm	

*L-arginine and L-ornithine should not be used by adolescents, juvenile diabetics, and pregnant or lactating women.

See the Age Reduction Supplement Guide in Chapter 9 for a list of supplement suppliers and complete instructions on the correct and safe use of supplements.

GROWTH HORMONE STIMULATORS

Much has been written lately about the benefits of growth hormones for tough, healthy bodies. Athletes have been known to pay large amounts of money for small amounts of growth hormone. The current fashion for sculpted muscles has made growth hormone practically a household word among weight-training enthusiasts and other fitness-minded people.

However, we are concerned here only with the effect of growth hormones on delaying aging. And in this they have a powerful role to play.

Growth hormones are produced by your body to stimulate DNA, RNA, and protein synthesis. (As already mentioned, this synthesis is critical to cell reproduction and repair.) These hormones help:

- Build strong muscles
- Trigger your metabolism to convert food to fuel instead of fat
- Increase lean muscle mass
- Improve the immune system
- Increase tissue repair rates
- Strengthen tendons and connective tissue
- Reverse bone mineral loss

Growth hormone supply is most abundant during adolescence for two reasons: Production is at peak levels to accommodate the growth spurt common to adolescence; and the factors that inhibit growth hormone release in later years have not yet developed.

Contrary to popular opinion, your *production* of growth hormone does not significantly decrease with age. You produce a sufficient supply of the stuff throughout life. However, several age-related factors inhibit its release.

The most important inhibiting factor is the antagonistic relationship between growth hormone, insulin, and the rise in free fatty acids. As I discussed in Chapter 12, your energy metabolism deteriorates with age. Your hypothalamus malfunctions and triggers improper insulin responses to your blood sugar levels. Preprogrammed genetic aging patterns and self-created aging factors such as overconsumption of fat and physical inactivity cause your cells to lose many of their insulin receptor sites. Since insulin is needed to bind glucose to cells, the reduced insulin supply creates a glucose intolerance. Your metabolism is forced to switch to free fatty acids as the primary fuel source. The cumulative effect of these breakdowns is the development of one or more of the degenerative diseases from which most of us die—cardiovascular disease, hypertension, diabetes, cancer, and atherosclerosis.

Your supply of growth hormones, which could stabilize your energy metabolism and delay aging, is trapped in the middle of this muddle.

The process works something like this: When your blood sugar level is normal, growth hormone is released without inhibition. However, growth hormone suppresses insulin release. So once growth hormone is released, your blood sugar level increases. Eventually this information gets back to the hypothalamus, which triggers an insulin response to restabilize blood sugar levels. If your hypothalamus is malfunctioning as a result of excess free fatty acids, it triggers an excessive insulin response, which in turn inhibits the release of growth hormone. (Although this may sound like a chicken and egg theory, it is the improper insulin response that inhibits growth hormone release, not vice versa.) See "Insulin-Response Improvers" in this chapter for possible ways to increase growth hormone *release*.

Diet is another important factor. Proteins contain amino acids—especially glycine, L-tyrosine, L-ornithine, and L-arginine—that stimulate growth hormone release. Fasting and a calorie-restricted diet increase growth hormone by temporarily eliminating the carbohydrates and sugars that depress growth hormone. Sugar produces insulin, which I've already mentioned is a growth hormone inhibitor. Other diet-related growth hormone inhibitors are excessive calories and large meals.

Strenuous exercise (such as weight lifting) has been shown to stimulate growth hormone release, especially in those under thirty. For those over thirty, the best way to encourage growth hormone release is to delay the shift in energy metabolism from glucose to free fatty acids as the primary energy source. Free fatty acids stimulate excessive insulin response. Together they inhibit growth hormone release and cause you to lose lean muscle mass and gain fat. Table 39, "Energy Enhancers," and Table 42, "Insulin-Response Improvers," included in this chapter, provide valuable information on how one may be able to delay these metabolic shifts.

Reducing excessive blood and body fats (*see* supplements listed for each in chapters 8 and 10, respectively) are necessary for the proper release of growth hormone. You might want to discuss with your doctor the possibility of taking a megadose (1000 to 3000 mg.) of nicotinic acid daily, which may lower triglycerides and increase growth hormone. Just taking megadoses of growth hormone–releasing amino acids is expensive and often worthless unless you control the metabolic shifts mentioned above.

For those interested in stimulating the natural release of growth hormone, the supplements listed in Table 41 below should prove useful.

As beneficial as growth hormone can be, I do not recommend growth hormone–stimulating supplements for adolescents, juvenile diabetics, or pregnant and lactating women. Growth hormone blocks insulin, which may cause diabetes in those prone to the disease.

TABLE 41

Possible Growth Hormone (GH) Stimulators

Supplement	Daily Amount	Effect
Daytime GH stimulators		
L-ornithine	2–5 gm	Amino acids release GH during the day. Use on
L-arginine	2–5 gm	an empty stomach and before exercise.
L-tyrosine	500–1500 mg.	
Vitamin B-6	20–30 mg.	
Vitamin C	500 mg.	
Nighttime GH stimulators		
L-ornithine	2–5 gm	Amino acids release GH while sleeping. Take
L-arginine	2–5 gm	immediately before sleep on an empty
L-glycine	4–8 gm	stomach.
Vitamin B-6	20–30 mg.	Vitamin cofactors to help GH release at night
Vitamin C	500 mg.	
L-carnitine	500–1000 mg.	Decrease triglycerides that release free fatty acids
Cod liver oil	2 tsp.	and suppress growth hormone
Insulin-response improvers	(*See* Table 42)	Prevent excessive insulin that suppresses growth hormone

See the Age Reduction Supplement Guide in Chapter 9 for a list of supplement suppliers and complete instructions on the correct and safe use of supplements.

- Use growth hormone stimulators between meals, before exercise, and at night before sleep.
- Before using L-tyrosine to release growth hormone, read the section entitled "Body Rhythms" in Chapter 6.

INSULIN-RESPONSE IMPROVERS

Your insulin responses deteriorate over time mainly due to cellular and neuroendocrinological aging. (*See* Chapter 2 for a complete discussion of these aging theories.)

As your muscle cells age they become less receptive to glucose as a source of fuel. This triggers a complicated set of metabolic shifts in which free fatty acids become the primary fuel source; the hypothalamus malfunctions and triggers the release of excess insulin and serotonin and insufficient dopamine; increased excess insulin inhibits growth hormone release and causes fat gain; triglycerides and cholesterol levels increase; and serotonin and dopamine imbalance hastens neuroendocrinological aging. The results of all these interactions are obesity, adult-onset diabetes, atherosclerosis, and cancer.

TABLE 42

Possible Insulin-Response Improvers

Supplement	Daily Amount	Effect
Dietary fibers		
Guar gum	2–3 gm*	Control the release of sugar from foods to
High methoxy pectin	300–600 mg.*	regulate insulin when taken ½ hour before
	*at each meal	meals
L-cysteine	500–1500 mg.	Stabilize blood sugar to control insulin
Vitamin C	1–2 gm	
Vitamin B-1	10–60 mg.	
B-complex vitamins		
	(*See* Age Reduction Supplement Guide in Chapter 9)	
Zinc	30–50 mg.	
GTF chromium	200–300 mcg.	
Glutathionine	50–150 mg.	
Herbs		
Stringbean pods	250–750 mg.	Help lower blood sugar to decrease glucose
Juniper berries	250–750 mg.	intolerance (*not* for hypoglycemia)
Jerusalem artichoke	250–750 mg.	
Goldenseal	250–750 mg.	

See the Age Reduction Supplement Guide in Chapter 9 for a list of supplement suppliers and complete instructions on the correct and safe use of supplements.

You can help delay these metabolic shifts by eating a high-fiber, low-calorie diet; avoiding sugars; exercising regularly; and possibly by using the supplements listed in Table 42.

- If you are hypoglycemic, do not use herbs to lower blood sugar.
- Mix guar gum and pectin with eight ounces of water or sugar-free beverages and drink at the beginning of the meal.

DIGESTION AIDS

The gradual degeneration of the digestive system is a normal part of aging. The process might begin in the mouth, where periodontal disease and tooth loss prevent proper chewing. The age-related decline in the sense of smell may depress the necessary cues to secrete the right enzymes that begin the process of digestion in the mouth. In addition, these same salivary glands and their ducts undergo fatty degeneration, reducing the flow of saliva and the potency of its enzymes to digest starches.

Stomach glands also atrophy and produce less of the pepsin activity and gastric acid needed to digest proteins. The tissue of the small intestines is damaged by cross-linkage and covered with putrid material left over from a poor diet. These factors inhibit the absorption of vitamins, minerals, and other nutrients.

Food is therefore slowly and incompletely digested, increasing the risk of bowel cancer, malnutrition, allergic reactions, and the accumulation of toxic wastes in your colon.

Some of the more common symptoms of digestive problems are:

- Bloating
- Flatulence
- Diarrhea
- Constipation
- Nausea
- Vomiting
- Heartburn
- Headaches
- Dizziness
- Tiredness
- Joint pains
- Skin reactions
- Breathing problems
- Food cravings
- Psychological disturbances

Many digestive problems (even age-related ones) can be eliminated simply by following the Age Reduction System's program for optimal nutrition. Vary your diet, and make sure it includes plenty of fresh fruits, whole grains, vegetables, yogurt. You may want to consider undergoing the Age Reduction System's two-week detoxification program.

If you often experience digestive problems, you may want to undergo laboratory testing to determine whether you need supplemental stomach acid. Radiotelemetry is a laboratory test in which you swallow a pH-sensitive radiotransmitter pill, an electronic sending device. You eat a specified test meal, and the device measures your secretion of stomach acid. Applied kinesiology, another testing technique, measures the involuntary loss of specific strength of specific muscles due to changes in physiological function—in this case, stomach acid deficiency.

You may want to try the supplements listed in Table 43 at the beginning of meals to aid the different phases of digestion.

TABLE 43

Possible Digestion Aids

Supplement	Daily Amount	Effect
Stomach aids		
Betaine HCl*	100–150 mg.	Hydrochloric acid (HCl) lowers stomach pH to
Glutamic acid HCl*	300–450 mg.	digest protein.
Pepsin	30–60 mg.	Works with HCl to digest proteins
Enzymes		
Aspergillum		
Protease	10–20 mg.	Predigests food in the stomach and digests food
Amylase	26–52 mg.	in the intestines
Lipase	5–10 mg.	
Cellulase	4–8 mg.	
Pancreatin (4×)	200–1000 mg.	Digests proteins, carbohydrates, and fats in the intestine
Bromelain	100 mg. (240 GDU units)	Digest proteins. Helpful for food allergies caused by incomplete protein digestion
Papain	10 mg. (300 MCU units)	
Chymotrypsin	10–20 mg.	
Intestinal Aids		
Lactobacilli	1–2 tsp. dry culture	Destroy toxins in lower bowels; relieve digestive
Acidophilus	*or*	complaints
Bulgaricus	1 Tbsp. liquid	
Bifidus	*or*	
Cancasicus	10,000,000 units	
Dietary fibers	(*See* Chapter 7)	Promote correct bowel regulation, relieve constipation, increase intestinal motility
Herbs		
Asafoetida	125–250 mg. ⎫	Chinese and American herbs that support
Wild yam	125–250 mg. ⎬ per	digestion
Cumin seed	125–250 mg. ⎭ meal	
Papaya leaves	125–250 mg.	
Antacids		
Magnesium oxide	1–2 gm per meal	Aluminum-free antacids. Counteract excess
Calcium carbonate	1–2 gm per meal	stomach acid

*Do not use hydrochloric acid if you have an ulcer.

See the Age Reduction Supplement Guide in Chapter 9 for a list of supplement suppliers and complete instructions on the correct and safe uses of supplements.

CELL AIDS

In Chapter 2, we discussed how your cells age. In this section we'll tell you how you may be able to delay that process.

The primary causes of cellular aging are free radicals, cross-linkage, accumulated wastes and toxins, and decreased cell repair and reproduction rates. Some of the more obvious symptoms of cellular damage are old-looking skin, arteriosclerosis, osteoporosis, immune system failure, and certain types of cancer. Damaged brain cells cause Alzheimer's disease. Damaged hypothalamic cells cause the hypothalamus to malfunction and induce neuroendocrinological aging.

Here are specific strategies for combatting each cause of cellular aging:

Free Radical Causes	Combat Strategies
Too much or too little oxygen	Live in a moderately elevated climate (3000–5000 feet). Exercise moderately but consistently.
Solar and other radiation	Wear a maximum-protection sunscreen outdoors; avoid unnecessary X rays, bright lights, and microwave exposure.
Air pollutants such as ozone, nitrous oxide, and toxic chemicals	Live and work in minimally polluted environments. Use air and water filters and air ionizers. Avoid smoke of all kinds. Refrain from exercising in highly polluted environments.
Inadequate levels of antioxidants such as vitamin E, selenium, vitamin C, and cysteine.	Increase antioxidant levels. (See "Artificial Antioxidants" in the Supplement Nutrient Guide in Chapter 9 for complete information.)
Inadequate levels of enzymes that deactivate free radicals, such as superoxide dismutase (SOD), glutathionine peroxidase, and catalase.	Increase enzyme levels. (See "Enzymes" in the Supplement Nutrient Guide in Chapter 9 for more information.)
Overconsumption of unsaturated fats	Decrease fat consumption. Protect unsaturated fats from oxidation by adding artificial antioxidants (50 mg. of BHA or BHT added to 10 fluid ounces of liquid fats prevents oxidation).

Cross-Linkage Causes	Combat Strategies
Presence of excess metals and other inorganic elements, free radicals	Perform aerobic exercises. Avoid smoking and drinking too much alcohol.
Presence of deteriorating organic matter in cells	Improve immune system to destroy organic invaders. Follow Age Reduction System's calorie-restriction program. Avoid smoking, drinking too much alcohol, or eating too much sugar. See "Enzymes" and "Protein-Digesting Enzymes" in the Age Reduction Supplement Guide (Chapter 9) for enzymes to dissolve cross-linkage.

Accumulated Wastes and Toxins Causes	Combat Strategies
Poor dietary habits	Follow Age Reduction System's recommendations for calorie restriction and detoxification. Eat the natural foods for longevity.
Exposure to toxic environmental elements	Live and work in minimally polluted environments. Follow Age Reduction System's recommendations for detoxification. Avoid smoking or drinking excess alcohol.

Each of the listed causes of cellular aging is exacerbated by the age-related slowdown in cell repair and reproduction rates. Balancing the neuroendocrine system and reducing negative stress help improve repair and reproduction rates. The supplements listed in Table 44 (pages 256–257) support healthy cells in a variety of ways.

TISSUE REJUVENATORS

Your body contains four tissue types: connective, skin, nervous, and muscular. Because tissues are composed of cells, the same factors that degenerate cells also degenerate tissues.

Tissues are particularly vulnerable to cross-linkage damage. Collagen and elastin, the substances that give tissues strength and elasticity, respectively, tend to cross-link; become dense and insoluble; prevent the absorption of water, oxygen, or nutrients; and finally break or fray.

Most of us associate the breakdown of collagen and elastin with flabby, dry, aging skin, but the same process occurs in your heart, lungs, muscles, organs, arteries, and ligaments. As you will see in the individual section on cardiorespiratory aids, tissue breakdown in these areas leads to arteriosclerosis, stroke, and heart disease.

Mucopolysaccharides are your body's primary tissue support system. These thick, gelatinlike substances— composed of proteins and carbohydrates—literally glue your body together. They lubricate your tissues and joints, maintain the elasticity of skin and blood vessels, prevent the formation of arteriosclerotic plaque, support tissue growth and repair, regulate blood fat levels, and act as tissue-regulating hormones.

Unfortunately, aging decreases your production of mucopolysaccharides. That's why it may be helpful to supplement your diet with natural mucopolysaccharides from other sources. (See Table 45 for more information.)

Supplemental mucopolysaccharides have also been used to:
• Treat migraine headaches

TABLE 44

Possible Cell Aids

Nutrients	Daily Amount	Antioxidant Free Radical Deactivator	Anti-cross-linkage Agent	DNA & Cell Repair Aid	Cell Membrane Stabilizer	Protein-Synthesizer Aid	Lipofuscin Decreaser	Hypothalamus Sensitivity Restorer	Life-extending Agent in Research
Water-soluble vitamins and relatives									
Vitamin B-1	10–60 mg.	X	X						
Vitamin B-2	10–35 mg.	X							
Vitamin B-3	20–40 mg.	X				X			
Vitamin B-5	40–100 mg.	X	X			X			X
Vitamin B-6	20–30 mg.	X	X		X	X			X
Vitamin B-12	10–50 mcg.					X			
Biotin	200–600 mcg.					X			
Folic acid	400 mcg.					X			
Vitamin C (ascorbic acid)	1–2 gm	X		X					
Hesperidin	100–1000 mg.	X				X			
Rutin	100–1000 mg.					X			
Choline	200 mg.–3 gm					X			
Myo-inositol	500–1500 mg.	X				X			
Fat-soluble vitamins and nutrients									
Ascorbyl palmitate	1–2 gm	X		X					
Vitamin A	5000–10,000 IU	X		X	X				
Beta carotene	40,000–160,000 IU	X		X	X				
Vitamin E	100–200 IU	X		X	X		X		
Vitamin D	400–1000 IU					X			
Soya lecithin	5–15 gm	X			X				
Minerals									
Selenium	250–300 mcg.	X			X				X
Manganese	5–20 mg.								
Zinc	30–50 mg.	X	X		X	X			
Chromium	250–300 mcg.					X			
Silica	200 mg.								
Magnesium orotate	1200–2000 mg.						X		
Amino acids									
L-cysteine	500–1500 mg.	X	X			X			X
L-methionine	100–200 mg.	X	X			X			
L-glutathionine	50–150 mg.	X	X			X			
L-tyrosine	500–2000 mg.	X						X	

Accessory Supplements	Daily Amount	Antioxidant Free Radical Deactivator	Anti-cross-linkage Agent	DNA & Cell Repair Aid	Cell Membrane Stabilizer	Protein-Synthesizer Aid	Lipofuscin Decreaser	Hypothalamus Sensitivity Restorer	Life Extending Agent in Research
Enzymes									
SOD (superoxide dismutase)	> 6000 mcg.	X							X
Catalase	> 100,000 units	X							
Glutathione peroxidase	12,000 units	X							
Protein-digesting enzymes									
Bromelain	240 or more GDU units		X						
Papain	300 or more MCU units		X						
Chymotrypsin	10 mg. or more		X						
Artificial antioxidants									
BHA	125–300 mg.	X							X
BHT	125–300 mg.	X							X
Thiodioproprionic acid	25–75 mg.	X							
Miscellaneous									
DMAE (dimethylaminoethanol)	100–300 mg.	X			X		X		X
DHEA (dehydroepiandrosterone)	(*See* Supplemental Nutrient Guide)			X					X
Coenzyme Q-10	10–30 mg.	X				X			X
Herbs									
Ginseng	200–1000 mg.	X		X	X	X		X	X
Aged garlic extract	800–1600 mg.	X							
Chaparral	1000 mg.	X							
Glandular									
Pineal extract	(*See* Supplemental Nutrient Guide)							X	X
Thymus extract								X	

See the Age Reduction Supplement Guide in Chapter 9 for a list of supplement suppliers and complete instructions on the correct and safe use of supplements.

TABLE 45

Possible Tissue Rejuvenators

Supplement	Daily Amount	Effect
Mucopolysaccharides		Stimulate tissue repair and help rejuvenate collagen and connective tissue
Chondroitan sulfate A	2–6 gm	
or		
Extract of trachea and aorta	2–6 gm	
or		
Compound plant extracts of *Chondrus crispus*	2–6 gm	
Ascorbic acid	1000–2000 mg.	Nutrients that play a role in forming healthy connective tissue
Silicon	100–200 mg.	
Glycine	2000–3000 mg.	
Vitamin B-6	20–30 mg.	
Manganese	5–20 mg.	
Zinc	30–150 mg.	
Calcium	600–1200 mg.	
L-cysteine	500–1500 mg.	
L-methionine	100–200 mg.	
Vitamin B-12	10–50 mg.	
Cod liver oil	2 tsp.	Contain prostaglandin precursors to regulate tissue functions
Evening primrose oil	1.5–3 gm	
Soya lecithin	5–15 gm	
Cell aids	(*See* Table 44)	Create healthy cells for healthy tissue

See Age Reduction Supplement Guide in Chapter 9 for a list of supplement suppliers and complete instructions on the correct and safe use of supplements.

- Treat osteoporosis and ulcers
- Speed recovery from broken bones and other injuries
- Relieve arthritis, diabetes, and hemorrhoids
- Treat acne and psoriasis
- Inhibit the development of tumors and arteriosclerosis

In addition to taking supplements, you can support your healthy tissues by following recommendations for cell aids, avoiding overexposure to sun and other environmental hazards, minimizing makeup and other "skin care" products, and eating the natural foods for longevity.

SKIN SAVERS

Your skin is easily the most noticeable gauge of your age. You earn every line, every wrinkle, every fold. Your face is an etching of your life. In some countries a person's face is said to assume "character" with age, to become more interesting, more revealing. In our youth-obsessed society, however, a wrinkle is a form of failure. Consequently, our skin-care industry is set up to dispense mostly misinformation designed to appeal to vanity and insecurity.

These are the bare facts about your skin and aging.

First, your skin is a tissue and thus is subject to all the cellular aging mechanisms already described. Skin cells cross-link with each other, making it difficult to absorb water, oxygen, or nutrients. Collagen and elastin lose their firmness and elasticity, so the skin sags. As cellular repair and reproduction slow down with age, old dry cells remain on your skin's surface longer, making it look tired and dull. In addition, cells that stay around longer accumulate more waste products and toxins, causing age spots and an uneven complexion. Although skin cells reproduce more slowly, they do reproduce throughout life. That's why old people seem to have so much more skin than they need. The ears and nose keep growing throughout life, too. Ever take a close look at your grandparents' ears? And finally, tiny capillaries near the skin's surface are burst by overexposure to sun.

Second, your skin has moisturization, hydrogenation, and nutrition processes of its own that are far superior to those offered by the so-called experts. Contrary to popular opinion, your skin breathes, eats, and drinks from the blood vessels located beneath the skin, not from the surface. So topically applied creams and moisturizers, while they may plump up old dry cells and prevent irrigation, do not actually moisturize your skin, although they may help prevent moisture from evaporating off the skin's surface. In fact, many moisturizers actually prevent your skin from moisturizing itself by clogging pores near the blood vessels.

Third, while the cell and tissue aids already discussed will help you prevent collagen and elastin breakdown, the current crop of collagen and elastin creams and potions will do nothing to prevent or reverse the process. Your skin is simply incapable of absorbing topically applied "extracts" into the molecular structure of the skin itself. What collagen and elastin creams are really useful for is applying a moisture barrier to your skin's surface. Even though you can't absorb much moisture from the air, dry, cold, windy weather and other environmental factors can cause you to lose it.

The best way to delay skin aging is to help your skin help itself—from the inside. Here's how:

- Eat a healthy diet that provides it with the necessary vitamins and nutrients.
- Drink lots of water.
- Get plenty of sleep. Most of your skin's cell-repair processes take place while you sleep.
- Hang upside down or lie with your feet higher than your head for at

least ten minutes a day to improve the blood supply to your facial skin (not to mention your brain).

- Keep your skin's surface clean by washing it twice daily with a mild, perfume-free soap and lots of water.
- Avoid using heavy creams or lotions that clog your pores at the blood vessel. (Those labeled "deep penetrating" are the worst.) If your skin is dry, apply as little lotion as you can.
- Avoid using makeup as much as possible. Organic products such as cosmetics and skin lotions set up a bacterial climate on the skin's surface that invites infection. If you do use makeup, be sure to cleanse your skin very carefully each day.
- Try exfoliating your skin once or twice a week. Under ideal conditions I wouldn't recommend using scrubs, but most of us are exposed to polluted environments that damage skin cells faster than the normal rate of cell replacement. By removing dead skin cells you encourage your skin to increase its cell repair and reproduction rates.
- Avoid exposing your skin to too much cold, dry, or windy weather. These conditions cause your skin to lose moisture. If you live in a dry environment, use a humidifier as often as possible.

TABLE 46

Basic Skin-Care Program

Step 1	
Clean skin and remove old dead cells.	I use a mild cleaner with papain enzymes and allantoin (derived from comfrey bark) to remove dead cells.
Step 2	
Protect skin against the sun and environment.	I apply a 90% pure, very light aloe vera moisturizer that contains a sunblock of SPF 15. Aloe soothes and heals skin without clogging the pores. It also contains RNA for protein synthesis enzymes to remove damaged tissues and the humectants NMF (natural moisturizing factor) and soluble collagen to hold in skin moisture.
Step 3 *(when necessary)*	
Soften dry skin.	I apply pure apricot kernel oil containing vitamin E and vitamin A to dry skin areas.
Step 4 *(optional)*	
Apply a mask once a week.	I use an enzyme-and-china-clay mask that makes skin look and feel better.

TABLE 47

Possible Skin Savers

Supplement	Daily Amount	Effect
Evening primrose oil	2–3 gm	Contain essential fatty acids for skin formation
Cod liver oil	2 tsp.	and repair. Cod liver oil contains vitamin A, which increases epidermal growth
Cell Aids		
Antioxidant and free radical deactivators	(*See* individual supplements)	Control free radicals' damaging of skin cells
Anti–cross-linkage agents		Attack cross-linkage in skin aging
Lipofuscin decreasers		Remove lipofuscins (liver spots) in old skin
L-cysteine	500–1500 mg.	Replace sulfur lost in skin aging
L-methionine	100–200 mg.	
Silicon	100–200 mg.	Create healthy, flexible skin
Mucopolysaccharides	2–5 gm	
Beta carotene	150,000–200,000 IU	Prevents ultraviolet sunlight damage
Vitamin B-1	10–60 mg.	Help synthesize essential skin fats
Vitamin B-5	40–100 mg.	
Biotin	200–600 mg.	
Pure water	1 quart	Replaces moisture in skin

See the Age Reduction Supplement Guide in Chapter 9 for a list of supplement suppliers and complete instructions on the correct and safe use of supplements.

- Always wear a sunscreen with a high sun protection factor rating when you know you are going to be exposed to the sun. The sun is the *primary* culprit in the breakdown of collagen and elastin, in cross-linkage damage, and in skin aging.

As a health-care expert and occasional public figure, my skin is often scrutinized for the flaws or clues that may reveal something about the credibility of the Age Reduction System. Although just the idea of being a role model should be enough to make anyone break out in acne, I've been blessed by my parents with a clear complexion. Since my fair skin tends to be dry, and since I'm not interested in participating in the premature aging that usually follows fair skin, I have devised the skin-care program given in Table 46, which is simple enough for even me to use every day. The supplements that I have found useful in preventing premature skin aging are listed in Table 47.

ORGAN AND GLAND REJUVENATORS

The same age-related processes that degenerate your cells and tissues also negatively affect your organs. The walls of your heart, lungs, kidneys, and liver stiffen, weaken, lose elasticity, become impermeable to water, oxygen, and nutrients. Your heart and lungs decrease their capacity to pump blood, inhale oxygen, and exhale carbon dioxide. Your liver may suffer up to a 50 percent decrease in its ability to process nutrients, neutralize toxins, synthesize cholesterol. Your kidneys gradually lose their ability to regulate and filter body fluids.

As your organs decline you are less able to supply your body with needed nutrients, water, and oxygen, while you are simultaneously more likely to accumulate unwanted toxins and wastes.

The fallout of this degenerative process is high blood pressure, arteriosclerosis, heart disease, stroke, and arthritis.

Your body has its own means of monitoring and protecting your organs. Prostaglandins—a family of fatty acid molecules—prevent blood clotting and arterial spasms, reduce your risk of heart attack, and improve the efficiency of your immune system. Recent studies indicate that a prostaglandin deficiency can trigger metabolic shifts, resulting in improper insulin response, increased autoimmune disease, abnormal blood clotting, and inflammation.

Prostaglandins are created from the essential fatty acids discussed in Chapter 8, "Optimal Nutrition for Age Reduction." Cod liver oil, evening primrose oil, lecithin, and soy oils are ideal sources of the essential fatty acids needed to create prostaglandins. (See supplements listed in Table 48 for correct amounts.)

Some of you may have inherited increased risk of certain types of organ failure. For example, kidney, liver, or heart disease may run in your family. To forestall the development of any of these diseases, you may want to consider undergoing organ-specific RNA therapy. Although still considered unorthodox in the United States, organ extract therapy has been used in Europe since the 1950s.

As you will recall from our discussion of cellular aging theories in Chapter 2, ribonucleic acid (RNA) acts as a messenger to carry the genetic information needed for protein synthesis. A high concentration of RNA is found whenever a cell is growing or dividing.

As you age, your concentration of RNA and your rate of cell reproduction decrease. Since cells are replaced more slowly, they have more time to accumulate toxins, become damaged, and mutate. The rate of cellular aging consequently increases.

Organ extract therapy supposes that by either introducing fresh young cells or RNA extracted from the same organs (in animals), one can increase the amount of RNA as well as the rate of cell repair and reproduction.

Research at the Pathological Institute of the University of Munich in Germany, begun in the mid-1950s and continuing up to the present, has indicated that the addition of RN-13 (RNA derived from thirteen different organs) to cell cultures can increase the growth of cells in those cultures by approximately 100 percent. Other European research with both animals and humans has produced similar results.

Most organ extract therapy is called "organ-specific." That's because RNA cells derived from a specific animal organ and intramuscularly injected into humans stimulate protein synthesis in the corresponding human organ rather than in other organs.

If you feel you are a potential candidate for organ failure or disease, you may want to explore the idea of RNA therapy further. More than forty types of organ-specific RNA (Regeneresen) therapy are currently being used by U.S. doctors in treatments costing $600 to $800. I believe that homeopathically prepared organ-specific RNA treatments can produce similar results for a fraction of the cost.

The Food and Drug Administration and American Medical Association do not recognize organ therapies as valid treatments. Locating organ-specific RNA and a doctor to administer it in the United States is difficult.

You can purchase organ-specific RNA from the Longevity Institute listed in Chapter 9 among the supplement suppliers. Try contacting the Life Extension Foundation, listed in the reference section, for a referral to

TABLE 48

Possible Organ Rejuvenators

Supplement	Daily Amount	Effect
Soya lecithin	5–15 gm	Produce prostaglandins, which regulate
Cod liver oil	2 tsp.	different organs
Evening primrose oil	1.5–3 gm	
Vitamin B-6	20–30 mg.	Support evening primrose oil in producing
Zinc	30–50 mg.	prostaglandins
Magnesium	600–1000 mg.	
Vitamin C	1–2 gm	
Cell aids	(*See* separate	Additional supplements that support your vital
Tissue rejuvenator	supplements)	organs
Homeopathic medicines	(*See* Chapter 12)	Specific medicines detoxify particular organs.
Longevity herbs	(*See* Age Reduction Supplement Guide in Chapter 9)	Balance and restore the energy in organs
Coenzyme Q-10	15–30 mg.	Increases heart strength, prevents abnormal heartbeats, lowers high blood pressure

See the Age Reduction Supplement Guide in Chapter 9 for a list of supplement suppliers and complete instructions on the correct and safe use of supplements.

doctors who may administer organ-specific RNA.

In addition to taking the supplements listed in Table 48, you may improve the health of your organs and delay aging by avoiding excess fats and alcohol and by reducing your exposure to chemical carcinogenic agents, radiation, and environmental toxins. (Overworking your lungs, liver, and kidneys to detoxify and filter out poisons is a key factor in the wear and tear that causes aging.)

Another way to protect your organs is to balance your autonomic nervous system, support your neuroendocrine system, and reduce negative stress. Each of these factors influences the release of enzymes, hormones, and chemicals critical to proper organ function, and their optimal health helps ensure yours.

BRAIN AND NERVE ENHANCERS

It is impossible to overemphasize the importance of a healthy brain and nervous system to longevity. Not only does the neuroendocrine system direct the metabolic processes that determine when and how you will grow old, it also dictates whether you will be sufficiently alert and functional to enjoy your later years.

More than any other human aspect, the brain and nervous system age as a result of both physiological *and* psychological factors.

The physiological causes are many. They begin, as does life itself, with the cell. As brain cells deteriorate—primarily from free radicals, cross-linkage, heavy metal poisoning, and other cell damaging factors—they cause the blood vessels to stiffen and collect arteriosclerotic plaque. (People between the ages of fifty and eighty often show up to 50 percent blockage of the arteries to the brain.)

Clogged blood vessels reduce the flow of oxygen, water, and nutrients to the brain. Decreases in energy metabolism and in consumption of glucose, the primary brain fuel, promote pathology. Starved for oxygen, glucose, nutrients, and energy, the brain and nerve cells degenerate further, transmitting fewer and less accurate signals at a slower pace.

Also contributing to the breakdown in cellular communication is the age-related decrease in the activity of neurotransmitters, chemicals that are essential for brain/nerve communication, behavior, and function.

The decrease and imbalance among neurotransmitters trigger a variety of metabolic shifts that can eventually lead to adult-onset diabetes, obesity, muscle deterioration, reproductive failure, organ damage, arteriosclerosis, immune system failure, senility, hypertension, psychic depression, low thyroid function, and increased risk of cancer.

The daytime rhythmic shift between the brain neurotransmitters dopamine and serotonin controls sleep, wakefulness, daytime energy, and nighttime repair processes.

Dopamine is necessary for:
- Movement
- Sexual activity
- Insulin regulation
- Physical energy
- Thinking
- Short-term memory
- Autonomic nervous system balance

Dopamine is metabolized into noradrenaline, the major neurotransmitter in the sympathetic nervous system, and adrenaline, the primary adrenal gland hormone.

Besides altering your sleep/wake cycle, an imbalance in serotonin changes body temperature, alters sexual behavior, contributes to Parkinson's disease, and sways the neuroendocrine balance.

The neurotransmitter acetylcholine is necessary for:
- Memory
- Cognitive functioning
- Learning
- Preventing senility
- Hand-eye coordination
- Parasympathetic nerve transmission

Other neurotransmitter amino acids, peptides, and nucleotides regulate different functions.

As cell communication breaks down, the brain falters in its ability to regulate the release of these chemicals and hormones. It triggers inappropriate responses to information—e.g., releases excess insulin, causes mood swings, overtaxes the liver and kidneys (which are charged with maintaining proper blood chemical balance), and induces premature neuroendocrinological aging.

The symptoms of the aging brain vary markedly among individuals. Some people remain mentally alert until death. Others experience a gradual decline in memory, learning abilities, and speed of thinking. In its advanced stages, the symptoms of brain aging are called senility or senile dementia and afflict about 4 percent of the adults over sixty-five years old. Alzheimer's disease, the most common illness causing senile dementia, occurs from an extensive destruction of brain neurons. Disorientation, forgetfulness, loss of bodily control, and the inability to perform simple tasks may require those suffering from advanced brain aging to be under constant care since they become unable to look out for themselves.

Recent research indicates that the rate of brain aging can be dramatically slowed (or hastened) by the kind and amount of work the brain is required to do. In some ways the brain is akin to a muscle—if you don't use it, it atrophies.

Marian Diamond, an anatomist at the University of Berkeley, reported in the *American Scientist* that rats in an isolated, deprived environment suffered brain cell loss. This is directly analogous to the loss of brain cells observed in post-mortem examinations of those elderly who were kept in isolation wards.

In contrast, Mark Rosenweigh, a researcher at the University of California, placed rats in an environment with plenty of toys, ladders, and other stimulating items. Their cerebral brain cortex (the part for learning and thinking) was thicker than that of animals deprived of such enriched environments.

Applying these proven results to humans, it seems likely that people who isolate themselves from others and avoid learning or having fresh experiences will age, especially neurologically, much more quickly than their active counterparts.

To keep your brain operating at peak effectiveness, you need to provide many different kinds of stimulation. Exercise, in addition to increasing the supply of oxygen to your brain, also causes it to fire neurons across specific pathways. Loving social interaction causes the brain to fire other pathways. Learning and processing new information requires the activity of yet another set of pathways. Just as a child's brain and I.Q. develop more quickly when he or she is surrounded by visual, auditory, kinesthetic, emotional, and intellectual stimulation, so does the same stimulation help retard brain aging.

Another way to protect the integrity of your brain and nervous system is to get plenty of rest and maintain balanced body rhythms. Sleep is the restorative phase that repairs damaged brain cells. Body rhythms govern the release of chemicals and hormones critical to proper neuroendocrinological functioning.

Make a habit of using both sides of your brain. The left side is for logical thinking, language, and analysis. The right side deals in imagination, rhythm, creativity, and intuition. Left-brain dominance prevails in our society. Develop your weak side. Perform arts, music, and visualization if you are left-brain dominant. Learn logical thinking or use a computer if you are right-brain dominant.

Practice meditation or hypnosis or spend time regularly in an isolation tank. Each of these techniques provides deep nourishment to the brain and nervous system and has been shown to improve learning abilities, memory, problem solving, and creativity.

If you feel you are already suffering from brain aging, you may want to consult with your doctor about two types of treatments. The anti-aging drugs Hydergine, EDTA, Piracetam, and Centrophenoxine treat different types of brain dysfunction (see Chapter 13 for details about each drug). Hyperbaric oxygen treatment, performed in two treatments a day for fifteen days, may also prove helpful. Elderly patients in nursing homes who have undergone this therapy have experienced a marked removal of

TABLE 49

Possible Brain and Nerve Enhancers

Supplement	Daily Amount	Effect
Phosphatidyl choline/lecithin DMAE (dimethylaminoethanol)*	5–15 gm 100–300 mg.	Forms acetylcholine, a neurotransmitter that improves memory, learning, and thinking
L-phenylalanine** L-tyrosine	200–1000 mg. 500–2000 mg.	Forms the neurotransmitter dopamine necessary for correct neuroendocrine function. Prevents depression and fatigue, enhances energy.
Vitamin B-6 Vitamin C	20–30 mg. 500 mg.	Vitamins to form dopamine
RNA	500–1000 mg.	RNA improves memory, nerves, and the transfer of information in synthesizing cells
Vitamin B-12	10–50 mcg.	Helps produce RNA
Cell aids	(*See* individual supplements given in this chapter)	Remove lipofuscins that destroy neurons; protect against free radicals and fight cross-linkage that damages nerve cells

Protein-digesting enzymes
  Bromelain
  Papain
  Chymotrypsin
	
	240–500 GDU
	300–600 MCU
	10 mg.
		Eliminate cerebral allergies that result from incomplete protein digestion

Herbs
  Rehmannia
  Hoelen
  Moutan
  Cinnamon
  Dioscorea
  Cornus
  Aconite
  Alisma
	
	5.0 gm
	3.0 gm
	3.0 gm
	1.0 gm
	3.0 gm
	3.0 gm
	1.0 gm
	3.0 gm
		Traditional Chinese "Rehmannia Eight" formula said to prevent senility. It also may be useful for degenerated kidneys, diabetes, climacteric disorders, skin problems, cataracts, glaucoma, failing eyesight, impotence, excretion difficulties.
		
		Should not be used by people with weak intestinal tracts, frequent diarrhea, and fever.

*DMAE should be taken initially in the lower recommended dosage. Increase at the rate of 50 milligrams every two weeks until you reach the maximum dosage. If you experience insomnia, headaches, or a stiff neck, reduce or eliminate the supplement. *Pregnant women should not use DMAE.*

**L-phenylalanine may raise blood pressure.

See the Age Reduction Supplement Guide in Chapter 9 for a list of supplement suppliers and complete instructions on the correct and safe use of supplements.

almost intractable senility symptoms and in some cases have been able to go home and function normally. Contact the American Academy of Medical Preventics, listed in the Age Reduction Resource Guide, for information and the names of doctors who perform these techniques.

And finally, you can help delay cellular brain aging by eating a healthy diet and possibly by taking the supplements listed in Table 49 to stimulate neurocircuitry as well as compensate for neurotransmitter decline.

MUSCLE IMPROVERS

Since muscles are composed of cells and tissues, they are equally vulnerable to the aging factors already discussed in those sections. The age-related deterioration of cells and energy metabolism means that as your muscles become intolerant to glucose as an energy source, they are also receiving less ATP (adenosine triphosphate), the universal energy molecule. Muscles are also susceptible to two other premature aging factors: decreased growth hormone supply and an unbalanced neuroendocrine system.

Growth hormone, as we discussed earlier, is produced and released by your body to stimulate DNA, RNA, and protein synthesis. It helps build strong muscles, strengthens tendons and other connective tissue, and improves your immune system. Growth hormone production and release is at its peak during adolescence; its release is gradually inhibited with age. Decreased growth hormone contributes to muscular deterioration and fat deposition.

An unbalanced neuroendocrine system reduces your supply of dopamine and noradrenaline (a neurotransmitter necessary for energy production, survival activities, and moving about). It also reduces brain levels of acetylcholine, a neurotransmitter needed to control voluntary and involuntary muscles properly. Acetylcholine loss is associated with lack of muscular coordination, tone, and control and poor reaction speed. Finally, an unbalanced neuroendocrine system helps to set into motion the excessive insulin–depressed growth hormone cycle (discussed above in the "Growth Hormone Stimulators" section) that causes you to convert food into fat instead of fuel for your muscles.

Your best protection against premature muscle aging is to follow a balanced fitness program throughout life. Exercising improves the supply of oxygen, water, and nutrients to muscle tissues and cells, stabilizes and improves energy metabolism, and significantly slows the loss of lean muscle mass, muscular coordination, and reaction speed that result from aging.

In addition, the supplements in Table 50 may help you stimulate growth hormone production and release, increase cell repair and reproduction, and stabilize your neuroendocrine system.

TABLE 50

Possible Muscle Improvers

Supplement	Daily Amount	Effect
Daytime growth hormone stimulators*	(Should be taken on an empty stomach, early in the day, and before exercise)	
L-ornithine	2–5 gm	Amino acids release growth hormone during the day. L-tyrosine also enhances energy.
L-arginine	2–5 gm	
L-tyrosine†	800–1000 mg.	
Vitamin B-6	20–30 mg.	
Vitamin C	400 mg.	
Nighttime growth hormone stimulators*	(Should be taken forty-five minutes to an hour before going to bed on an empty stomach)	
L-ornithine	3–6 gm	Amino acids release growth hormone while sleeping and aid falling asleep.
L-glycine	4–8 gm	
Vitamin B-6	20–30 mg.	Vitamin cofactors help growth hormone release.
Vitamin C	400 mg.	
L-carnitine**	500–1000 mg	Increase growth hormone by decreasing free fatty acids that otherwise suppress it. L-carnitine also enhances the release of ATP (adenosine triphosphate), fights muscle wasting, improves energy transfer.
Cod liver oil	2 tsp.	
Insulin-response improvers	(*See* section in this chapter)	Prevent excessive insulin that suppresses growth hormone
Cytochrome C**	500–1000 mg.	Increases oxygen availability to the mitochondria. Aids muscular reaction, reduces fatigue, and helps endurance training
Inosine**	300–600 mg.	Improves oxygen-carrying capacity of blood to muscles to reduce muscular fatigue from activity
Vitamin B-5 (pantothenic acid)**	40–100 mg.	Produce ATP (adenosine triphosphate) for all energy processes, endurance, and stamina.
Vitamin B-6 (pyridoxine)	20–30 mg.	

*Growth hormone stimulators should not be used by adolescents, juvenile diabetics, and pregnant or lactating women.

†Before using L-tyrosine to release growth hormone, read "Resetting Your Internal Time Clocks" in Chapter 6.

**Use these supplements one-half hour before exercise.

See the Age Reduction Supplement Guide in Chapter 9 for a list of supplement suppliers and complete instructions on the correct and safe use of supplements.

Supplement	Daily Amount	Effect
DMG (dimethylglycine)**	50–250 mg.	Controls lactic acid buildup during exercise. Enhances stamina, power, and endurance.
Octacosanol**	50–200 mcg.	A wheat germ concentrate that improves reaction time, oxygen use, endurance, and stamina. Reduces cholesterol.
Coenzyme Q-10	15–30 mg.	Prescribed to increase muscular energy and strengthen heart contractions in people with a history of heart problems
Energy enhancers	(See separate supplements previously listed)	Increase ATP for greater physical and chemical energy. May improve endurance and stamina.
Brain and nerve enhancers	(See separate supplements previously listed)	Enhance brain function and nerve transmissions that regulate muscular activities
Protein supplements	—	Predigested and free form amino acids of the correct amino acid ratio help build muscles
Water or electrolyte solution	As needed hourly during exercise and upon completion	Replace fluids lost from perspiring during exercise that weakens and dehydrates your body
Water-soluble nutrients	(See Chapter 9, Supplemental Nutrient Guide)	Replace nutrients lost through exercise, stress, and perspiration
Caffeine	200–300 mg.	Increase fat metabolism for energy while exercising
Protein-digesting enzymes Bromelain Papain Chymotrypsin	240–1000 GDU 300–1000 MCU 10–20 mg.	Stimulate muscle repair of bruises and reduce muscle inflammation and soreness

**Use these supplements one-half hour before exercise.

SUPPORTERS FOR YOUR SKELETAL SYSTEM

As your skeletal system ages, your bones become weak and brittle. Your spinal discs give in to the force of gravity and compress against each other, causing a loss in height and frequent back problems. Your jaw loses bone mass, creating pockets around the teeth that cause periodontal disease. The connective tissue that forms joints deteriorates (as discussed earlier) and causes inflammations. A breakdown in calcium metabolism causes calcium to be leached from the skeletal system and deposited in the cells of muscles and other soft tissues, leading to arteriosclerosis and other sclerotic diseases. A negative calcium balance plays a role in cardiovascular disease, hypertension, and strokes. (See below for a discussion of factors leading to the breakdown of calcium metabolism.) Post-menopausal women are particularly susceptible to bone loss, since after menopause they no longer produce the hormone estrogen, which protects against bone loss.

You can substantially reduce and delay calcium imbalances and skeletal system aging by making some simple changes in your diet and life-style.

Eat a diet that is rich in calcium and magnesium (e.g., dairy products, dark green leafy vegetables, broccoli, and whole grains). Calcium is an essential bone mineral, while magnesium is necessary to keep calcium in the skeletal system and out of soft tissue cells.

Avoid eating phosphorus-rich foods such as soft drinks, dairy substitutes, food preservatives, toothpaste. Most Americans consume too much phosphorus, which increases the risk of calcium metabolism breakdown. The correct daily amount of calcium, magnesium, and phosphorus is from 600 to 1000 milligrams of each.

Avoid eating salt-rich foods. Salt inhibits the exchange of sodium and calcium across cell membranes and causes calcium to accumulate in smooth muscle cells.

Also avoid eating too much protein (it leaches calcium from the bones), drinking too much alcohol, or smoking too many cigarettes.

Avoid nutrient supplements containing phosphorus and the standard 2:1 ratio of calcium/magnesium.

Brush your teeth and floss daily.

Exercise regularly. It helps prevent bone mineral loss.

Discover mineral imbalances with hair analysis, intracellular element measurements, and bone densitometer testing. Intracellular element measurements directly measure the mineral content of cells by using a scanning electronic microscope with X-ray fluorescence. The Digital Bone Densitometer works by radiographic measurements of bone. Both these devices detect osteoporosis and tendencies toward arteriosclerosis, cancer, and other diseases.

If you suffer from arthritis, rheumatism, or other skeletal problems, consult with your doctor about taking these supplements.

Factors Causing Bone Calcium Loss

Dietary Factors
- More dietary phosphorus than calcium
- Insufficient dietary calcium (less than 600 to 1000 milligrams daily)
- Less dietary magnesium than calcium

- Excess sodium (salt)
- Excess protein (see Chapter 8)
- Excess vitamin D (more than 15,000 IU daily) from supplements, vitamin D–enriched dairy products, fish, concentrated liver oils, flour, margarine, cereals, and canned sardines
- Vitamin C inadequacy (less than 100 milligrams a day)
- Chronic coffee drinking (more than two cups daily)

Life-style Factors

- Stress
- Excess alcohol drinking (more than three drinks daily)
- Overexposure to toxic metals, especially lead, mercury, cadmium, and aluminum. (If you believe you may be overexposed, undergo hair analysis testing.)
- Chronic use of antacids containing aluminum (many commercial preparations contain aluminum, so read labels)
- Stimulant and diuretic drugs
- Living in a chronically clouded environment
- Spending most daylight hours indoors

Metabolic Factors

- Liver disease
- Kidney disease
- Lack of estrogen in women
- Insufficient stomach acid (test with radiotelemetry or EAV)
- Low thyroid activity
- Abnormal vitamin D metabolism
- Glucose intolerance and high blood sugar
- Parathyroid gland problems
- Insufficient cell energy
- Damaged cell membranes

TABLE 51

Possible Skeletal Supporters

Supplement	Daily Amount	Effect
Calcium	600–1200 mg.	Provide elements to build strong bones and joints
Magnesium	600–1000 mg.	
Silicon	100–200 mg.	
Zinc	30–50 mg.	
Vitamin C	1000–2000 mg.	Promote the formation of healthy tissues and bones.
Vitamin D	400–1000 IU	(Vitamin B-6 also aids Carpal tunnel syndrome.)
Vitamin B-6	20–30 mg.	
Folic acid	400 mcg.	

Supplement	Daily Amount	Effect
Mucopolysaccharides	(*See* tissue aids listed earlier in this chapter)	Enhance tissue and bone formation
Vitamin B-5	40–100 mg.	Reduces inflammation of osteoarthritis

See the Age Reduction Supplement Guide in Chapter 9 for a list of supplement suppliers and complete instructions on the correct and safe use of supplements.

Post-menopausal women should consider estrogen replacement therapy (ERT). (See "Female Sexual System Rejuvenators," later in this chapter.)

MALE SEXUAL SYSTEM REJUVENATORS

The male sexual system deteriorates gradually throughout life, mainly as a result of the age-related breakdowns of other parts of the body. Since there is no preprogrammed switch-off point for the male sexual system, most men in good health can enjoy sex throughout life. However, the system is susceptible to both physiological and psychological aging factors.

Physiological causes include brain and nervous system degeneration, malnutrition (particularly deficiencies in thiamine, niacin, vitamin B-12, and vitamin E), alcoholism, obesity, unbalanced body rhythms, diabetes, hormonal imbalances, and hypoglycemia.

The male sexual system is highly dependent on a balanced neuroendocrine system for proper functioning, since the parasympathetic system creates erections and the sympathetic system causes ejaculations. Those with an advanced degree of neuroendocrinological imbalance or aging are likely to suffer from impotence.

Drugs that depress the male sexual system include:
• Anti-hypertensive agents
• Corticosteroids
• Stimulants
• Cocaine
• Barbiturates
• Hallucinogens
• Depressants
• Estrogens
• Anti-ulcer agents.
• Marijuana, which, in addition to depressing the sexual system, decreases sperm mobility
Consuming too much L-tryptophan or serotonin-rich foods such as

TABLE 52

Possible Male Sexual System Improvers

Supplement	Daily Amount	Effect
Selenium	200–300 mcg.	Normalize testosterone production;
Zinc	30–50 mg.*	increase sperm count and motility: help
L-carnitine	400–800 mg.	problems of impotence in some men
L-arginine	4 gm	
GABA	100 mg.	Compensate for low sex drive among men
L-tyrosine	500–1500 mg.	who have excess prolactin hormone
Dragon Bone	3.0 gm	Traditional Chinese "Lotus Stamen"
Oyster shell	3.0 gm	formula for impotence and involuntary
Lotus stamen	6.0 gm	emissions
Tribulus	6.0 gm	
Euryale	6.0 gm	
Lotus seed	3.0 gm	
Cinnamon	4.0 gm	Traditional Chinese "Cinnamon and Dragon
Ginger	4.0 gm	Bone" formula for loss of sexual vigor.
Dragon Bone	3.0 gm	Best suited for weak men with delicate
Peony	4.0 gm	constitutions.
Oyster shell	3.0 gm	
Jujube	4.0 gm	
Licorice	2.0 gm	
Vitamin E	100–200 IU	Supplements that help benign prostate
Evening primrose	3–4 gm	hypertrophy, an enlargement of the
L-glutamic acid	175–525 mg.	prostate gland that causes decreased
L-alanine	180–540 mg.	and painful urination, insomnia,
L-glycine	145–435 mg.	dribbling, and physical and mental
		irritation. This problem is common in
		elderly men.
Muscle aids and energy enhancers	(*See* individual supplements in previous corresponding list)	Increase energy, endurance, and stamina for sex

See the Age Reduction Supplement Guide in Chapter 9 for a list of supplement suppliers and complete instructions on the correct and safe use of supplements.

unripe bananas may contribute to excess serotonin, a sexual system depressant. This may be counteracted by ingesting the amino acid L-tyrosine, which converts into dopamine, a sexual system stimulant.

Even something as simple as frequently wearing tight pants can decrease blood circulation in the pelvis and interfere with the ability to achieve erection.

Psychological factors that damage the male sexual system include depression, stress, performance anxiety, low self-esteem, and a poor body image.

The symptoms of an aging sexual system are depressed desire, difficulty becoming aroused, the need for increased recovery time, decreased amount of sperm ejaculated, shorter orgasm, sagging testes, and degeneration of the sex glands and tissues.

Grim as this sounds, it is almost entirely avoidable. Centenarians are documented as having good sex throughout life, and you can, too.

The best way to prevent premature sexual system aging is to improve the state of your mind. Relax. The point of sex is pleasure, not performance. As you get older you may want to ejaculate less often and enjoy sex more often. A fifty-year-old man probably should not ejaculate more than once every three days, but having sex every day without orgasm will do wonders for self-esteem, satisfaction, and the prospects for longevity. The ancient Chinese developed special techniques to control ejaculation and extend lovemaking. You may want to explore these. My male clients who master these techniques tell me they receive excellent ratings as lovers.

An understanding lover who doesn't pressure you to perform is essential for good sex. Impotence from performance anxiety is a common problem of men with demanding lovers.

If your sexual desire is dampened by negative stress or excessive fatigue, take better care of yourself. Learn how to cope with stress. Get enough sleep. Eat a healthy diet and exercise regularly to increase energy, improve body image, and keep sexual mechanisms functioning.

If you believe your sexual problems spring from psychological factors beyond your control, you may want to consult a therapist or other counselor.

You may also find you can support your sexual system and prevent premature aging by taking the supplements listed in Table 52.

FEMALE SEXUAL SYSTEM REJUVENATORS

Since female sexual systems are cyclical rather than continual, delaying the shift from one cycle to the next is an important longevity factor for women. Evolution becomes officially attentive to the female sexual system at puberty, when the onset of ovulation makes it possible to bear children. Evolution loses interest at the onset of menopause, when the childbearing years are over. In its own self-interested way, evolution simply turns off the now unnecessary sexual system—hormones and all—and goes about its other business.

Unfortunately, in this case your self-interest and that of evolution do not coincide. The act of switching off your sexual system is one of the key metabolic shifts of aging. So, by stabilizing your ovulation and menstruation cycles, you can also add years to your life.

The first symptoms of sexual system deregulation usually occur in your mid-thirties. The frequency of ovulation and menstruation decreases. At the onset of menopause, ovulation and menstruation cease altogether. Your body stops producing estrogen and progesterone, causing mood swings, hot flashes, and other discomforts. Cellular, tissue, and organ aging affect your vagina, vulva, cervix, uterus, and ovaries. Your sexual apparatus shrinks, stiffens, loses flexibility and elasticity. Intercourse can become painful.

Many of the factors that hasten premature sexual system aging in men are equally degenerative to women.

Physiological factors include hormonal imbalances, circulatory difficulties, obesity, unbalanced body rhythms, environmental toxins. Drugs that decrease your sexual drive, increase frigidity, and induce sexual system aging are:

- Heart drugs
- High blood pressure medication
- Tranquilizers
- Sedatives
- Antidepressants
- Antihistamines
- Anti-ulcer drugs
- Steroids
- Bromides
- Appetite suppressants
- Anticonvulsant drugs
- Alcohol
- Speed
- Marijuana
- Cocaine and other illegal drugs

Birth control pills that contain excessive amounts of synthetic estrogens and testosterone-based progesterones are the worst offenders among drugs that age the sexual system. To understand why, you must realize that birth control pills trick your body into believing it's pregnant; and pregnancy itself mimics the metabolic process of aging.

When you become pregnant your immune system is temporarily depressed. (That's because its energy and attention have been diverted to protect the fetus and prevent its expulsion as a foreign body.) Depressed immunity is a key factor in aging. During pregnancy your body gains fat, loses muscle, and secretes excess insulin. Each of these processes is necessary for a healthy pregnancy; each is also part of the aging process. Some pregnant women even become diabetic, an unmistakable metabolic shift of aging. Steroid contraceptives decrease carbohydrate utilization and increase triglycerides, free fatty acids, and body fat. They accelerate the development of diabetes and atherosclerosis. Oral contraceptives increase risk of some kinds of cancer and stroke. Fortunately, an increasing number of physicians are prescribing oral contraceptives with very low amounts of hormones. This may work to benefit the female system rather than age it.

Sexual system malfunction and aging is also caused by psychological factors. Negative stress, depression, anxiety, low self-esteem, and poor body image tend to depress sexual activity, which in turn causes your physical sexual apparatus to decay and wither. Remember that nature doesn't keep what isn't being used.

TABLE 53

Possible Female Sexual System Rejuvenators

Supplement	Daily Amount	Effect
Iron	10 mg.	Prevents anemia, a common problem for women between the ages of puberty and menopause and especially during pregnancy.
Folic acid	400 mcg.	Works with iron to prevent anemia
Vitamin B-12	10–50 mcg.	
Vitamin B-6	20–30 mg.	
Copper	1.5–2.5 mg.	
Vitamin C	1–2 gm	
L-tyrosine	500–1500 mg.	Helps delay female sexual aging by increasing dopamine in the hypothalamus
Vitamin E	100–200 IU	Increase pelvic blood flow to the clitoris and prevent pelvic congestion, which decreases sexuality and orgasm ability
DMG (dimethylglycine)	50–100 mg.	
Zinc	30–50 mg.	Compensate for nutrient loss in oral contraceptive users.
Vitamin B-6	20–30 mg.	
Folic acid	400 mcg.	
Evening primrose oil	3–4 gm	Help relieve premenstrual tension when started 2 to 3 days before its onset, also dysmenorrhea (painful menstruation). In clinical research, 500 mg. of vitamin B-6 used under doctor's supervision appeared to relieve premenstrual syndrome (PMS).
Cod liver oil	2 tsp.	
Calcium	400 mg.	
Magnesium	800 mg.	
Vitamin B-6	20–30 mg.	
Zinc	30–50 mg.	

The first step in delaying sexual system aging is to stabilize the menstrual cycle and prevent premature menopause. The second step is to replace the hormones no longer produced after menopause so that the aging effects associated with menopause are avoided or reduced.

There are several ways you can prevent premature menopause. Eating a healthy diet, keeping your body fat low, and exercising regularly will rejuvenate your sexual mechanisms. Keeping your body rhythms synchronized is important for delaying sexual aging. (See Chapter 6 for details.) Learning how to cope with negative stress and getting enough sleep will increase your sexual appetite—consistent and rewarding sex is critical to keeping your sexual system functioning properly. You may want to seek professional help if you feel unable to overcome any sexual problems.

Estrogen/progesterone replacement therapy is extremely valuable if you are over thirty-five. It's possible that, by stabilizing your estrogen/progesterone levels *before* menopause and increasing brain dopamine, you can actually delay menopause. During and after menopause, estrogen/progesterone replacement therapy can be used to treat hot flashes, vaginal dryness and atrophy, depression, anxiety, nervousness, and insomnia. It also may help reduce the risk of breast cancer, osteoporosis, and heart attack in post-menopausal women. This therapy increases glucose tolerance, controls cholesterol, and delays the metabolic shifts of aging. It has the opposite effect from high amounts of synthetic estrogens in oral contraceptives.

One word of caution: If you decide to use estrogen/progesterone therapy, make sure your doctor provides a *balance* of the two hormones. Use of estrogen alone has been associated with conditions such as endometrial cancer. In addition, I recommend that you request natural estrogen estradiol rather than conjugated estrogens. Besides being safer, estrogen estradiol has the added benefit of lowering total blood cholesterol and increasing the ratio of HDL to LDL cholesterol, which will help protect you from heart disease. You should also use progestin type of progesterone.

Other supplements that may help maintain the integrity of your sexual system and delay aging are listed in Table 53.

ANTI-AGING DRUGS

Using drugs to slow or prevent aging may be extraordinarily valuable in the future, but the current crop of anti-aging drugs are of limited use today. The problem is that our understanding of aging mechanisms (as well as the entire human organism) is so limited that what works in theory may prove disastrous in reality. In addition, we have not yet developed adequate testing procedures to be able to prescribe the correct drugs for extending life.

An effective analogy for this problem is science's ability to create salt water "identical" to sea water. Based on sophisticated chemical analysis, we have every reason to believe we can exactly duplicate the chemical composition of salt water. However, for some reason salt-water fish can't live in the synthesized duplicate.

I don't use "chronotherapy" drugs myself and rarely recommend them to my younger clients for these reasons:

- It's easy to become mesmerized by the life extension promise these drugs provide and then to tend to overdose.
- The synthetic products on which these drugs are based may cause your metabolism to react by creating toxic by-products.
- Synthetic drugs may also unbalance your vital energy, ultimately shortening your life.
- The negative side effects of some of the more powerful "chronotherapy" drugs may overwhelm their potential benefits.
- Individual drug interactions with nutrients, supplements, other drugs, and metabolic processes are frequently unknown.

I do believe that, under professional supervision and the right conditions, especially in the elderly, "chronotherapy" drugs are useful. L-dopa, for example, has proven invaluable in treating Parkinson's disease, an accelerated form of aging that causes rigid paralysis in the elderly. Other drugs whose benefits may outweigh the side effects are aspirin, Hydergine, vasopressin, EDTA (ethylenediamine tetracetate), and GH-3 (Gerovital).

Caution: Do not under any circumstances experiment with any of the powerful drugs discussed in this section unless you are under the supervision of a doctor trained in gerontologic pharmacology. The data here is supplied for your information only.

Aspirin
Action: An analgesic and anti-inflammatory drug.
Effects: Normally used to reduce pain from inflammation and rheumatoid arthritis. However, when used daily in low doses, aspirin has been shown to decrease risk of heart attack by thinning the blood and avoiding blood clotting. As a cortisol antagonist, it may delay aging by reducing stress-related disorders. It also appears to prevent lipofuscin deposits and strengthen cell membranes in humans.
Side effects: Excessive amounts cause hearing loss, prolonged bleeding, nausea, dizziness, excitability, and, in the elderly, the common loss of high-pitch hearing.

Gerovital (GH-3)
Action: A Rumanian anti-aging drug, an expensive version of buffered procaine. GH-3 (available in the United States in eleven states) breaks down in the body and forms PABA (a B vitamin) and DEAE (diethylaminoethanol), a relative of DMAE (dimethylaminoethanol) that helps synthesize the neurotransmitter acetylcholine. GH-3 is a MAO (monamine oxidase) inhibitor, as well as a cortisol inhibitor.
Effects: GH-3 appears to have a temporary effect in relieving depression, improving intelligence, enhancing concentration, and promoting general well-being. According to research conducted at the University of Southern California, GH-3 may slow cellular aging through its beneficial effect on neurotransmitters. As a cortisol antagonist, it may delay aging by reducing stress-related disorders. It also appears to prevent lipofuscin deposits and strengthen cell membranes in humans.
Side effects: Unknown.

Hydergine
Action: A non-hallucinogenic derivative of lysergic acid (LSD), Hydergine accumulates in the brain to increase protein synthesis and brain cell metabolism, modulate nerve control, and stabilize EEG readings.
Effects: Doctors use Hydergine to treat senility-related symptoms such as lack of alertness, poor memory, confusion, and depression. It may also prevent hypoglycemia's mental symptoms, such as inability to concentrate, irritability, insecurity. Hydergine has been found to reduce mental deterioration from cerebral arteriosclerosis and to increase I.Q. in healthy people of all ages.
Side effects: Hydergine overdoses may cause headaches, facial flushing, indigestion, nausea, vomiting, low blood pressure, weakness, or coma. The most common side effect is nasal congestion.

L-Dopa
Action: L-dopa is an amino acid precursor to the neurotransmitter dopamine. As L-dopa passes through the blood-brain barrier (a membrane that protects the brain from toxic elements), it is converted into dopamine. L-dopa is an antioxidant and growth hormone releaser. Bromocriptine is similar to L-dopa, but with fewer side effects.

Effects: Doctors use L-dopa to control the rigidity, tremors, and abnormal gait symptomatic of Parkinson's disease. However, its anti-aging properties are related to righting the imbalance of dopamine/serotonin that occurs with—and perhaps induces—aging. It has extended life-span in experimental research. It has also increased sexual drive, restored ovulation in menopausal women, and relieved depression.

Side effects: Although rare, there are more than 100 potential side effects to using L-dopa. The most common are muscle twitching, spastic eyelids, diarrhea, nausea, weakness, rapid and irregular pulse, confusion, agitation, vomiting, dry mouth, moodiness, and uncontrolled body movements.

Levamisole

Action: Levamisole is an agent used to destroy worms. It also mildly stimulates the immune system.

Effects: Although still experimental, it appears to prevent hypersensitivity reactions and improve immune responses.

Side effects: Unknown.

Biguanide drugs

Action: There are three types of biguanide drugs: Phenformin, Metformin, and Buformin. All are anti-hypoglycemic drugs that lower blood sugar levels, possibly by inhibiting liver formation of sugar carbohydrates. Biguanide drugs also inhibit free fatty acids and oxygenation, and they lower blood cholesterol and triglycerides. It is postulated that biguanide drugs extend life by increasing hypothalamic/pituitary sensitivity to feedback, thereby reducing premature aging disorders such as obesity, diabetes, and atherosclerosis.

Effects: Phenformin has been used successfully to reduce the incidence of diabetes mellitus and cancer, restore female ovulation, strengthen the immune system, and prevent bone demineralization. In experiments with animals, Phenformin has delayed preprogrammed arteriosclerosis and extended life-span.

Side effects: Adverse reactions to biguanide drugs are severe. In individuals with diabetes, Phenformin may increase mortality from cardiovascular disease. These drugs should not be used by anyone who has kidney problems or has ever suffered congestive heart failure. On rare occasions, biguanide drugs may overescalate your level of lactic acid, causing lactic acidosis. Other side effects include metallic taste, appetite loss, diarrhea, and cramps.

Centrophenoxine

Action: Restores nerve synapse communication, elminates age pigments, and stabilizes cell membranes.

Effects: Treats mental deterioration—memory loss, confusion, and intellectual impairment. Available in Europe, but not in the United States.

Side effects: Unknown.

Dilantin (diphenylhydantoin)

Action: Dilantin increases intercellular potassium concentration by altering the hypothalamic/pituitary sensitivity to feedback. It inhibits the normal aging process by influencing the central aging clock that governs metabolic shifts.

Effects: Doctors prescribe Dilantin to prevent epileptic seizures and restore regular heartbeat. However, in experiments with animals it has succeeded in inhibiting the formation of arteriosclerosis and extending life-span. In experiments with humans it has decreased the incidence of cancer.

Side effects: The most common adverse reactions are dizziness, drowsiness, constipation, nausea, and vomiting. Other less common side effects include jerky eye movements, slurred speech, low blood pressure, and coma.

Physostigmine and Arecoline

Action: These drugs inhibit cholinesterase, the enzyme that destroys acetylcholine, a brain neurotransmitter. Age-related loss of acetylcholine is associated with reduced mental function.

Effects: Experimental research indicates physostigmine and arecoline improve memory in the elderly. Unfortunately, these drugs lose half of their potency in less than one hour after administration. Tetrahydroamine, a largely untested but potentially useful related drug, also acts as a cholinesterase inhibitor, but is effective for six to twelve hours. On balance, supplemental lecithin, choline, and DMAE (dimethylaminoethanol) are the safest and surest methods for increasing acetylcholine.

Side effects: Hallucinations, muscular twitching, weakness, nausea, diarrhea, bronchial spasms, heart palpitations.

PCPA (parachlorophenylalanine)
Action: An experimental drug that decreases brain serotonin.
Effects: Increases male sexual activity along with testosterone.
Side effects: Unknown.

Sulfadiazine
Action: Sulfadiazine is used to prevent and cure bacterial infections.
Effects: Physicians prescribe sulfadiazine to treat dysentery, meningococcal infections, urinary tract infections, and certain streptococcal infections. In experiments with geriatric patients, small daily doses have rejuvenated tissue and sexual function and improved hearing, vision, and general health. (NOTE: This experiment used vitamin B-5 and magnesium ascorbate—a buffered form of vitamin C and magnesium—in combination with sulfadiazine drugs.)
Side effects: A mild side effect is the depletion of intestinal lactobacilli, which can be counteracted by supplementing B vitamins. Other and potentially dangerous adverse effects include fever and damage to kidneys, liver, skin, nerves, bone marrow, and blood system. In one study 57 percent of the patients experienced at least some of these side effects.

Testosterone
Action: Offsets the age-related loss of the male sex hormone testosterone.
Effects: Increases libido, erections, ejaculation, and sexual pleasure.
Side effects: Edema, skin changes, sore mouth, abnormal liver functions.

Vasopressin
Action: Vasopressin is a posterior pituitary hormone that helps the kidneys absorb water. Age-related loss of kidney hydration is associated with memory loss and behavioral abnormalities.
Effects: Doctors use vasopressin to treat elderly patients (particularly in the fifty-five to sixty-five age range) for memory and behavior problems. It is also useful for treating the early stages of Alzheimer's disease.
Side effects: Adverse reactions include nasal congestion, irritation, heartburn, tremor, dizziness, headache, cramps, nausea, and numerous other problems.

Isoprinosine
Action: Dramatically increases immunity, helps repair a damaged immune system.
Effects: European drug sold under the name of Immunovir may help prevent AIDS in individuals exposed to the virus. Treats pre-AIDS and AIDS patients. Used to treat herpes, influenza, and hepatitis. Anticancer possibilities. Has extended test animals' life-span.
Side effects: Unknown.

Piracetam and Pramiracetam
Action: Stimulate ATP (adenosine triphosphate) in brain cells for energy. Increases cholinergic activity.
Effects: Improves thinking, learning, and memory. Treats Alzheimer's disease and senility.
Side effects: Unknown.

Epilogue

This chapter heading summarizes the Age Reduction System's purpose: to add an epilogue to your life.

In novels, the epilogue gives you a chance to find out how life turned out for the characters you loved . . . or loved to hate.

In real life, an epilogue is an opportunity to actualize the wisdom you've accumulated along the way. Instead of being driven by the concerns of youth—getting ahead, raising a family, creating a string of accomplishments—you will, if you're fortunate, be blessed by the benefits of age—greater self-acceptance and understanding, a recognition of essential values, freedom from the tyranny of others' opinions. I'm not suggesting that these are the only, or even the most important, benefits of reaching old age. I am suggesting that each of life's phases has its own rewards and that few of us would choose, with hindsight, to return to a younger age.

However, for an epilogue to be worthwhile, you must be physically, mentally, and emotionally capable of participating in it. That's why the Age Reduction System is designed not just to add years to your life but life to your years.

The Age Reduction System offers a set of guidelines, ideas, and techniques that have proven successful in bridging the gap of the average life-span—69 years—to the maximum life-span—110 years.

The rigidity of absolute "truth" is the antithesis of the Age Reduction System's approach. I don't believe longevity can be achieved by slavishly following someone else's rules. Even the best ideas can become bad ones when they cease to respect individuality.

You are an utterly unique, one-of-a-kind original. There has never been anyone quite like you before, and there will never be anyone quite like you again. Your energy; metabolism; nutrient requirements; responses to stress, weather, environment; DNA codes; and countless other aspects are as unique as your fingerprints.

Trying to reduce to a set of textbook rules the complicated, elusive energy that animates you is about as practical as trying to catch a moonbeam in your hand.

The temptation, however, is great. Since the days of the Industrial Revolution, our society has emphasized standardization. We want humans to be as predictable as machines. As a result, we put a lot of consequence on "what's normal."

So What's Normal?

Normal is the label that "qualified observers" stamp on statistical calculations of the tendencies of large populations in standardized conditions. What is normal bears little resemblance to what is real, for several reasons.

First, it is impossible for the observer to be objective about what he is observing. He brings to the act of observation his own preconceptions and prejudices, which can substantially pervert his judgment. Remember, for example, that if the same standards for diabetes were applied to both thirty-year-olds and sixty-five-year-olds, nearly all the older subjects would have diabetes. Since this idea is unacceptable to scientists, they simply changed the standards for what qualifies as a "normal" insulin response in older people.

Second, while definitions of "what's normal" may be useful in developing broad policies for masses of people, they contain a wide margin of error for the individual. For example, protein requirements may vary among individuals by as much as 200 to 300 percent. Vitamin requirements may vary by 1000 percent. Sensitivity to weather, drugs, environmental hazards, and stress also vary dramatically.

Third, the fountain of information about health and longevity is, as yet, little more than a trickle. What's considered "normal" or benign now may later be discovered to be dangerous. In the 1950s, housewives were told that sugar was good for their children, that it provided a valuable source of energy. Now we know that refined sugar is a deadly enemy. In 1983 we thought that blood cholesterol levels of 220 to 260 milligrams were "normal" for middle-aged Americans. In 1984 we discovered that these cholesterol levels are actually *elevated* and are a *direct cause* of heart disease. We've now established new standards for "normal" blood cholesterol levels: less than 200 milligrams for Americans over thirty.

Your health and longevity are directly related to your ability to understand and accommodate to your unique mental, physical, and emotional needs. The Age Reduction System is designed to assist you in this process of self-discovery.

Designing Your Own Age Reduction System

In working with my clients I have usually found that two or three elements in their lives loom largest as threats to longevity. I might identify the problems as stress- or environment- or diet-related. Humans are nothing if not complicated. So I often use a computer to analyze the almost infinite variables and arrive at a reasonable course of action.

My computer profiles have been used by a great many of my clients. If you would like to be a part of that data base or learn more about your own metabolic fingerprint, you can do so by writing or calling:

Age Reduction System Computer Profile Program
P.O. Box 85152, Department MB159
San Diego, CA 92138
215-815-7788

Bibliography

The Age Reduction System has provided you with a solid foundation on which to build a long, healthy life. If it has also lit a fire under you to find out more about what makes you tick or to investigate further some peculiarity of your own, you may find this guide useful. It is not always easy to sift the facts of longevity from the chaff of speculation, hyperbole, and downright dangerous misinformation.

The bibliography here includes the books and articles, organized by subject area, that were instrumental in creating the Age Reduction System.

AGING

BOOKS

Blumenthal, Herman. *Handbook of the Diseases of Aging.* New York: Van Nostrand Reinhold Co., 1983.

Comfort, A. *The Biology of Senescence.* New York: Elsevier, 1979.

Dilman, V. M. *The Law of Deviation of Homeostasis and Diseases of Aging.* Boston: John Wright, 1981.

Finch, C. F., and L. Hayflick. *Handbook of the Biology of Aging.* New York: Van Nostrand Reinhold, 1977.

Florini, J. *Handbook of Biochemistry in Aging.* Boca Raton, Florida: CRC, 1981.

Kenney, R. *Physiology of Aging, A Synopsis.* Chicago: Year Book Medical Publishing Company, 1982.

Kent, Saul. *Your Personal Life-Extension Program.* New York: William Morrow & Co., 1985.

Masoro, E. *Handbook of Physiology in Aging.* Boca Raton, Florida: CRC, 1980.

Pelletier, K. R. *Longevity, Fulfilling Our Biological Potential.* New York: Dell, 1981.

Regelson, W. *Intervention in the Aging Process, Part A: Quantization, Epidemiology and Clinical Research.* New York: Alan R. Liss, 1983.

Strehler, B. L. *Time Cells and Aging.* New York: Academic Press, 1977.

Walker, R. F., and R. L. Cooper. *Experimental and Clinical Interventions in Aging.* New York: Marcel Dekker, 1983.

PERIODICALS AND ARTICLES

Burnet, "A Genetic Interpretation of Aging." *Lancet,* 2:827:480–483, 1973.

Kent, S., ed. *Antiaging News.* Hollywood, Florida: Life Extension Foundation, 1982–1985.

Palmore, E. B. "Predicting Longevity, A Follow-up Controlled for Age." *Gerontologist,* 9:4:247–250, 1969.

——. "Physical, Mental and Social Factors in Predicting Longevity." *Gerontologist,* 9:2:103–108, 1969.
——. "Longevity Predictions Implication for Practice." *Prost. Med. Journal,* 50:11:160–169, 1971.
Schock, N. "The Physiology of Aging." *Scientific American,* 100–110, January 1962.

BIOENERGY: ACUPUNCTURE, HOMEOPATHY
BIOILLUMINESCENT PHOTOGRAPHY

BOOKS

Barnothy, M. F. *Biological Effects of Magnetic Fields* (Vol. 1 and 2). New York: Plenum, 1964, 1969.
Burr, H. S. *The Fields of Life.* New York: Ballantine, 1972.
Diamond, John. *BK: Behavioral Kinesiology.* New York: Harper and Row, 1979.
McGarey, William. *Acupuncture and Body Energies.* Phoenix, Arizona: Gabriel Press, 1974.
National Health and Medical Research Council. *Acupuncture.* Appendix 10: *Shanghai Institute of Physiology,* Oct. 24, 1973. Canberra, Australia: Australian Government Publishing Service, 1974.
Omura, Y. *Acupuncture Medicine.* Tokyo: Japan Publications, 1982.
Ostrander, S., and L. Schroeder. *Psychic Discoveries Behind the Iron Curtain.* New York: Bantam, 1970.
Vithoulkas, G. *The Science of Homeopathy.* New York: Grove Press, 1980.
Walther, David S. *Applied Kinesiology.* Pueblo, Colorado: Systems D.C., 1976.

PERIODICALS AND ARTICLES

Dale, R. "The Origins and Future of Acupuncture." *American Journal of Acupuncture,* 10:2:101–121, 1982.
Gibson, R. G., *et al.,* "The Place for Non-pharmaceutical Therapy in Chronic Rheumatoid Arthritis: A Critical Study of Homeopathy." *British Homeopathic Journal,* July 1980.
Khoe, W. "Homeopathic Detoxification Combined with Electroacupuncture According to Voll." *American Journal of Acupuncture,* 9:4:319–325, 1981.
Kuraishy, Tariq. "Ultramolecular Medicine, A Hybridized Approach to Homeopathy and Electrodiagnosis." *Journal of the Society of Ultramolecular Medicine.*
Nelson, William. Personal Communication, September 1984 and May 1985.
Taubles, G. "The Ultimate Theory of Everything." *Discovery,* April 1975.
Ustianowski, P. A. "A Clinical Trial of Staphysagria in Post Coital Cystitis." *British Homeopathic Journal,* July 1980.
Voll, Reinhold. "Verification of Acupuncture by Means of Electroacupuncture According to Voll." *American Journal of Acupuncture,* 6:11:6 & 5, 1978.
Young, D. K. "Uncovering Stress (and a Whole Lot More)." *Health and Healing,* 1:2, 1984.
——.*Health and Healing,* 1:1, 1983.

BODY RHYTHMS, SLEEP

BOOKS

Drucker-Colin. *The Function of Sleep.* Academic Press, 1979.
Ehret, C., and L. Scanlon. *Overcoming Jet Lag.* New York: Berkley Books, 1983.
Minors, D. S., and J. M. Waterhouse. *Circadian Rhythms and the Human.* Boston: Wright DSG, 1981.
Samis, H. V., and Capoblanco. *Aging and Biological Rhythms.* New York: Plenum, 1978.
Williams, K. *Sleep Disorders, Diagnosis and Treatment.* John Wiley and Sons, 1978.

PERIODICALS AND ARTICLES

Inouye, S., and H. Kawamura. "Persistence of Circadian Rhythms in a Mammalian Hypothalamic 'Island' Containing the Supurachiasmitic Nucleus." *Proceedings of the National Academy of Science, USA,* 76:5962–5966, 1979.

Rusak, B., and I. Zucker. "Neural Regularities of Circadian Rhythms." *Physiology Review,* 59:449–526, 1979.
Samis, H., and Zajac-Batell. "Aging and Temporal Organization." In *Experiment and Clinical Interventions in Aging,* eds. R. Walker and R. Cooper. New York: Marcel Dekker, 1983.

CELL DAMAGE AND REPAIR

BOOKS

Cutler, R. "Nature of Aging and Life Maintenance Processes." In *Interdisciplinary Topics in Gerontology.* Basel: Karger, 1976.
Halstead, B. *Hyperbaric Oxygen Therapy.* Colton, California: Golden Quill Publishers, 1978.
Jakoby, W. B. *Enzymatic Basis of Detoxification.* New York: Academic Press, 1980.
Saifer, P., and M. Zellerbach. *Detox.* Los Angeles: Jeremy Tarcher, 1984.

PERIODICALS AND ARTICLES

Bjorksten, J. "The Crosslinkage Theory of Aging as a Predictive Indication and Possibilities and Limitations of Chelation as a Means for Life Extension." *Rejuvenation,* 8:3, September 1980.
———. "The Crosslinkage Theory of Aging." *Journal of the American Geriatrics Society,* 16:4:408–427, 1968.
Harman, D. "Free Radical Theory of Aging." *Journal of Gerontology,* 23:4, October 1968.
———. "Free Radical Theory of Aging: Dietary Implications." *American Journal of Clinical Nutrition,* 25:8:839–843, 1978.
Hayflick, L. "The Biology of Human Aging." *American Journal of Medical Science,* 265:6:432–455, 1973.
Orgel, L. E. "Aging of Clones of Mammalian Cells." *Nature,* 243:441–445, June 22, 1973.
Sheldrake, A. R. "The Aging Growth and Death of Cells." *Nature,* 250:381–385, August 2, 1974.
Strehler. "The Mechanisms of Aging." *Body Forum,* 34–45, March 1979.
Summerfield, F. "Free Radicals, DNA Damage and Aging." *Anti-Aging News,* 5:4:37–42, 1984.

CENTENARIANS

BOOKS

Davies, David. *The Centenarians of the Andes.* London: Barrie and Jenkins, 1975.
Georgakas, D. *The Methuselah Factors.* New York: Simon and Schuster, 1980.
Leaf, A. *Youth in Old Age.* New York: McGraw-Hill, 1975.
Salvador, M. *Vilacamba Tierra de Largos.* Quito, Ecuador: Casa de Cultura, 1972.

PERIODICALS AND ARTICLES

Connor, W., *et al.* "The Plasma Lipids, Lipoproteins and Diet of the Tarahumara Indians of Mexico." *American Journal of Clinical Nutrition,* 31:1131–1142, July 1978.
Leaf, A. "Observation of a Peripatetic Gerontologist." *Nutrition Today,* 4–12, September 1973.
———. "Unusual Longevity, The Common Denominators." *Hospital Practice,* 75–86, October 1973.
Mazess, R. "Bone Mineral in Vilacamba, Ecuador." *Journal of Roentgenology,* 1302:671–674, 1978.
Mazess R., and S. Forman. "Longevity and Age Exaggeration in Vilacamba, Ecuador." *Journal of Gerontology,* 34:1:94–98, 1979.
Otto, A. S. *Life Lines,* 1979.

CLINICAL TESTING

BOOKS

Corbett, J. *Laboratory Tests in Nursing Practice*. Norwalk, Connecticut: Appleton Century Crofts, 1982.

Passwater, R., and E. Cranton. *Trace Elements, Hair Analysis and Nutrition*. New Canaan, Connecticut: Keats, 1983.

Sauberlich, H. E., *et al*. *Laboratory Tests for the Assessment of Nutritional Status*. Cleveland, Ohio: CRC, 1977.

PERIODICALS AND ARTICLES

Cameron, John. "Precision and Accuracy of Bone Mineral Determination by Direct Photon Absorptionmetry." *Journal of Investigational Radiology*, 3:141–150, 1968.

Smith, E., *et al*. "Physical Activity and Calcium Mineral Increase in Aged Women." *Medical Science Sports and Exercise*, 13:1:60–64, 1981.

DISEASE, DEVELOPMENT, MEDICINE, AND PHYSIOLOGY

BOOKS

Cheraskin, E., W. M. Ringsdorf and J. W. Clark. *Diet and Disease*. New Canaan, Connecticut: Keats, 1968.

Falker, F., and J. Tanner. *Human Growth*. New York: Plenum Press, 1978.

Fleckenstein, A. *Calcium Antagonism in Heart and Smooth Muscle*. New York: John Wiley and Sons, 1983.

Kushi, M. *The Cancer Prevention Diet*. New York: St. Martin's Press, 1983.

Oliver. *Clinical Sexuality*. New York: J. B. Lippincott, 1974.

Pelletier, K. *Holistic Medicine*. New York: Dell, 1979.

Sinclair, David. *Human Growth After Birth*. London: Oxford University Press, 1978.

Williams, R. J. *Biochemical Individuality*. Austin, Texas: University of Texas Press, 1956.

PERIODICALS AND ARTICLES

Abraham, G. E. "Premenstrual Tension, Cure Problems." *Obstetrics and Gynecology*, 4:12:5–38, 1980.

Dull, R., and R. Peto. "Mortality in Relation to Smoking 20 Years Observation on Male British Doctors." *British Journal of Medicine*, 2:1525–1536, 1976.

Garrison, R. J., *et al*. "Cigarette Smoking and HDL Cholesterol." *Atherosclerosis*, 30:17–25, 1978.

McCarran, D. A., *et al*. "Does a Lack of Calcium Cause Hypertension?" *Science*, 225:205–206, 1984.

Schwartz, Klaus. "Silicon, Fibre and Atherosclerosis." *Lancet*, 454–457, February 1977.

DRUGS AND PHARMACOLOGY

BOOKS

Bailey, Herbert. *GH3*. New York: Bantam, 1977.

Clinical Guide to Drugs. Hershey, Pennsylvania: Internal Communications, 1981.

Davies. *Textbook of Adverse Drug Reactions*. Oxford University Press, 1978.

Goodman, L. S., and A. Gilman. *The Pharmacological Basis of Therapeutics*. New York: Macmillan, 1978.

Hathcock, J., and Julius Coon. *Nutrition and Drug Interrelations*. New York: Academic Press, 1978.

Martin, Eric. *Hazards of Medication*. New York: J. B. Lippincott, 1978.

PERIODICALS AND ARTICLES

Bantus, R. T., *et al.* "Profound Effects Combining Choline and Piracetam on Memory Enhancement and Cholingenic Function in Aged Rats." *Neurobiology of Aging,* 2:105–111, 1981.

Budoff, P., and S. Sommers. "Estrogen-Progesterone Therapy and Premenopausal Women." *Journal of Reproductive Medicine,* 22:241–247, 1979.

Bunch, J. W., *et al.* "Inhibition of Platelet Cyclooxygenase by Oral Aspirin." *Clinical Research,* 25:513A, 1977.

Cotzias, G., *et al.* "Levodopa Fertility and Longevity." *Science,* 196:541–549, 1977.

Geldstein. "Mode of Action of Levamisole." *Journal of Rheumatology,* Suppl. 4:143–147, 1978.

"Index of Nutritional Abnormalities Induced by 50 Commonly Prescribed Drugs." La Jolla, California: IMA Publications Inter-Marketing Associates, Inc., 1978.

Judd, H. L., *et al.* "Estrogen Replacement Therapy." *Obstetrics and Gynecology,* 58:267, 1981.

Lewis, D., *et al.* "Protective Effects of Aspirin Against Acute Myocardial Infarction and Death in Man with Unstable Angina." *New England Journal of Medicine,* 309:396, 1983.

Pick, R., *et al.* "Aspirin Inhibits Development of Coronary Atherosclerosis in Cynomalges Monkeys (Macaca Fascicularis) Fed an Atherogenic Diet." *Journal of Clinical Investigation,* 68:158–162, 1979.

Sapsie, Alfred. "Cortisol Antagonist Role of Aspirin." Personal Communication, May 1985.

Weingartner, H., *et al.* "Effects of Vasopressin on Human Memory Function." *Science,* 211:601–603, 1981.

ENVIRONMENT, ECOLOGY, CLIMATE, AND WEATHER

BOOKS

Aging and the Geochemical Environment, Panel on Aging and the Geochemical Environment in Relation to Health and Disease. U.S. National Committee for Geochemistry National Research Council, 1981.

Faust, V. *Biometeorology.* Stuttgart, Germany: Hippokniten Publishing, 1977.

Gofman, J. *Radiation and Human Health.* New York: Pantheon Books, 1983.

Ott, John N. *Health and Light, The Effects of Natural and Artificial Light on Man and Other Living Things.* Old Greenwich, Connecticut: Devin Adair, 1973.

Peterson, W. F. *Man Made Weather.* Springfield, Illinois: C. C. Thomas, 1959.

Rogers, E. S. *Human Ecology and Health.* New York: Macmillan, 1960.

Sulman, F. *Health, Weather and Climate.* Basel, Switzerland: S. Karger, 1979.

Waldbutt, G. *Health Effects of Environmental Pollutants.* St. Louis: C. V. Mosby, 1978.

Winter, Ruth. *Cancer Causing Agents, A Preventive Guide.* New York: Crown, 1979.

PERIODICALS AND ARTICLES

Peterson, F. "Drug Sensitivity and the Meteorologic Environment." *New Int. Clinics,* 17:1:255–269, 1972.

Tromp, S. "The Relationship of Weather and Climate to Health and Diseases," *Scientific Foundations of Environmental Medicine,* eds. G. Howe and J. Loraine. London: William Heinemann, 1974.

EXERCISE, FITNESS, AND BODY COMPOSITION

BOOKS

Behnke, A., and J. Wilmore. *Evaluation and Regulation of Body Build and Composition.* Englewood Cliffs, New Jersey: Prentice-Hall, 1974.

Larson, L. *International Guide to Fitness and Health.* New York: Crown, 1973.

———. *Fitness, Health and Work Capacity International Standards for Assessment.* New York: Macmillan, 1974.

McArdle, W., F. Katch, and V. L. Katch. *Exercise Physiology.* Philadelphia: Lea & Feabiger, 1981.

PERIODICALS AND ARTICLES

Bjorntorp, P., *et al.* "Physical Training in Human Obesity and Effects of Long-Term Physical Training on Body Composition." *Metabolism,* 22:1467–1475, 1973.

Bloom, M. "Fitness in America: Is America Keeping Up?" *Medical World News,* 2:87, December 1978.

Deuries, H., and G. Adams. "Comparison of Exercise Responses in Old and Young Men." *Journal of Gerontology,* 27:344–348, 1972.

Kanvonen, M. "Endurance Sports, Longevity and Health." *Annals of the New York Academy of Science,* 301:653–655, 1972.

Kholsa, T. "Longevity of Athletes." *Lancet,* 2:790:1318, 1972.

Langery, G. "Athletic Activity and Longevity." *Lancet,* 2:1771:286, 1972.

Leaf, A. "On the Physical Fitness of Men Who Live to a Great Age." *Executive Health,* 13, 1972.

Leon, A., and H. Blackburn. "The Relationship of Physical Activity to Coronary Heart Disease and Life Expectancy." *Annals of the New York Academy of Science,* 301:561–578, 1977.

Morgan, W. P. "Anxiety Reduction Following Acute Physical Activity." *Psychiatric Annals,* 9:3:141–147, 1979.

Polednak, A., and A. Damore. "College Athletes' Longevity and Cause of Death." *Human Biology,* 42:11:28–46, 1970.

Rose, C. L., and M. L. Cohen. "Relative Importance of Physical Activity for Longevity." *Annals of the New York Academy of Science,* 301:671–702, 1972.

Sharfstein, L. "20 Year Cal Study of 1 Million Finds Exercise Prolongs Life." *Medical Tribune.* December 12, 1979.

Thompson, P. D. "Exercise, Diet, or Physical Activities as Determinants of HDL-Levels in Endurance Athletes." *Atherosclerosis,* 46:333–339, 1983.

HEALTH AND LIFE-STYLE

BOOKS

Geller H., and G. Steele. *The 1974 Probability Tables of Dying in the Next Ten Years from Specific Causes.* Indianapolis: Methodist Hospital, 1979.

Pelletier, K. *Holistic Medicine,* New York: Dell, 1979.

Robbins, L. C. *How to Practice Prospective Medicine.* Indianapolis: Methodist Hospital, 1970.

PERIODICALS AND ARTICLES

Belloc, N. B. "Relationship of Health Practices and Mortality." *Preventive Medicine,* 2:67–81, 1973. .

Belloc, N. B., and L. Breslow. "Relationship of Physical Health Status and Health Practices." *Preventive Medicine* 1:409–421, 1972.

Libow, L. S. "Interaction of Medical, Biological and Behavioral Factors on Aging, Adaptation and Survival, An 11 Year Longitudinal Study." *Geriatrics,* 29:11:25–88, 1974.

Scharffenberg, J. A. "Health Consequences of a Good Lifestyle." *American Association for the Advancement of Science,* 1981,

The Prevention Index, Part 1, Emmaus, Pennsylvania: Rodale Press, 1985.

HERBS

BOOKS

Heinerman, John. *Science of Herbal Medicine.* Oren, Utah: Biworld Publishers, 1979.

Hsu, Hong-Yen. *Commonly Used Chinese Herb Formulas with Illustrations.* Long Beach, California: Oriental Healing Arts Institute, 1980.

Keys, J. D. *Chinese Herbs, Their Botany, Chemistry and Pharmacodynamics.* Rutland, Vermont: Charles E. Tuttle, Inc., 1976.

Morton, J. *Major Medicinal Plants. Botany, Culture and Uses.* Springfield, Illinois: Charles C. Thomas, 1977.

Otsuka, K., *et al. Natural Healing with Chinese Herbs.* Long Beach, California: Oriental Healing Arts Institute, 1982.

Tenashi, B., and Hong-Yen, Hsu. *Chinese Herbal Medicine and the Problems of Aging.* Long Beach, California: Oriental Healing Arts Institute, 1984.

Yeung, Hin-Che. *Handbook of Chinese Herbs and Formulas.* Vol. I and II. Los Angeles: Hin-Che Yeung, 1985.

PERIODICALS AND ARTICLES

Bittles, A., *et al.* "The Effect of Ginseng on Lifespan and Stress Responses in Mice." *Gerontology,* 25:3:125–131, 1979.

Shaw, J. "Aging Process and Anti-Aging Effects of Chinese Herb Medicines." *International Journal of Chinese Medicine,* 1:1:45–49, 1984.

Sun, Yan, *et al.* "Immune and/or Augmentation of Local Graft Versus Host Reaction by Traditional Medicinal Herbs." *Cancer,* 52:70–73, 1983.

IMMUNITY

BOOKS

Burnet, F. M. *Immunology, Aging and Cancer, Medical Aspects of Nutrition and Selection.* San Francisco: W. H. Freeman and Company, 1976.

Kay, M. B., *et al. Handbook of Immunology in Aging.* Boca Raton, Florida: CRC Press, Inc., 1981.

Walford, R. L. *The Immunologic Theory of Aging.* Baltimore: Williams & Wilkins, 1969.

PERIODICALS AND ARTICLES

Beaumont, J. I. "Autoimmune Hyperlipidemia." *Atherosclerosis,* ed. R. L. Jones. Berlin: Springer-Verlag, 1970.

Berkein, A., and B. Benacernaf. "Depression of the Reticuloendethelial System Is Phagocytic Function by Injected Lipids." *Proceedings of the Society of Experimental British Medicine,* 128:793–795, 1968.

Chandra *et al.* "Serum Thymic Factor Activity in Deficiencies of Calories, Zinc, Vitamin A and Pyridozine." *Clinical Experimental Immunology,* 42:332–335, 1980.

Stein *et al.* "Influence of Brain and Behavior on the Immune System." *Science,* 191:435–40, 1976.

Waldford, R. "Immunologic Theory of Aging, Correct Status." *Federal Proceedings,* 33:9:2020–2027, 1974.

Waldford, R., *et al.* "Long Term Dietary Restriction and Immune Function in Mice, Response to Sheep Red Blood Cells and to Mitogens." *Mech. Aging Dev.,* 2:443–451, 1974.

NEUROENDOCRINE SYSTEM, BRAIN, AND NERVES

BOOKS

Amaducci, L., *et al. Aging of the Brain and Dementia.* New York: Raven Press, 1980.

Enna, S. J., *et al. Brain Neurotransmitters and Receptors in Aging and Age-Related Disorders.* New York: Raven Press, 1981.

Everitt, A. V., and J. A. Burgess. *Hypothalamus, Pituitary and Aging.* Springfield, Illinois: Charles C. Thomas, 1976.

Gellhorn, Ernest. *Autonomic Imbalance of the Hypothalamus.* Minneapolis: University of Minnesota Press, 1957.

Horn, A. S., *et al. The Neurobiology of Dopamine.* New York: Academic Press, 1979.

Johnson, R. H., and J. M. Spalding. *Disorders of the Autonomic Nervous System.* Philadelphia: F. A. Davis Co., 1974.

Osborne, Neville. *Biology of Serotonergic Transmissions.* New York: John Wiley and Sons, 1982.
Terry, R. D., *et al. Neural Aging and Its Implications in Human Neurological Pathology.* New York: Raven Press, 1982.

PERIODICALS AND ARTICLES

Astaldi, G., *et al.* "Growth Hormone and Lymphocyte Activation." *Lancet,* 2:709, 1972.
Cann, D. "Endorphins in Contemporary Medicine." *Contemporary Therapy,* 9:3:40–45, 1983.
Cryer *et al.* "Cessation of Growth Hormone with Secretion with Acute Elevation of Free Fatty Acids Concentration." *Metabolism,* 21:867–873, 1972.
Denckla, W. D. "Interaction Between Age and the Neuroendocrine System and Immune Systems." *Federal Proceedings,* 37:5:1263–1267, 1978.
Diamond, M. *The American Scientist.* January–February 1978.
Finch, C. E. "The Regulation of Physiological Changes During Mammalian Aging." *C. Rev. Bul.,* 51:49–83, 1976.
———. "Neuroendocrine Mechanisms and Aging." *Federal Proceedings,* 38:2:178–187, 1979.
French, J. D. "The Reticular Formation." *Scientific American,* May 1957.
Merimee, T. J., and S. E. Fineberg. "Growth Hormone Secretion in Starvation, a Reassessment." *Journal of Clinical Endocrinology,* 39:385–386, 1974.
Quabbe, H. J., *et al.* "Growth Hormone, Glucagon, and Insulin Response in Depression of Plasma FFA and the Effects of Glucose Infusion." *Journal of Clinical Endocrinology and Metabolism,* 44:383–391, 1977.
Rabinowitz, D., *et al.* "Effects of Human Growth Hormone on Muscle and Adipose Tissue Metabolism in the Forearm of Men." *Journal of Clinical Investigation,* 44:51–61, 1965.
Rosenweig, M. R., *et al.* "Direct Contact with Enriched Environment Is Required to Alter Cerebral Weight in Rats." *J. of Comp. and Phys. Psyc.,* 88:360–367.
Roth, G. S. "Receptor Changes and the Control of Hormone Action During Aging." *Aging, Cancer, and Cell Membranes,* eds. Berek *et al.* New York: Thieme-Stratton, 1980.

NUTRITION AND DIET

BOOKS

Birch, G. C., and K. J. Parker. *Dietary Fiber.* New York: Applied Science Publishers, 1983.
Blackburn, G., J. Grant and R. Vernan. *Amino Acids, Metabolism and Medical Applications.* Boston: John Wright, 1983.
Bowes, A. *Food Values of Portions Commonly Used.* Philadelphia: Lippincott, 1980.
Burkitt, D. B. "Diseases of Affluence." *Nutrition and Killer Diseases,* ed. John Rose. Park Ridge, New Jersey: Noyes, 1982.
Diet, Nutrition and Cancer. Washington, D.C.: National Academy Press, 1982.
Harris, R. S., and H. V. Loesecke. *Nutritional Evaluation of Food Processing.* New York: John Wiley and Sons.
Moment, G. *Nutritional Approaches to Aging Research.* Boca Raton, Florida: CRC Press, 1982.
Passwater, Richard. *Evening Primrose Oil.* New Haven, Connecticut: Keats, 1981.
Roe, D. *Drug Induced Nutritional Deficiencies.* Westport, Connecticut: AVI Publishing, 1976.
Spiller, G. *Nutritional Pharmacology.* New York: Alan Liss, 1982.
———. *Topics in Dietary Fiber Research.* New York: Plenum Press, 1978.

PERIODICALS AND ARTICLES

Bessman, S. P. "Justification Theory." *Nutrition Reviews,* 37:209, 1978.
Brin, M. "Dilemma of Marginal Vitamin Deficiency." (Proceedings of the 9th International Congress of Nutrition, Mexico 4:1972). Basel, Switzerland: Kanger, 1975.

Carlson, A., and F. Hoelzel. "Apparent Prolongation of Lifespans of Rats by Intermittent Fasting." *Journal of Nutrition,* 31:363, 1976.

Cheek, D., *et al.* "Cellular Growth, Nutrition and Development." *Pediatrics,* 45:2:315–334, 1970.

Crapper *et al.* "Aluminum and Other Metals in Senile (Alzheimer) Dementia." *Alzheimer's Disease and Related Disorders,* eds. R. Kitzman and K. L. Bick. New York: Raven Press, 1978.

DiMagno, E. P. "Exocrine Pancreatic Replacement Therapy." *New England Journal of Medicine,* 296:1318, 1977.

Dyerbeng *et al.* "Alpha Linolenic Acid and Eicospentaenoic Acid." *Lancet,* 1:26:199, 1980.

Fernandes, G., *et al.* "Nutritional Inhibition of Genetically Determined Renal Disease and Autoimmunity with Prolongation of Life in KdKd Mice." *Proc. Natl. Sci. USA,* 75:2888–2892, 1978.

Fernstrom, J. D. "Modification of Brain Serotonin by the Diet." *Annu. Rev. Med.,* 25:1–8, 1974.

Goodhart, R. S. *How Well Nourished Are Americans?* (I–II). New York: National Foundation Vitamin Report for 1961–1963.

Gordon, G. "New Dimensions in Calcium Metabolism." *Anti-aging News,* 4:10:109–118, 1984.

Hanson, F. "Nutrition and Immunity: The Influence of Diet on Autoimmunity and the Role of Zinc in the Immune Response." *American Review of Nutrition,* 2:151–172, 1982.

Hardinge, M. G., *et al.* "Nutritional Studies of Vegetarians. Dietary Levels of Fiber." *American Journal of Clinical Nutrition,* 6:523, 1958.

Hemmings, W., and E. Williams. "Transplant of Large Breakdown Products of Dietary Protein Through the Gut Wall." *Gut,* 19:715, 1978.

Hinai *et al.* "Eicosapentaenoic Acid in Platelet Function in Japanese." *Lancet,* 11:1132, 1980.

"It's Not Fishy: Fruit of the Sea May Foil Cardiovascular Disease." *Journal of the American Medical Association,* February 1982.

Jakubowski, J. A., and N. G. Ardlie. "Modification of Human Platelet Function by a Diet Enriched in Saturated Fat or Polysaturated Fat." *Atherosclerosis,* 31:335–344, 1978.

McCay, C. M. "Retarded Growth, Life Span, Ultimate Body Size and Changes in the Albino Rat after Feeding Diet Restricted in Calories." *Journal of Nutrition,* 18:1–13, 1939.

Recommended Dietary Allowances, 9th rev. ed. Washington, D.C.: National Academy of Sciences, 1980.

Ross, M. "Nutrition and Longevity in Experimental Animals." *Nutrition and Aging,* ed. M. Winnick. New York: John Wiley and Sons, 1976.

Ross, M. H. "Length of Life and Calorie Intake." *American Journal of Clinical Nutrition,* 25:834–838, 1972.

Saynor, R. "Effect of a Fish Oil in Blood Coagulation." *Throm. Hgln.,* 46:65, 1981.

Sen, D. P., *et al.* "Hypocholesteronic Effect Induced in Rats by Oil-Sardine Fish and Sardine Oils Having Different Degrees of Unsaturation." *JAOCS,* 54:297–303, July 1977.

Shahani, K., *et al.* "Role of Dietary Lactobacilli in Gastrointestinal Microecology." *American Journal of Clinical Nutrition,* 33:2448, 2457, 1980.

Siess, W., *et al.* "Platelet Membrane Fatty Acids, Platelet Aggregation and Thromboxane Formation During Mackerel Diet." *Lancet,* 3:15:441–444, 1980.

Weindruch, R. H., *et al.* "Influence of Controlled Dietary Restriction on Immunological Function and Aging." *Federal Proceedings,* 38:6:2007–2016, 1979.

Worthington, B. "Dietary Fiber/Questions Related to Dietary Fiber." *Contemporary Developments in Nutrition,* ed. B. Roberts. St. Louis: C. V. Mosby, 1981.

STRESS, MEDITATION, AND RELAXATION

BOOKS

Benson, Herbert. *The Relaxation Response.* New York: Avon, 1975.

Check, D. B., and LeCron, L. *Clinical Hypnotherapy.* New York: Grune and Stratton, 1968.

Davis, M., *et al.* *The Relaxation and Stress Reduction Workbook.* Richmond, California: New Harbinger, 1980.

Friedman, M., and R. A. Rosenman. *Type A Behavior and Your Heart.* New York: Alfred A. Knopf, 1974.

Kutash, Irwin, and L. B. Schlesinger, *Handbook on Stress and Anxiety.* San Francisco: Jossey Bass, 1980.

McKay, M., *et al. Thought and Feeling, the Art of Cognitive Stress Intervention.* Richmond, California: New Harbinger, 1981.

Orme-Johnson, D., and J. Farrows. *Scientific Research on the Transcendental Meditation Program.* New York: MIU Press, 1977.

Pelletier, Kenneth. *Mind as a Healer, Mind as a Slayer.* New York: Delta, 1977.

Selye, Hans. *The Stress of Life.* New York: McGraw-Hill, 1956.

PERIODICALS AND ARTICLES

Bahrke, M. S., and P. Morgan. "Anxiety Reduction Following Exercise and Meditation." *Cognitive Therapy and Research,* 2:4:323–333, 1978.

Benson, H., and L. H. Hartley. "Decreased VO_2 Consumption During Exercise with the Elicitation of the Relaxation Response." *Journal of Human Stress,* 38–42, June 1978.

DeSilva, R., and B. Lown. "Ventricular Premature Beats, Stress and Sudden Death." *Psychosomatics,* 19:11:649–661, 1978.

Donlon, P., A. Meadow and E. Amsterdam. "Emotional Stress as a Factor in Ventricular Arrythmias." *Psychosomatics,* 20:4:233–240, 1979.

Engel, G. L. "Psychological Factors in Instantaneous Cardiac Death." *New England Journal of Medicine,* 294:12:664–665, 1976.

Sapsie, A. "Stress, Cortisol Interferon and Stress Diseases—I: Cortisol as the Cause of Stress Disease." *Medical Hypothesis,* 13:31–44, 1984.

Soloman, G. "Emotional Stress, the Central Nervous System and Immunity." *Annals of the New York Academy of Science,* 164:2:335–343, 1969.

SUPPLEMENTS

BOOKS

Challer, J. *Vitamin C Updated.* New Canaan, Connecticut: Keats, 1983.

Frank, B. *Nucleic Acid and Antioxidant Therapy of Aging and Degeneration.* New York: Rainstone Publishing, 1977.

Graham, Judy. *Evening Primrose Oil.* New York: Thorson, 1984.

Heinz, A., *et al. Marine Algae in Pharmaceutical Science.* New York: Walter de Gruyter, 1979.

Sheldon, S. *The Complete Guide to Antiaging Nutrients.* New York: Simon and Schuster, 1985.

PERIODICALS AND ARTICLES

Abraham, G., and G. Goei. "Effect of a Nutritional Supplement Optivite on Symptoms of Premenstrual Tension." *Journal of Reproductive Medicine,* 28:527–581, 1983.

Abraham, G., and J. Hargrove. "Effect of Vitamin B-6 on Premenstrual Tension Symptomatology in Women with Premenstrual Tension Syndromes: A Double Blind Crossover Study." *Infertility,* 3:155, 1980.

Aksenova, N., *et al.* "Influence of Ribonucleic Acids from the Liver on Implantation of Growth of Transplantable Tumors." *Nature,* 196:443–444, 1962.

Anderson *et al.* "The Effects of Weekly Dosages of Ascorbate on Certain Cellular and Hormonal Immune Responses in Normal Volunteers." *American Journal of Clinical Nutrition,* 33:71–76, 1980.

Ansanuma *et al.* "Reduction of the Incidence of Wasting Disease in Neonatally Thynectized CBA-W Mice by the Injection of Thymosin." *Endocrinology,* 86:600–610, 1970.

Beisel, W. "Single Nutrients and Immunity." *American Journal of Clinical Nutrition,* 35:417–468, 1982.

Belizan, J., *et al.* "Reduction of Blood Pressure with Calcium Supplementation in Young Adults." *Journal of the American Medical Association,* 249:1161, 1983.

Ben-David *et al.* "Anti-Hypercholerolenic Effect of Dehydroepiandrosterone." *Proceedings of the Society for Experimental Medicine,* 125:1136–1140, 1967.

Benjamin, H. S., *et al.* "Allium Sativum (Garlic) and Atherosclerosis: A Review." *Lancet Nutrition Research,* 3:119–128, 1983.

Bjellhe, E. "Dietary Vitamin A and Human Lung Cancer." *International Journal of Cancer,* 15:561, 1975.

Cathcart, R. "Vitamin C Titrating to Bowel Tolerance, Anascorbemia and Acute Induced Scurvy." *Medical Hypothesis,* 7:1358, 1981.

Chan, P., *et al.* "Growth Suppression of Human Leukemia Cells in Vitro by L-Ascorbic Acid." *Cancer Research,* 40:1062, 1980.

Chandra, R., and D. Dayton. "Trace Element Regulation of Immunity and Infection." *Nutritional Research,* 2:721–733, 1982.

Coronary Drug Project Research Group. "Clofibrate and Niacin in Coronary Heart Disease." *Journal of the American Medical Association,* 231:360, 1975.

DiRossa, M. "Biological Properties of Carrageenan." *Journal of Pharm. Pharmacology,* 24:89–102, 1972.

Disorbo, D., and L. Nathanson. "High-Dose Pyridoxal Supplemental Culture Medium Inhibits the Growth of a Human Malignant Melanoma Cell Line." *Nutrition and Cancer,* 5:10, 1983.

Duchateau, J., *et al.* "Beneficial Effects of Oral Zinc Supplementation on the Immune Response of Old People." *American Journal of Medicine,* 70:1001–1004, 1981.

Edes, T., *et al.* "Intestinal and Hepatic Mixed Function Oxidase Activity in Rats Fed Methionine and Cysteine Free Diets." *Proc. Sec. For Exp. Biol.,* 162:71, 1979.

Ferris *et al.* "Senile Dementia: Treatment with Deanol." *Journal of the American Geriatric Society,* 222:241–244, 1977.

Finley, E., and F. Cerklewski. "Influence of Ascorbic Acid Supplementation on Copper Status in Young Adult Men." *American Journal of Clinical Nutrition,* 37:553, 1983.

Gelenberg *et al.* "Tyrosine for the Treatment of Depression." *Journal of Psychiatry,* 137:5:622–628, 1980.

Goldstein. "Thymosin: Basic Properties and Clinical Potential in Treatment of Patients with Immunodeficiency Disease and Cancer." *Appl. Cancer Chemotherapy Antibiot. Chem.,* 24:47–59, 1978.

Griffin, A., and S. Clark. "Roles of Selenium in the Chemoprevention of Cancer." *Advances in Cancer Research,* 29:419–442, 1979.

Hargrove, J., and G. Abraham. "Effect on Infertility in Women with Premenstrual Tension Syndrome." *Infertility,* 2:315, 1980.

Hartoma, R., *et al.* "Zinc, Plasma Androgens and Male Sterility." *Lancet,* 2:1125–1126, 1977.

Hochschild, R. "Effect of Dimethylaminethanol p-chlorophenoxyacetate on the Lifespan of Male Swiss Webster Albino Mice." *Experimental Gerontology,* 8:173–183, 1973.

Isidori, A., *et al.* "A Study of Growth Hormone Release in Man after an Administration of Amino Acids." *Current Medical Research and Opinion,* 7:7:475–481, 1981.

Jecjcebhoy, K., *et al.* "Chromium Deficiency, Glucose Tolerance, and Neuropathy Reversed by Chromium Supplementation in a Patient Receiving Long-Term Total Paratenal Nutrition." *American Journal of Clinical Nutrition,* 30:531–538, 1977.

Johnson, M., and R. Vaughn. "Death of Salmonella Typhimurium and Escherichia Coli in the Presence of Freshly Reconstituted Dehydrated Onion and Garlic." *Applied Microbiology,* 17:903–909, 1969.

Mathews, R., *et al.* "Beta Carotene Therapy for Erythropoeitic Protoporphyria and Other Photosensitivity Diseases." *Archives of Dermatology,* 113:1229, 1977.

Morrison, L. "Therapeutic Applications of Chondroitan-4-Sulphate, Appraisal of Biological Properties." *Folia Angeologica,* September 1977.

Muller, D., *et al.,* eds. "Vitamin E and Neurological Function." *Lancet,* 225–227, January 29, 1983.

Murata, K. "Inhibitory Effects of Chondroitan Polysulphate on Lipemia and Atherosclerosis in Connection with Its Anticoagulant Activity." *Naturwissenschaften,* 49:1, 1962.

National Cancer Institute. *Selected Abstracts of Vitamin A and Cancer Biology.* Bethesda, Maryland: National Cancer Institute, 1979.

Nockels, C. "Protective Effects of Supplemental Vitamin E Against Infection." *Federation Proceedings, Federation of the American Society of Experimental Biology,* 38:2134–2138, 1978.

Odens, M. "Prolongation of Life Span in Rats." *Journal of the American Geriatrics Society,* 21:450, 1973.

Oeuriu, V., and E. Vochitu. "The Effect of the Administration of Compounds Which Contain Sulfhydryl Groups on the Survival Rates of Mice, Rats and Guinea Pigs." *Journal of Gerontology,* 20:417–418, 1965.

Offenbacher, E., and Xavier PiSonder. "Beneficial Effect of Chromium-Rich Yeast on Glucose Tolerance and Blood Lipids in Elderly Subjects." *Diabetes,* 29:919–930, 1980.

Oherich. "Sperm Swim Singly after Vitamin C Therapy." *Journal of the American Medical Association,* 249:2747, 1983.

Peters, B., and H. Levin. "Effects of Pysotigmine and Lecithin on Memory in Alzheimer's Disease." *Annals of Neurology,* 6:219–221, 1979.

Peto, R., *et al.* "Can Dietary Beta Carotene Materially Reduce Human Cancer Rates?" *Nature,* 290:201–208, 1981.

Salonor, J. "Association Between Cardiovascular Death and Myocardial Infarction and Serum Selenium in a Match-Pair–Longitudinal Study." *Lancet,* 2:175–179, 1982.

Salway, J., *et al.* "Effect of Myo-Inositol on Peripheral Nerve Function in Diabetes." *Lancet,* 2:1282–1284, 1978.

Schaumburg, H., *et al.* "Sensory Neuropathy from Pyridoxine Abuse." *New England Journal of Medicine,* 309:446, 1983.

Schroeder, H. A., and A. Mitchener. "Selenium and Tellurium in Rats, Effect on Growth Survival and Tumors." *Journal of Nutrition,* 101:1531–1540, 1971.

Schwartz, A. "Dehydroepiandrosterone, An Anti-Obesity and Anticarcinogenic Agent." *Nutrition and Cancer,* 3:46–53, 1981.

Seelig, M. "The Requirement of Magnesium by the Normal Adult." *American Journal of Clinical Nutrition,* 14:342–390, 1964.

Siegel, B. "Enhanced Interferon Response to Murine Leukemia Virus by Ascorbic Acid." *Infection and Immunity,* 10:409–410, 1974.

Sprince, H., *et al.* "Protective Action of Ascorbic Acid and Sulfur Compounds Against Acetaldehyde Toxicity; Implications in Alcoholism and Smoking." *Agents and Actions,* 5:2:164–173, 1975.

Sued *et al.* "Tyrosine Administration Reduces Blood Pressure and Enhances Brain Norepinephrine Release in Spontaneously Hypertensive Rats." *Proceedings of the National Academy of Science,* 76:3511–3514, 1979.

Tatu, M., *et al.* "Glucose Tolerance and Plasma Insulin in Man During Acute and Chronic Administration of Nicotinic Acid." *Acta Med. Scandia.,* 186:247,253, 1969.

Van Fleet, J., *et al.* "Effect of Selenium–Vitamin E on Adriamycin-Induced Cardiomyopathy in Rabbits." *American Journal of Veterinary Research,* 39:997–1010, 1978.

Wurtzman, R. "Behavioral Effects of Nutrients." *Lancet,* 1145–1151, May 21, 1983.

Reference and Resource Guide to Associations and Organizations

The Reference and Resource Guide lists the publishers and health organizations that publish health education material, supply names of local, reliable health professionals, and sponsor seminars and workshops.

ACUPUNCTURE

Acupuncture Education Center
13757 N.E. Third Court, Suite 210-A
North Miami, Florida 33161
(305) 945-5359

Gives acupuncture seminars, distributes literature, provides doctor referral service.

AGING

American Aging Association, Inc. (AGE)
Attn.: Denham Harman, M.D.
University of Nebraska Medical Center
Omaha, NE 68105

Publishes newsletter on aging for scientists and laymen.

Huxley Institute for Biosocial Research
1114 First Avenue
New York, NY 10021
(212) 759-9554

Distributes information to lay persons and professionals about the aging mind, nutrition, orthomolecular medicine, and other topics. Publishes a newsletter, provides referral service of health professionals, involved in preventive medicine.

International Association on the Artificial Prolongation of Human Specific Lifespan
Fabiolaan, 12 Krokke-Zoute, B 8300
Belgium

Publishes *Rejuvenation* (in English), which contains information about extending life.

Linus Pauling Institute for Science and Medicine
2700 Sand Hill Road
Menlo Park, CA 94025

Provides information on vitamin C and preventive medicine. Funds research on aging, publishes a quarterly newsletter.

Life Extension Foundation
2835 Hollywood Boulevard
Hollywood, FL 33020
(800) 327-6110

Publishes *Antiaging News.* Sells popular books on aging, provides referral lists of life extension doctors.

ECOLOGY AND ENVIRONMENT

Human Ecology Action League (HEAL)
505 North Lake Shore Drive
Chicago, IL 60611
(312) 329-9097

Finances environmental health research, educates about environmental risks. Provides information about foods, drugs, water, and toxic chemicals that affect health. Distributes publications and the newsletter *Human Ecologist.*

Society for Clinical Ecologists
4045 Wadsworth Boulevard
Wheat Ridge, CO 80033
(303) 424-5515

Publishes newsletter, provides referral service for locating a clinical ecologist in your area.

Soil and Health Foundation
33 East Minor Street
Emmaus, PA 18049
(215) 967-5171

Promotes research in environment and medicine, assists members in improving their own health, provides hair and drinking water analysis, publishes a newsletter.

HERBS

Oriental Healing Arts Institute
1945 Palo Verde Avenue, Suite 208
Long Beach, CA 90815
(213) 431-3544

Provides books, literature, and information about Chinese medicine and herbs.

HOLISTIC HEALTH, HEALERS, AND PREVENTIVE MEDICINE

American Holistic Medical Association
Route 2 Welsh Coulee
La Crosse, WI 54601
(608) 706-0611

Educates about holistic health principles. Publishes quarterly newsletter, provides doctor referral service for your area.

American Healers Association
P.O. Box 213
Princeton, NY 08540

Provides information on nonmedical healers, offers referral list of certified healers in your area.

American Academy of Medical Preventics
6151 West Century Boulevard
Suite 1114
Los Angeles, CA 90045
(213) 645-5350

Educates professionals and lay persons about degenerative diseases, chelation therapy, and atherosclerosis. Holds workshops and seminars, provides doctor referral lists, publishes quarterly newsletter.

Orthomolecular Medicine Society
2698 Pacific Avenue
San Francisco, CA 94115
(415) 346-5692

Scientific research organization provides referral information about doctors utilizing orthomolecular medicine across the country.

HOMEOPATHY

National Center for Homeopathy
1500 Massachusetts Avenue, N.W. #41
Washington, DC 20052
(202) 223-6182

Distributes newsletter and other literature, teaches classes, provides doctors referral service.

International Foundation for Homeopathy
1141 N.W. Market
Seattle, WA 98107
(206) 324-8230

Teaches homeopathy, gives seminars, publishes bimonthly newsletter, provides doctors referral service.

United States Homeopathic Association
6560 Backlick Road
Springfield, VA 22150
(703) 569-5311

Publishes monthly newsletter, distributes information and books to lay persons and professionals, provides doctors referral service.

NUTRITION

Northwest Academy of Preventive Medicine
15650 North East 29th Street
Bellevue, WA 98008
(206) 747-9660

Educates professionals, publishes journal and newsletters, provides referral service.

International College of Applied Nutrition (ICAN)
P.O. Box 1000
San Gabriel, CA 91776
(818) 286-3123

Society of professionals involved in different aspects of nutrition. Publishes a journal and newsletter, provides doctor referral service.

Price Pottenger Nutrition Foundation
P.O. Box 2614
La Mesa, CA 92041
(619) 582-4168

Conducts educational programs for lay persons and professionals, disseminates books and other literature about good nutritional practices.

Index

A

Acetaldehyde, toxic effects of, 86,
   106
Acetylcholine, 32, 129, 141, 265,
   268
   and aging, 30
   effect of alcohol on, 86
Achromycin, 88
Acidophilus, 162, 169
Acne, and cortisol level, 52
Aconite, 102, 144, 267
Actinomycin, effect of, on body
   cycles, 87
Activated charcoal, 141, 151, 162
   and detoxification, 112, 113
Acupuncture, 8, 227–231
   resource guide to, 297
Acupuncture Education Center,
   229, 297
Acupuncture energy doctor, 79
Adamenko, Vickor, 232
Adaptive systems, testing for, 34
Adrenal gland, 100, 182

Adrenaline, 24, 74, 100, 102, 184,
   210, 265
   and obesity, 185
   and stress, 51, 60
Adult-onset diabetes. *See* Diabetes
Aerobic exercise, 213–214. *See
   also* Exercise
   and metabolism, 12
   target heart rates for, 214–215
   weight loss from, 205
Aerobic rebound, 222
Age Reduction Diet, 176–207. *See
   also* Nutrition; Nutritional
   supplements
   benefits from, 178
   beverages in, 203
   and body weight, 187
   caloric restriction in, 177
   cautions, 189, 190
   complex carbohydrates in,
      199–201
   condiments in, 204
   desserts and sweeteners in,
      203–204